T0296669

Western Medical Thought from Antiquity to the Middle Ages

Western Medical Thought
from Antiquity
to the Middle Ages

∾∾∾

Edited by Mirko D. Grmek

Coordinated by Bernardino Fantini

Translated by Antony Shugaar

HARVARD UNIVERSITY PRESS
Cambridge, Massachusetts
London, England
1998

PRINTED IN THE UNITED STATES OF AMERICA

Originally published as *Storia del pensiero medico occidentale 1:*
Antichità e medioevo, © 1993 Gius. Laterzo & Figli Spa, Rome and Bari.

Library of Congress Cataloging-in-Publication Data

Storia del pensiero medico occidentale. English
Western medical thought from antiquity to the Middle Ages /
edited by Mirko D. Grmek ;
coordinated by Bernardino Fantini ;
translated by Antony Shugaar.
p.   cm.
Includes bibliographical references and index.
ISBN 0-674-40355-X (alk. paper)
1. Medicine, Ancient.   2. Medicine, Medieval.
I. Grmek, Mirko Dražen.   II. Fantini, Bernardino.   III. Shugaar, Antony.
R135.S83513   1999
610'.9—dc21   98-8462

Contents

Western Medical Thought from Antiquity to the Middle Ages

~ 1 ~

Introduction

MIRKO D. GRMEK

The chief objective of this work is to provide a historical reconstruction of the gradual transformations and apparently sudden alterations in medical theory and practice in the so-called Western civilizations. By Western civilizations, we are referring first to the Mediterranean basin, later to the countries of western and northern Europe, and, most recently, to nations on every continent, foremost among them North America. In this reconstruction, we consider fundamental the relationships that link medical knowledge to mentalities, philosophy, and various forms of science and technology.

The Origins of Medical Historiography

Ever since the establishment of medical skill as a distinct art, its practitioners have reflected on that art's origins, its historical progress, and the current state of medicine—both as a profession and as a scientific discipline.

One of the earliest Western medical texts, the Hippocratic treatise *De prisca medicina*, begins with a historical explanation of the establishment of medical *techne*. According to the author of this treatise, writing in the fifth century B.C., medicine was discovered—just as the culinary art had been discovered before it—through a series of attempts, judged *a posteriori* as either failures or successes, a method that modern epistemologists describe as trial and error.[1]

According to another Hippocratic treatise, *De arte,* a polemical rebuttal of detractors of the medical art, the art in question had been discovered only recently; once the correct approach was adopted, however, it had quickly attained perfection, and medicine had become a complete and organic discipline.

This sunny view was not shared by the school of Aristotle, at least as far as theoretical aspects were concerned. A peripatetic doxography, fragments of which are preserved in "Anonymous of London" (Anonymus Londinensis), reviewed the differing opinions on the causes of diseases.[2] The concept of the imperfection of medicine in the classical age is expressed here quite clearly, but the idea of historical progress appears only as an insubstantial shadow. The author reviews the doctrines of ancient and more recent physicians, making a praiseworthy effort at objectivity and critical detachment; he completely ignores, however, the matter of historical perspective.

In the literature that has survived, the oldest accounts of medical history, properly speaking, come from the Roman world and date from the beginning of the Christian era: they are found, first of all, in the works of the Latin encyclopedists, Celsus and Pliny the Elder, and later in the various treatises by Greek physicians, such as Soranus of Ephesus and Galen.

Celsus's *De medicina* opens with a historical overview:

> Just as agriculture promises nourishment to healthy bodies, so does the Art of Medicine promise health to the sick. Nowhere is this art wanting, for the most uncivilized nations have had knowledge of herbs, and other things to hand for the aiding of wounds and diseases. This Art, however, has been cultivated among the Greeks much more than in other nations—not, however, even among them from their first beginnings, but only for a few generations before ours. Hence, Aesculapius is celebrated as the most ancient authority, and because he cultivated this science [*scientia*], as yet rude and vulgar, with a little more than common refinement, he was numbered among the gods . . . At first the science of healing [*medendi scientia*] was held to be part of philosophy [*scientiae pars*], so that treatment of disease [*morborum curatio*] and contemplation of the nature of things [*rerum naturae contemplatio*] began through the same authorities . . . But it was, as some believe, a pupil of

Democritus, Hippocrates of Cos, a man first and foremost worthy to be remembered, notable both for professional skill [*ars*] and for eloquence [*facundia*], who separated this branch of learning from the study of philosophy [*studium sapientiae*]. After him Diocles of Carystus, next Praxagoras and Chrysippus, then Herophilus and Erasistratus, so practiced this art that they made advances even towards various methods of treatment [*in diversas curandi vias*].

Medicine was divided during this time, according to Celsus, into three parts (dietetics, pharmacology, and surgery). While the earliest dietitians still claimed that the theoretical study of nature was an indispensable part of medicine, certain of their successors—who called themselves Empirics, noteworthy among them Serapion, Apollonius, Glaucias, and Heraclides of Tarentum—insisted on basing medical practice solely upon clinical experience.

"But after those mentioned above," Celsus continues, "no one troubled about anything except what tradition had handed down to him until Asclepiades changed in large measure the way of curing [*medendi ratio*]. Of his successors, Themison, late in life, diverged from Asclepiades in some respects."[3]

Thus, Celsus presents the history of medicine as a progression, which basically unfolded in Greece, beginning with the establishment of a sophisticated medical knowledge by Aesculapius, and the break from philosophy brought about by Hippocrates, continuing with the contributions of the Alexandrian anatomists and the Empirics, all the way up to the innovations—which were still quite recent for him—of the methodic sect. He describes a progression, certainly, but not progress in the modern sense of the term. Celsus recognized the importance of the successive improvements that were brought to bear in the treatment of diseases, but he did not therefore think that the theoretical medicine of his time was necessarily superior to medicine of the past.

For many centuries historical interest in the field of medicine centered on the authorities of the past. Certain authors used historical citations as a ploy to gain greater acceptance of their own ideas. In the writings of Galen, and especially in his commentaries on the Hippocratic collection, the frequent historical digressions provide fine examples of the use of history, philology, and rhetoric in defense of a specific system of medicine. If Galen idealized the figure of Hippocrates and extolled the worth of the medical treatises of the classical age, he did so to combat more effectively doctrines opposed to his own.

In the Middle Ages, respect for authorities and reliance on the canonical texts imposed by the dominant religions led physicians—entirely
won over to Galenism—to replace historical inquiry with legend. They
used the heritage of the past solely for purposes of teaching and rhetoric.

During the thirteenth century, in the Arab cultural world, Ibn Abi
Usaybi'a inaugurated a new genre of medical history: the biographies of
great doctors.[4] His method differed from mere hagiography, for his interest in the lives of men of science served chiefly to catalog their works and
to encourage a greater familiarity with their ideas on the principles of
medicine and on medical ethics. Another new development can be observed in the work of Ibn Abi Usaybi'a: his writings composed the first
medical historical study to aspire to universality, which is to say, he included the achievements of illustrious physicians not only of all periods
but of the entire known world.

In European medicine, a systematic biographical approach began
with the fifteenth-century humanists (for example, Giovanni Tortelli with
his *De medicina et medicis*),[5] and flourished greatly following the invention
of the printing press. From Symphorien Champier and Conrad Gessner
to Johann Antonides van der Linden, authors compiled increasingly exhaustive biobibliographical collections; these works, however, never rose
above the level of the scholarship of collectors. Interest focused on listing
rather than evaluating.

The Scientific Revolution

The orientation of medical historiography shifted at the end of the seventeenth century when the development of diplomatics and the new directions in ecclesiastical and political history combined with the remarkable
breakthroughs in philosophy and the extraordinary achievements of science and technology to create what we know as the "scientific revolution."
During this period, the earliest "modern" manuals of the history of Western medicine appeared, written in French by the Genevan physician
Daniel Le Clerc[6] and in English by the London physician and parliamen-
tarian John Freind.[7] The use of "vulgar" languages in the compilation of
texts that aspired to scientific respectability was a clear indication of a
profound change in attitudes.

Le Clerc resolved to apply the methodological precepts of Francis
Bacon to the study of medical history. His diligent collection of historical
"facts" and his arrangement of those facts in rigorous chronological order

would make it possible to draw from them, "inductively," conclusions of a more general nature. He attempted a division into periods that was proper to the discipline, and wished to establish links, discover rules, and identify associations of lasting significance. The vastness of the undertaking forced Le Clerc to break off work midway through; the daunting obstacle was the analysis of the huge body of work by Galen. All the same, Le Clerc added to the second edition of his manual a rough outline of the development of medicine after Galen, up to the middle of the seventeenth century. His insistence on the importance of Paracelsus's work was a significant new contribution. An advocate of critical empiricism, Le Clerc rejected pagan legends and made a concerted effort to establish facts through reliable documents.

John Freind's historical account ends with the Renaissance, a period that he extolled greatly. The Middle Ages were included, of chronological necessity, but were treated with considerable disdain. An admirer of Newton and an adept of iatrophysics, Freind recognized that great aesthetic satisfaction could be obtained from reading ancient medical texts, but he only truly valued these literary documents of the past when he felt they might still be scientifically sound. Believing that something untrue was no longer worth knowing, Freind chose from among ancient medical texts and documents, examining them in the light of his own doctrinaire convictions. He, along with most of his contemporaries, felt that the ultimate purpose of all historical analysis—at least, in the realm of the history of science—was to distinguish, amid a mass of apparently chaotic information, the steps of progress that had led to the current state of knowledge.

The key word—progress—had finally been uttered. The Enlightenment was dazzled by this concept. It stands as a clear presence in medical historiography. The concept powerfully influenced the articles on medical history in the *Encyclopédie* and guided the decisions of Albrecht von Haller in the assembly of his great biographical and bibliographic anthologies.

The Pragmatic Approach and the Romantic Illusion

Beginning in the late eighteenth century, the leading role in the study of medical history fell to German-speaking scholars. They maintained their leadership of the field until the catastrophic rise of National Socialism in the 1930s.[8] Inspired by the rebirth of German philosophy, and especially by the critical thought of Kant, Philipp Gabriel Hensler outlined in 1783 a program for a new medical historiography. Shortly thereafter, Johann

Daniel Metzger and Johann Ackermann underscored the practical aspects of medicohistorical studies. They deplored biographies and called for a critical exegesis of the "sources." Despite good intentions and handsome methodological formulations, the actual results were at first quite disappointing. There was one substantial exception, however: Kurt Sprengel, a physician, professor of pathology, botanist, and, above all, polyglot and polymath, achieved—through a prodigious effort—Hensler's program. The false modesty found in the title of his work ("Essay of a Pragmatic History of Medicine")[9] should not deceive the reader, as to either the importance of this undertaking, or the ambitions of its author. For that matter, in the French edition, the title no longer includes the words "essay" and "pragmatic," for, in the view of the French translator, Sprengel wished to "provide a complete and philosophical history of Medicine, considered as an art and as a science."

How should we understand the word "pragmatic"? Sprengel provides no explanations or justifications for his use of the word, but it is possible to discern two accepted meanings in the German of Sprengel's time. On the one hand, the word emphasized the practical aspect of something: a history that was described as "pragmatic," therefore, was intended to improve the reader's understanding of the present. On the other hand, this adjective had a philosophical connotation: any history to which it was applied—whether in medicine or in other fields of culture—would necessarily strive to demonstrate that progress is an inherent component, and that historical development has a "sense."

In the superb introduction, Sprengel declares that the history of medicine "does not limit itself to recounting the life stories of renowned physicians, nor to listing and critiquing the works that have been published on the art of healing, in general, and on each of its various branches, in particular." It was necessary, then, to distinguish—as was too seldom done—between the "history of medicine" proper and the "literature of medicine." "The former examines specifically the succession of prevailing systems, the methods upon which the treatments of diseases have been based, the revolutions that have swept the realms of theory and practice." A history of the art of healing, as described above, is accompanied by histories of anatomy, physiology, the natural sciences, and pharmacology, as well as histories of physics and chemistry.

Since only the march of civilization can explain the origin, the progress, and the decline of the sciences in general, it is necessary to observe with great care the progressive development of the human spirit—if we wish to make the history of medicine truly useful and instructive—so that we may properly grasp the different medical doctrines; understand the purpose behind the efforts made to attain the truth, whether successful or not; and amend the system that we ourselves have chosen . . . The history of civilization and of the progress of the human soul would seem to be the true foundation of the history of the sciences in general, and of medicine in particular.

In a certain sense, again according to Sprengel, philosophy is "the mother of medicine, and the betterment of the one is inseparable from that of the other." By combining the history of the two disciplines, we can learn "in each century, the precise extent of knowledge, the opinions that prevailed, and the spirit of art . . . The more attention we devote to the history of medicine, the better we will be able to judge the prevailing opinions of each century in accordance with the spirit that predominated, in that century, in the schools of philosophy." First and foremost, Sprengel exhorted, it was necessary "to grasp the ideas of each author just as one of his contemporaries might have done." The historian must uncover "positive facts," "drawing [them] as much as possible from the original sources," and then assemble them "in such a way as to form a concatenation that joins clarity with accuracy."

Sprengel's manual is a milestone of medical historiography, both for its sheer mass of information and for the way it links ideas and historical events. Here, the traditional succession of "the great physicians" is replaced by a presentation of "schools of thought" and the study of intellectual derivations. This procedure is certainly quite seductive, but it leads to insufficiently solid interpretations. The need to "explain" everything too often exposes the historian to the temptation to judge the past.

The influence that Kant's abstract and critical intellectualism had upon Sprengel was accompanied by the influence of the idealism of his contemporary, Hegel. Sprengel rejected *Naturphilosophie,* although he continued to seek out the "profound meaning" of events. German historians of medicine who lived in the period from the late eighteenth to the early nineteenth centuries were fascinated by the belief that there must be a hidden meaning to history, a higher order that connects the past, the present, and the future. The historical development of medicine was, in their view, much like the development of the human spirit and even the more general development of organic nature, the progressive manifestation of a sort of absolute reason.

Sprengel's book is the first general history of medicine to devote equal attention and space to the modern era and to antiquity and the Renaissance. Nonetheless, the age of the "decline of the sciences," which separates the medicine of Galen from the "reestablishment of Hippocratic medicine in the sixteenth century," receives only passing mention. The Romantics, among them Johann Friedrich Blumenbach, were the first to "discover"—or perhaps to create as a concept—the Middle Ages of medicine.

The manuals written by Justus Hecker[10] and Heinrich Haeser[11] are worthy representatives of Romantic historiography. Beginning from the very title of his work, Hecker boasted that it was based solely on an exegesis of the source materials, while Haeser insisted on the quality of his work as a tool of learning. The former offers a program of medical historical research, inspired by the philosophy of Schelling, while the latter is a perfect achievement of that same philosophy. For the first time, we find here a systematic and in-depth body of research on the history of pathology. Although Haeser's style is often honeyed and his narrative is *schwärmerisch*, or exalted, with a sometimes unmerited admiration for the knowledge, ideas, and technical achievements of bygone eras, it must be said that his power of "contextual" understanding is remarkable, his learning enormous, and his documentation impeccable. Haeser's work served as the model for that *Quellenforschung* on which German medical historiography was to so pride itself. It has been said, rightly enough, that Haeser's manual was the precursor of all later manuals of medical history, and that, to this day, no other book has made it truly obsolete.

In Italy, the history of medicine had two pioneers: Salvatore De Renzi[12] and Francesco Puccinotti.[13] Both resembled the German Romantics, as much for their reliance on sources and their interest in the Middle Ages (in particular, their reassessment of the school of Salerno) as for their fondness of "Hippocratism" and their resistance to new experimental medicine. They attributed a profound significance to the historical development of medicine. De Renzi made explicit reference to Giambattista Vico, who theorized a recurring cyclical development of history. Vico, in De Renzi's words, "singled out in the history of science the true source of the progress of knowledge and the improvement of the human species." Puccinotti, by contrast, relied on the teachings of the church, and found in the history of medicine an expression of divine wisdom.

The Positivist Approach

The "scientistic" reaction to the ideologies and aims of the Romantics was slow and episodic at first, but it became more radical over the course of the nineteenth century; in the end it succeeded in discrediting its adversaries. The great clinician Karl August Wunderlich openly attacked the historical views of Haeser during his university lectures.[14] Instead of delving into the meaning of the historical concatenation of medical doctrines, Wunderlich described "discoveries," traced their origins, mapped their impact, and organized them in a well-articulated series. He focused with particular interest on "scientific medicine"; he therefore devoted special attention to physiology and the other sciences whose university designation had shifted from "auxiliary" to "fundamental."

Wunderlich considered the past to be nothing more than a narrow path leading up to the experimental medicine of his times. In considering the teachings of the school of Salerno, for example, he saw merely an oddity; amusing and distracting in its whimsy, rather than instructive in terms of its contribution to the history of medical thought. There were few ancient physicians indeed who found favor in Wunderlich's eyes; if he was generally scornful, however, he made up for it in his outspoken praise of a few medical giants, such as William Harvey and Hermann Boerhaave. In short, Wunderlich reduced the history of medicine to a sort of lay hagiography; all that counted was the "discoveries" that sprang from the brains of a few select greats.

While Johann Hermann Baas[15] also broke away from the Romantic school of historiography and from the "sympathetic" method, he did so by taking a path that ran in the opposite direction from that taken by Wunderlich. He wrote a history of doctors meant to be read by doctors. He was far more interested in the problems of the practical art of healing, professional institutions, and medical ethics than he was in anatomical or physiological discoveries. He judged the past by the yardstick of the present, but more from the point of view of practical medicine and less from that of the cutting-edge sciences. Translated into English by Henry E. Handerson, Baas's manual exerted a great influence over English-speaking physicians and historians; in particular, it won over readers with its empirical and sociological approach.

Wunderlich's work of history does not withstand a detailed critical examination. To be successful, the "scientistic" approach would have had to master completely, with more conscientious professionalism, the techniques of historical research. In short, it could not alter the working perspective of a medical historian, save by providing certain methodological acquisitions, notably those concerning heuristics and hermeneutics of sources.

The most important contributions came from France. Auguste Comte founded the positivist school of philosophy there, and François Magendie inaugurated experimental physiology. Émile Littré—physician, eminent philologist, disciple of Comte—preached positivist historiography by word and by example.[16] His critical edition, his translation, and his commentary on the complete works of Hippocrates marked a turning point.[17]

The university teachings of Charles Daremberg, summed up in a manual, offer a perfect illustration of the new spirit that permeated research into the history of medicine in France.[18] What with being an adept of Comte's positivism, Daremberg was so influenced by the work of Littré and Ernest Renan that he felt it was his sacred duty to "apply to history the method that has now made it the strength and glory of science, the method that had transformed all other forms of history, except the history of medicine." He specified in the preface that he wrote for his manual: "it is the general development of medicine; it is the determination of laws that guided this development, brilliant or obscure circumstances, constitutional or secondary circumstances that hindered it or advanced it; it is the study of the methods that from time to time guided the developments of science, doctrines, or systems."

In the foreword to the French edition of the work of Sprengel, the translator, Antoine Jourdan, thought it worthwhile to recall—treating it as a "widely recognized truth"—the opinion of Paul-Joseph Barthez, that "a man endowed with the necessary strength of judgment and wisdom can contribute much more to the genuine progress of a factual science than a man who is chiefly occupied in trying to help this science through experimental efforts." The chief conclusion (in fact, the premise) of Daremberg's historical research was that "the history of medicine is the demonstration, century by century, of the powerlessness of theories and the power of facts, of the meaninglessness of systems *a priori,* and of the irresistible and beneficial—however slow—action of the method of observation and experimental method in the establishment of the laws of pathology and of therapy in general."

Thanks to "progress," the past should, and indeed must, be subjected to the judgment of the present; to achieve that, however, it was necessary to carry out an "objective" reconstruction of the events of times gone by, that is, a "scientific" study of the written documents. "If facts are the very substance of science, then texts are also the substance of history." The *Quellenforschung*, then, had not been deposed: quite the contrary. The critical requirements of the new positivist approach were so stringent that all work done on ancient sources now had to be redone: "The field is immense," Daremberg exclaimed to himself, "and scarcely cleared."

Didactic Syntheses

To twentieth-century scientists working directly on the "advancement of the sciences," and even to doctors fighting disease, who daily try to improve the health of individuals or communities, perhaps nothing seems more pointless than historical study. Too many self-proclaimed historians of medicine, sadly, prove them right.

> As it is practiced, medical history is nothing more than an amused and very unsystematic inventory of singular things of bygone times; it is an amiable and anecdotal erudition, to which the veteran practitioner dedicates his "well-deserved" retirement, with a somewhat confused mingling of Latin class and the joys of his internship; the chief subjects of interest are lurid details and the "curiosa" that are forbidden to outsiders.[19]

The medical history by the prolific Augustin Cabanès,[20] still popular, offers an example of this genre. Medical and paramedical magazines currently publish a great bounty of articles of this sort.

Nevertheless, a serious and honorable profession has been established, from the late nineteenth century on, under the name "history of medicine"; there are university chairs, specialized institutes, learned societies, congresses, and prizes. In this official context, numerous works on the general history of Western medicine have been published over the last hundred years. Most of the authors have followed a method that they considered eclectic but that is in fact a sort of "soft" positivism combined with a sociological approach. They never tire of presenting the historical development of medicine as either a series of biographies or a monumental staircase leading up to the modern state of knowledge.

The manual by Julius Pagel (1898), wholly rewritten by Karl Sudhoff,[21] is a prudent synthesis, a paragon of the history—both critical and condensed—of medical literature. Sudhoff's ambition was to describe, with the greatest possible precision and objectivity, "the development of medical efforts to the extent that a study of the sources [*Quellenforschung*] offers us reliable knowledge."

The work of Max Neuburger fits into the same tradition.[22] The author declares that his attention is focused on "the connection between general culture and medicine, and the development of medical thought." In fact, his method consists of a systematic rereading of ancient medical literature. This handsome work is studded with personal observations, often quite pertinent ones. Sadly, he stopped with the Middle Ages.

For those who wish to limit their reading to "cold hard facts," with a great abundance of information cast in a discreetly positivist light, I recommend the manual by the American military physician Fielding H. Garrison.[23] In a single volume, it covers all cultures and all historical periods. The biographical, bibliographic, and institutional information is set forth parallel to the history of discoveries and doctrines.

The manuals written by Arturo Castiglioni in Italy[24] and Paul Diepgen[25] in Germany are particularly successful in combining the history of medical literature with the general history of civilizations.[26] The manual by Charles Singer basically treats medical history as equivalent to the history of the biomedical sciences.[27]

The increase in the number of publications since the end of the nineteenth century makes it difficult for a single person to edit a text that offers a competent treatment of the medicine of all civilizations and all ages. The first major history of medicine written by many authors was edited by Theodor Puschmann, Max Neuburger, and Julius Pagel.[28] This collection contains contributions of varying worth, but on certain subjects it is still a reference work to be considered. As for three other projects with a similar underlying conception,[29] one is sure to profit by consulting their majestic volumes if one is in search of specific information, but the lack of a shared choice of methodology is regrettable. The only sign of editorial consistency among these publications seems to be found in the iconography.

Between the Imperialism of the Historians of Science and the Separatism of the Historians of Medicine

Nowadays, a certain number of medical historians and virtually all historians of science consider the history of medicine to be a branch of the general history of the sciences. Paul Tannery defined the latter as the overall history of scientific thinking, considered in its social and philosophical context. Tannery wished to apply to this specific field the recommendations of the historian Leopold von Ranke. An objective and rigorous reconstruction of "what actually happened" *(wie es eigentlich gewesen)* was the stated objective of the authors of historical works that relied on both analytical research and synthetic appreciations.

Inspired by these ideals, George Sarton undertook a major investigation of the history of science; he dreamed of writing a manual that would be "truly synthetic and complete."[30] The pursuit and popularization of this discipline was for Sarton "a work of faith: faith in human progress, faith in the highest ideal that humanity has ever set up for itself, the progressive conquest of truth and justice." At the end of the First World War, this Belgian pacifist hoped to found a "new humanism" that would replace nationalist aspirations with the objectivity and universality of scientific thought; he advocated a harmonious union of sciences and letters and the reconciliation of idealism with common sense and scientific experience. Sarton believed that the history of science (in the singular, in contrast to Tannery's preference for "scienc*es*") could serve as a sort of bridge between peoples, and between scientific and literary cultures.[31]

According to Sarton (1918), "the history of science aims to establish the genesis and sequence of scientific events and ideas, while taking into account all of those intellectual exchanges and influences that the very progress of civilization constantly puts into play."

Although Sarton was a mathematician by education, he accorded major standing to life sciences and technologies; in a way, he annexed medicine as a part of science in the general sense.

The manuals of general history of science that proliferated in the twentieth century regularly gave considerable space to the history of medical ideas. The scientific territory covered in these works was so vast, and the bodies of expertise required were so varied that it became necessary to have a number of authors work together on each project.[32] Manuals of biological history give major space to scientific ideas of medical interest, nevertheless winnowing considerably.[33]

While there are entire chapters that would fit equally well into a history of medicine or a history of science, the latter does not fully contain the former. So we should hardly be surprised to learn that the "imperialist" campaign of certain historians of science provoked a strong reaction from professional historians of medicine. The outcry against the opinions of

Sarton was spearheaded by the Swiss physician and sociologist Henry E. Sigerist. He affirmed that medicine is not a branch of science and never will be; if one insists on calling medicine a science, then it is a social and not a natural science.[34]

Sigerist described medicine as the set of activities designed to prevent disease, cure disease, and allow the sick to resume a normal life. He thus brought new elements into the medical historical debate, elements that largely emerged from the context of scientific ideas.[35]

This situation was encouraged by institutional structures: each of the two disciplines had its own university chairs, institutes, associations, journals, and congresses. In institutional terms, the history of medicine preceded the general history of sciences.

Between Social History and the History of Ideas

During the international congress of the history of science held in 1931 in London and organized by Charles Singer, an ideological clash took place between the chairman and the Soviet delegation, led by Nikolai I. Bukharin and seconded by John Bernal and a few other illustrious British scholars. Singer was a fierce scientist and a vitalist; he met with the opposition of partisans of a sociological and materialist approach.

The sociological approach has become quite fashionable. We can hardly deny its many successes, especially in the fields of the history of public health and the history of medical practice in certain countries.[36] Its Marxist variant enjoyed considerable institutional development, more the result of political factors than of methodological merit. The level of medical history publications following the Marxist approach was generally quite low; they often made simplifications and misreadings that verge on pure ideological propaganda.

The rift between "pure" and "applied" science was sharpening and widening. Whereas the development of applied science was evidently determined, or at least influenced, by social factors, numerous historians felt that the issue of pure science was pretty much independent of those factors. The situation of medicine was an ambiguous one: it essentially belonged to the applied sciences, but it is possible to claim the existence of a theoretical part—the fundamental biomedical sciences—that does "pure" scientific research.

The "global" vision of medicine led Sigerist to take a stand not only against Sarton but also against his master, Sudhoff. Sigerist meant to limit the history of medicine neither to the field of scientific theories and practice nor to the field of medical literature as a whole. From the very beginning of his career, he had planned to write a manual that "would be different from all the others," and in particular different from Sudhoff's manual: in place of the opinions of physicians, he wanted to describe the fate of the patients. His interest, therefore, shifted from medical texts to documents of social history, from what the physicians thought to what the patients felt, from medical doctrines to problems of public health. In a number of works, Sigerist worked to "place medicine in the larger context of history as a whole." But he waited too late to begin work on his manual: he did not begin writing it until he was old enough to retire, and he died before he had completed the volume on classical Greek medicine.[37]

There was a time when virtually all of the authors of manuals of medical history and professors of that field were either physicians themselves or at least scientists. With the elimination of the classical languages from the cultural baggage of physicians and the development of nineteenth-century *Quellenforschung*, the work of philologists became increasingly important. The sociological orientation of the twentieth century opened the door to professional historians without medical training. The career of the American historian Richard H. Shryock offers a clear illustration of this break in the stranglehold of physicians on the field. Shryock's book on the history of modern medicine sets a standard in the study of the complex array and interplay of scientific and social factors.[38]

The new directions in historiography as a whole threw a spotlight brighter than ever on the history of medicine. The study of everyday life in all social classes and the quantitative approach—as they were practiced by Fernand Braudel and the Parisian school of the *Annales*, in particular, adepts of historic demography—and the new wave of epidemiologists worked together to give new importance to medical historical research and to offer new challenges to historians of medicine. Moreover, the sociology of contemporary medicine, a relatively new discipline, required historical references and immediately established a problematic relationship with the history of medicine. In the United States, the triumph of the sociology of sciences—for instance, the research undertaken by Robert K. Merton—gave a decidedly sociological twist to a technically refined history of medicine that yielded impressive results.

Alongside the "event-oriented" history there was a growing attention to "long-term" history, focusing on the enduring features of a civilization, less exclusively sociological in orientation. And it was through the history of mindsets that the history of "social facts" linked up with the history of ideas. This body of history has hardly become obsolete, and in fact it has recently enjoyed new popularity.

It is fair to question the strict social determinism of "pure" or "hard" sciences. Explanations of the psychological sort (particularly those that reduce the genesis and development of scientific ideas to the "genius" of "great minds") or of the epistemological sort (based on the internal logic of the development of ideas) are still seductive, for it seems difficult, if not impossible, to derive the content of scientific theories from social conditions alone.

The term "external" is used to describe the sociological approach, while the term "internal" is used for the history of concepts, theories, and methods, independent of the social setting. This terminology had to disappear with a tacit truce between "externalists" and "internalists," ending a conflict that raged following the polemic between Henry Guerlac and Alexandre Koyré at a symposium at Oxford in 1961.[39] Without doubt, this is a false problem, an artificial distinction that has created many misunderstandings: except in their extreme forms, which are in any case difficult to defend, these two approaches are complementary, not contradictory.[40]

If the sociological history of science reflects the "new stakes" of history in general, the history of scientific ideas is closely tied with epistemology. The history of science, it has been said, is the "workshop of epistemology," the mine from which epistemology takes its ore by the carload, the "facts" that support its theoretical scaffolding. Now, the epistemological standpoints tend to influence historical presentation, rather than being inspired by it.

History of science with a philosophical bent found its synthetic expression in the major manuals published under the direction of Ludovico Geymonat and Paolo Rossi, but the fundamental debate was carried on in the context of specialized studies. From the English-speaking world came the clash between Karl Popper and Thomas Kuhn; the French-speaking world proffered the new theoretical grids of structuralism and the historical analysis of scientific concepts. Unlike their English-speaking colleagues, who were chiefly attracted by physics, astronomy, and chemistry, many French epistemologists seem to have had a predilection for the biomedical sciences. Georges Canguilhem and Michel Foucault, for example—although neither of them have published works covering the whole of the history of medicine—certainly influenced the methodology of that discipline.

The Three Directions of Medical Historiography

Although the division of the historiography of medicine into internal and external currents is an artificial one, another tripartite division certainly does exist, both in theory and in institutional reality. Medical historical research and teaching often adopts three distinct directions: "scientific" (either iatrocentric or biocentric), "historical" (either sociological or philological), and "philosophical."

Iatrocentric historiography is history written by and for physicians. It is chiefly aimed at medical students. Biocentric historiography focuses on the study of strictly scientific ideas, concentrating more particularly on anatomy, physiology, biochemistry, and general biology than on clinical medicine. The masters of this historiography tend to have a university education or personal experience in the field of biomedical science. Their work is generally characterized by an unfortunate triumphalism, based on the belief that the present is better than the past and that the history of thought has a largely pedagogic purpose. The history of medicine, in this view, should do nothing more than present a better way of learning and understanding current ideas.

Many historians and philosophers denounced this approach as a serious methodological misstep. Reference was made to the "Whig interpretation" of scientific history, an expression coined in 1963 by George W. Stocking; the term is borrowed from a particular trend in political history. "Whiggism" was a radical and revolutionary current that justified opposition to authority, praised progress, and confirmed, even glorified, the present.[41] Examples of Whiggism (also known as "presentism") abound in works of popularization, in encyclopedia articles, and in the historical introductions to works of contemporary science.

In the critique of presentism, the point of no return was reached in the book by Thomas Kuhn on the structure of scientific revolutions.[42] The historian, Kuhn explained, should study the past "per se" and thus "set aside," in some sense "forget," the science of his or her own time. Justified in its essential concern, this anti-Whig current, the main body of which is known as "contextualism," occasionally exaggerates, adopting dogmatic positions that offend common sense. An entirely nonpresentist history is impossible, for historians cannot entirely forget who they are, nor what they know. Even if it were possible, would such a history be desirable? It exists, in a way, in the literature that was written in the period under study, but this is the material of history, not history proper. As Marc Bloch noted in his work *Apologie pour l'histoire*, "A misunderstanding of the present inevitably grows out of an ignorance of the past. But it is perhaps no less pointless to try to understand the past if one knows nothing of the present."

Admittedly, the tendency to select and reinterpret historical problems in the light of modern concerns and standards may lead to serious misinterpretations, especially in evaluating the relative importance of a theory or a practice in a given historical context. At the same time, the continuing relevance of history and its perennially "contemporary" nature lie in precisely this capacity to present a new view of the past at any time, in the light of new questions and new interests. If the risks of misinterpretation can never be entirely eliminated, they are at least limited by the critical approach of the historian and by his or her awareness of the fact that, in any study of the traces of the past, the historian always relies on a "theory," which can be contradicted by the emergence of new historical data or by a new interpretation of data already established.

Historians, then, try to avoid the traps of presentism without necessarily abandoning the advantages offered by the knowledge of their own time. In the field of philology, the task is certainly fascinating, but there are no major methodological innovations, and the work fits into the tradition of the fight against anachronism. Sociological history culminated in the "constructivism" of our times, which strives to place all scientific concepts and theories in a social context.[43] What has emerged from this development is a "history of medicine without the medicine."[44]

Philosophers, lastly, are happy to maintain the history of ideas as their own fief. Scientific theories are born exclusively from other theories (we could state it in a paraphrase of the celebrated adage of Virchow: "omnis theoria e theoria"); the concatenation of ideas, whether or not they are conditioned by the social circumstances, can and indeed must be understood in the light of epistemological analysis. But the history of scientific ideas should not be confused with the philosophy of science. The former's specific domain is the study and explication of the origin and transformations of the structures of scientific knowledge.[45] Naturally, this definition can be applied—*mutatis mutandis*—to the narrower history of biomedical ideas. It accords an enormous field of endeavor to philosophers, without handing over exclusive rights.

Like all other disciplines that are given the name of science, the history of medicine (just like the history of science) is a theoretical elaboration of information concerning an external reality. It shares with general science the thorny problem of the relations between theories and facts. To interpret the documents that are traces of the past in the present, the historian relies on a "historical theory," just as a physicist or a biologist makes use of a scientific theory to interpret an "experimental fact." History is a rational reconstruction of the past; it is not an objective mirror of what actually happened in the past. History establishes links and offers "explanations"; in turn, these explanations require philosophical and ideological schemes of interpretation, schemes that imply general ideas on the nature of knowledge, and on how knowledge is obtained and communicated to others.

The Objective and the Principles of This Work

The differences described in the preceding pages produced a great variety of approaches in the manuals of medical history. The approaches have included the reconstruction of discoveries and theories; the description of professional practices of the past; the history of specialization, schools, and institutions; an analysis of the social consequences of the development of medical knowledge or of medical practice; the study of the impact of the medical art on the pathocenosis, or "community of diseases" (particularly major effects over the past two centuries); and so on. This sort of narrow-focus history still has enormous importance, but nowadays the tendency is to bring these various aspects together, to establish syntheses designed to merge all the different methodologies and the various theoretical interests into a single collective effort. The resulting vision of historical reality is far more complete; it leads to a better understanding of the historical flow of knowledge and medical practice, as they relate to cultural, social, and economic factors.

This work fits into the context of that collective effort to create a synthesis. It is meant to embrace, by and large, the entire course of Western medical thought, revealing its complexity and describing the close links between it and the biological and social reality of human populations.

The historiography of medicine, much like the historiography of science in general, cannot be reduced to a complacent or nostalgic contemplation of the past. More and more, it is a militant profession, fundamental to a better understanding and advancement of scientific ideas, helping to enrich philosophical thought, assisting in the broadening of sociology and the general history of humankind, and allowing us better to master methods of research and offering a critical appreciation of medical problems. Is it not an intellectual necessity to understand the biomedical problems of our own time? And what better method than through their history is there to grasp their content and their meaning? In a time like the one in which we live, characterized by an explosive expansion of biomedical knowledge and a growing socioeconomic impact of medicine and health care policies, one is perhaps more anxious to look into the future than into the past. The new problems that arise each day might lead one to think that looking backward is useless. Still, a historian can easily demonstrate that, alongside the gaps and the occasionally revolutionary nature of new events, there are major historical continuities. And as we rummage among the great figures of the past in search of the roots of modern medical thought, thus studying its workings in order to better understand the creative act of the researcher and appreciate the daily work of the practitioner, we historians may feel—apart from the thrill of discovery— also the satisfaction described by Thucydides: "But whoever shall wish to have a clear view both of the events which have happened and of those which will some day, in all human probability, happen again in the same or a similar way—for these to adjudge my history profitable will be enough for me."[46]

Instead of treasuring up "facts," we have attempted to undertake something that was at once more modest and more ambitious: there was no particular attempt to compile long lists of names, dates, titles of books, and discoveries that mark the history of the medical art; rather we tried to compile a summary of the key ideas.

In an overall vision of the past of civilized humanity, we have attempted to determine both the variety of influences on the development of medical thought and the impact of that thought on the other branches of knowledge and human behavior in different historical periods. It therefore became necessary to take into account the links between the socioeconomic conditions as a whole and the social situation of the physician, in particular, and in another area, the scientific ideas, the beliefs, and the practices involved in the practice of medicine. Reference to the pathocenosis of the various eras was included to convey a better understanding of the nosological theory and the shifts in the field of medical interests; hence the obligation to retrace the general outlines of the constantly changing body of diseases upon which the "medical gaze" came to rest. Nevertheless, highly technical aspects of medicine are treated only in passing. The same is true of institutional aspects of medicine. The history of hospitals, for example, is examined only to the extent that these institutions expressed or influenced the medical thought of the time.

To create this intellectual history of the medical art in its relations with culture in general, we assembled an international group of experts, masters of the appropriate methods for the various eras and problems. Physicians and biologists, historians and sociologists, philologists and philosophers have all worked together in a setting that, we hope and trust, will ensure a unified whole without dimming the focus of each individual gaze.

~ 2 ~

The Birth of Western Medical Art

JACQUES JOUANNA

The second half of the fifth century B.C. marked a decisive step forward in Western medical thought. It was the moment we consider the "birth" of both medical literature and the art of medicine.[1]

We speak of the birth of medical literature in that the earliest surviving writings of Greek physicians, handed down under the name of Hippocrates, date from this period. This does not mean, of course, that these writings were the first examples of a body of literature in a nascent state. The phenomenon is quite similar to that of other literary genres "born" in the fifth century, among them history, tragedy, and rhetoric. Hippocrates is considered the father of medicine in much the same way that Herodotus is considered the father of history. In reality, however, the physician from Kos came from a long line of physicians, who proclaimed themselves descendants of Aesculapius; Hippocrates' grandfather is believed to have been the author of a number of medical works.[2] As for the treatises that have survived under the supposed authorship of Hippocrates, some of them make reference to an older tradition. The most celebrated example is the *De diaeta acutorum,* which speaks of "ancient" authors, referring in particular to the authors of the *Cnidian Maxims.*[3] More than a birth, then, perhaps we should speak of the earliest flourishing. Should we assume that this flourishing corresponded to a passage from the oral tradition to the written form? Certainly, the contemporaries of Hippocrates were impressed by the vast amount of medical literature that appeared in this period. "Physicians have written much," wrote Xenophon, at the turn of the fourth century B.C.[4] The emphasis by the author of a surgical treatise, attributed to Hippocrates, on the difficulty of setting forth an operation in writing suggests that the tradition of writing was not very old at that point, and that it stood up badly in comparison with oral teaching.[5] All the same, we must reject the simplistic view of a revolution coming about merely through a transition from oral to written communication. Oral communication, in fact, continued to be practiced as medical literature flourished. When the Hippocratic author of *De prisca medicina* decries certain tendencies toward modernization in medicine, he numbers among his adversaries both those of his contemporaries who expressed themselves orally and those who set forth their arguments in writing.[6] Even prior to its flourishing in the second half of the fifth century B.C., medicine had already produced a written literature. In a period prior to the appearance of that medical literature which survives to the present day, the collective work of the *Cnidian Maxims* had not only been published but had enjoyed a second edition.[7]

The Conditions of the Establishment of the *Technai*

If we consider medicine as an art, then it is no longer wrong to speak of its birth. In this period medicine first established itself as a *techne*. This Greek term defines two concepts that, at the time, were inseparable: art and science. Physicians were not content merely to describe diseases, to predict their course, and to enumerate the remedies. They also wondered about the ultimate purpose of their art and about its methods, as well as about its place with respect to the other arts and sciences. Their ideas were, variously, convergent or contradictory. With respect to the purpose of the art of medicine, all agreed that medicine should be useful to the sick, or not harmful, at the very least. When the question turned to whether a physician should tend all of the sick, or only those whom he considered to be curable, answers became contradictory. As for the procedures of the art, the earliest medical writings have the merit of pointing out that there is no medical art without method. Even so, physicians might then differ as to what they understood by method. Some authors felt the need to establish new principles, while others opted for the continuity of a tradition established long before. As for the place of medicine among the other *technai*, physicians were aware that medicine belonged to the category of arts that have man as their subject; they differed, however, when called upon to decide whether the science of man should precede medicine, or whether it is not indeed the product of medicine.

The variety of problems raised by physicians in thinking about their art, and the liveliness of the debates that arose, can be understood only in the context of the intense intellectual activity that marked all aspects of human endeavor in the second half of the fifth century. It is true that as early as the sixth century, the scientific spirit had developed in the Ionian world, with the philosophers of Miletus—Thales, Anaximander, and Anaximenes. These philosophers were chiefly concerned with cosmology. But Pythagoras of Samos, in the same period, had interests that went beyond cosmology, touching such matters as the soul of man and the nature of the life of the body. Pythagoras spread Ionian philosophy to Magna Graecia, following his arrival in Croton, in southern Italy; more-over, he had ties to the school of medicine of Croton. It was not until the middle of the fifth century, however, that the subject of humanity became the central theme, chiefly owing to the efforts of sophists, historians or ethnographers, and also physicians. It was then that Greek man discovered the sheer power of his own reason, putting that reason into discussion precisely when he discovered its power, in a remarkable climate of intellectual enthusiasm. During this period the rules of scientific knowledge were established. We thus see the constitution of an entire series of *technai*, all from the middle of the fifth century and the turn of the fourth. In other words, a number of works established the rules of the art, in a vast array of different areas: the art of oratory, medicine, dietetics, cooking, gymnastics, wrestling, horsemanship, architecture, sculpture, painting, and music.[8]

Simultaneously with the birth of these arts, we begin to see discussions, often impassioned ones, as to their very existence or concerning the methods to be applied. The sophists were certainly no strangers to this sort of debate. The earliest sophist, Protagoras, had written a work, still widely read in the time of Plato, in which he set forth the objections to be brought against specialists, both in art in general and in each art in particular.[9] Medicine too came under fire, but these objections, brought to bear by those "who have made an art of vilifying the arts,"[10] contributed indirectly to an enrichment of the thinking of the physicians, who were forced to find responses to these criticisms.

In spite of all these conditions, which explain the constitution of the *technai* in the second half of the fifth century B.C., it is unlikely that we should still possess so many medical treatises from this period had there not lived a physician whose reputation outshone those of his colleagues. All of the medical writings that constitute, in our view, the birth of Western medicine, crystallized around his name. Perhaps Hippocrates, eminent though he may have been, was but one of the physicians who contributed to this first flourishing of Greek medicine. Still, the fact remains that the written production that preceded him had been lost, as has the production that directly followed him.

Hippocrates between Legend and Reality

Hippocrates was already famous in his own lifetime. According to Plato, a young contemporary of his, he was considered the physician par excellence, just as Phidias of Athens or Polyclitus of Argos were the sculptors par excellence.[11] Hippocrates was celebrated for his teaching and for certain of his theories.[12] Aristotle, too, called Hippocrates great not in size but in talent.[13]

Later biographical sources, not all equally reliable, blend the authentic with the legendary, in proportions that are not always easy to determine.[14] In dealing with these biographical sources, we must guard certainly against excessive credulity but likewise against exaggerated skepticism. Not all the biographical works are purely fruit of the imagination, as some have chosen to believe. Inscriptions have provided in some cases felicitous confirmation of certain of the most ancient literary documents.

Born in 460 B.C. on the island of Kos, which was in that period part of the Athenian confederation, Hippocrates came from an aristocratic family renowned for its medical knowledge. His family claimed descent from Aesculapius through his son, Podalirius. The Asclepiads comprised three branches, which—beginning in the city of Syrna in Caria (modern-day Bayir in Turkey), where Podalirius was supposedly shipwrecked on his way back from the Trojan War—spread over a precise geographical area: the island of Kos, the peninsula of Cnidus, and the island of Rhodes. After the branch of the family on Rhodes died out, only the Asclepiads of Kos and Cnidus remained celebrated.[15] Hippocrates, himself a pupil of his grandfather, also named Hippocrates, and of his father, Heracleides, was heir to a long medical tradition. He gave new brilliance to that tradition, first in Kos, and later, after he had left his native island, in Thessaly, where he died.

Stories of his life, of greater or lesser plausibility, have been well known from Roman times onward: Hippocrates' visit to Democritus of Abdera, who was believed mad by his fellow townsfolk because he laughed at everything; Hippocrates' refusal to travel to Persia to put an end to a pestilence in the barbarian army, despite the tempting offers of the great king, Artaxerxes. These are the two best-known anecdotes, spread through the *Letters* attributed to Hippocrates. They are also the stories that have inspired writers and painters: La Fontaine wrote a fable based upon the supposed madness of Democritus, cured by Hippocrates *(Démocrite et les Abdéritains)*. Pieter Lastman, Rembrandt's teacher, portrayed the scene of Hippocrates coming to see Democritus. Anne Louis Girodet de Roussy instead painted the scene in which Hippocrates rejected the offers of the envoys of the king of Persia. These two anecdotes supposedly took place during the early part of Hippocrates' career, when he still lived on Kos.

Two other stories concern the later part of his career, in northern Greece. It is said that he was summoned by the Macedonian king, Perdiccas II, who appeared to be stricken with phthisis, following the death of his father, Alexander I. Hippocrates unexpectedly diagnosed a case of lovesickness, over the courtesan of the young king's late father. A similar story is told of the great physician of Hellenistic times, Erasistratus. On another occasion, Hippocrates is said to have refused once again to treat barbarians: this time, it was the barbarians neighboring northern Greece, the Illyrians and the Paeonians, who had been stricken with pestilence. While rejecting the request of the barbarian envoys, however, Hippocrates supposedly—through wiles—obtained the climatic information required to predict the progress of the disease into Greece, thus enabling him to prescribe appropriate treatment. He then came to the aid of the Greek populations, sending his sons and his disciples to northern Greece, and himself traveling all the way to Athens—after treating the Thessalians— and to the Peloponnesus, passing through Delphi. The existence of this pestilence has long been considered quite doubtful; neither its progress nor its timing coincides with the so-called plague of Athens described by Thucydides. And yet, Delphic epigraphy has preserved in two inscriptions, on the one hand, evidence of Hippocrates' passage through Delphi and, on the other hand, proof of the existence of religious privileges enjoyed by Hippocrates' family in Delphi, a circumstance mentioned in the earliest biographical documentation concerning the account of the pestilence.[16]

This information provided by biographical sources concerning the

Thessalian period of the life of Hippocrates can be supplemented by multiple references in the Hippocratic collection itself. In the treatises entitled *Epidemiae*, we find, for the first time in the history of medicine, a number of individual files on single patients, with a description—in some cases, day by day—of the development of the disease. The geographic origin of these patients is given in some cases, allowing us to follow on a map the places in which either Hippocrates or the physicians of his circle practiced medicine. Special mention should be made of the city of Abdera and, above all, of the island of Thasos. Generally, the cities mentioned were in Thessaly and northern Greece (Macedonia, Thrace) and on the Propontis, now the Sea of Marmara. Places outside this area are uncommon. The northernmost city in which there is documentation of the presence of a Hippocratic physician was Odessos, on the western coast of the Pontus Euxinus (Black Sea), modern-day Varna, in Bulgaria.[17] Toward the south of Thessaly, there is documentation for Athens and the island of Salamina; in the Peloponnesus, for Elis and Corinth; and in the Aegean Sea, for the islands of Skyros and Delos. In the entire work, however, there is only one mention of a patient from Kos.[18] This indicates that the clinical work of the Hippocratic school dates, on the whole, from the period following Hippocrates' departure from Kos, and that its development should be linked to Hippocrates' career and that of his disciples in Thessaly and in mainland Greece.

Although he did leave Kos, Hippocrates, after becoming famous, never broke off contact with his birthplace. Indeed, he was considered a stalwart patriot: according to the earliest biographical documentation,[19] he weighed in on the side of Kos during a dispute between it and Athens toward the end of the Peloponnesian War. Following Hippocrates' death, although he was buried in Thessaly, between Larissa and Gyrton, his homeland maintained a strong memory of him, to the point that Hippocrates was heroized. Each year, the city of Kos officially celebrated the anniversary of his birth, with the offering of sacrifices. And the small bronze coins that circulated at Kos, dating from Roman times, bearing either a bust of Hippocrates or a depiction of him seated, are a clear demonstration that the inhabitants of Kos considered him one of the island's claims to glory. This is also shown by a mosaic dating from Roman times, preserved in the Museum of Kos. It depicts an aged Hippocrates and an inhabitant of the island welcoming a still-young Aesculapius as he lands on the island.

The Medical Teachings of Hippocrates and the
Medical Schools in the Cities of Greece

Hippocrates' reputation derived from his teaching, above and beyond his practice of medicine. With the advent of urban civilization, medical teaching, like most other activities, was circumscribed to the city itself. Thus it was that, in the sixth century, according to Herodotus, the most renowned physicians were those of the city of Croton, in southern Italy, followed by those of Cyrene, a Greek colony in Cyrenaica (Libya).[20] Since, however, the city-state itself had not organized any medical education, nor established credentials authorizing the practice of medicine, the teaching that was done in the cities tended to remain closely bound up with aristocratic and family structures. The transmission of medical knowledge still regularly took place, during Hippocrates' time, within families, as had been the case during Homer's lifetime.

Hippocrates himself received his medical education within the Kos branch of the Asclepiad family. When Hippocrates initiated his two sons, Thessalos and Dracon, into the study of medicine, he was doing nothing more than perpetuating a family tradition. They perpetuated this same tradition by teaching medicine to their own sons, who both bore the name of their grandfather. Prior to our Hippocrates in this family, founded by Aesculapius and Podalirius, there had been only one other person by that name; following him, Byzantine scholarship reports five Hippocrates, while an inscription from Kos, recently published, allows us to add a sixth![21]

At first handed down only within the narrow family circle of the Asclepiads, medical teaching later opened out to include disciples from outside the family. Galen wrote: "With the passing of time, it seemed wise to admit to the practice of this art not only the members of the family, but outsiders as well."[22] This extension of education could not have happened had not the master received certain assurances on the part of disciples from outside the family. These assurances are expressed quite precisely in the famous Hippocratic oath,[23] which entailed a specific associative contract. In fact, this oath was taken by disciples from outside the family when they were selected to receive the teaching of the master. The contract specified the duties of the new disciple and provided moral and financial assurances to the teacher of medicine. The disciple paid a certain sum and promised to see to his master's material needs in case of mishap. The Hippocratic oath, which has rightly acquired an exemplary value because of the ethical undertakings of the second part, can be understood properly only within a specific social context and a given time. From this point of view, the oath appears closely bound up with a revolutionary opening of a medical school originally reserved solely for the members of a family.

When did this opening occur? According to a commentary on the oath, attributed to Galen, and known solely through the Arabic translation,[24] it was Hippocrates himself who decided to open the teachings to outsiders, owing to the dangerously small number of family members able to perpetuate the medical tradition on Kos. Even if we accept that the opening may have occurred prior to Hippocrates, the fact remains that with him it attained an unprecedented scale. Plato, in his *Protagoras*, indicated that it was possible to learn medicine from Hippocrates in exchange for payment.[25]

Of all of Hippocrates' disciples from outside the Asclepiads of Kos, Polybus was the closest to him. This Polybus, who should not be confused with the historian Polybius from the Hellenistic period, married Hippocrates' daughter and succeeded him as the head of the school of Kos when Hippocrates left for Thessaly.[26] Hippocrates' disciples were evidently not all natives of Kos. The Eastern origins of one of them, Syennesis of Cyprus, lead us to think that he must have become a disciple while Hippocrates still lived on Kos.[27]

The number and stature of Hippocrates' disciples—biographers mention ten others, the best known of whom was Dexippus of Kos—justify the traditional sense of "school," though it should remain clear to the reader that in this period a shared education did not necessarily result in a shared doctrine among the disciples, as was the case among the medical sects of Hellenistic and Roman times. Medical knowledge of the classical era was not ordered in a system, any more than philosophical knowledge was. The term *schole*, in the fifth century, was used to indicate a center located in a city, in which a master, in the context of a family tradition that might date back centuries, provided teaching to his sons and disciples, either belonging to the family or associated with the school. In this sense, it is possible to say that there was a school of Kos, as distinct from the school of Cnidus.

At Cnidus, too, medical knowledge was handed down from father to son in the family of the Asclepiads. Ctesias, a physician and historian who belonged to this branch of the Asclepiads, clearly refers to the family tradition in a fascinating passage concerning the risks involved in administering hellebore in the times of his father and grandfather.[28] Each of these schools had its own celebrities: Euriphon was for Cnidus what Hippocrates had been for Kos. We cannot be sure, however, that the teaching was organized in the same manner in the two cities. From Kos, in fact, we have no collective work that can be compared to that from Cnidus, the so-called *Cnidian Maxims.*

Concerning the relations between these two communities of physicians, antiquity provides us with certain documentation that clearly shows their mutual antagonism. Not all the documentation is equally reliable. For instance, there is no basis for the tradition according to which Hippocrates set fire to the building housing the archives of Cnidus.[29] Nevertheless, thanks to Galen, we can read an example of a specific criticism made by an Asclepiad of Cnidus, Ctesias, concerning the way in which an Asclepiad of Kos, Hippocrates, reduced a dislocation of the hip.[30] In more general terms, Galen speaks of a rivalry between the two branches of the Asclepiads of Kos and Cnidus. In his view, this rivalry was positive,[31] though that certainly did not exclude polemics. Indeed, Galen interpreted the polemic of the author of *De diaeta acutorum* against the *Cnidian Maxims* as being a polemic by Hippocrates himself against the Cnidians.[32]

The issue of the medical schools has given rise in recent decades to many disputes among experts. Some have gone so far as to question their very existence. It was in this period of radical revisionism that an inscription from Delphi concerning the Asclepiads of Kos and Cnidus was brought to the attention of scholars of Hippocrates.[33] Since this inscription states that there was an "association" *(koinon)* between the Asclepiads of Kos and Cnidus—something not previously known—some deduced from it that the existence of two separate medical schools might once again be open to question. Others concluded that the school of Kos might merely have been a professional "association" of physicians.[34] Actually, this inscription—which was intended to preserve through an oath the religious privileges enjoyed at Delphi by the family of the Asclepiads, excluding all those who were not true Asclepiads by paternal lineage—was set forth by an aristocratic organization, and not by a professional organization at all. It was meant to preserve the family's religious privileges at a time when the opening of the medical schools to disciples from outside the family might have led to usurpation of the title.

Even more than the opening of the medical schools, the reputation of the school of Kos may actually have been established primarily by Hippocrates' departure for Thessaly. Given that the geography of the Hippocratic collection corresponds to this second part of Hippocrates' career, it is somewhat paradoxical to speak always of the school of Kos when referring to Hippocrates. It might be more appropriate to speak of the Hippocratic school. Nonetheless, the school of Kos, properly speaking, hardly disappeared when Hippocrates left his native island. We have evidence both of the continued transmission of medical knowledge within the family of the Asclepiads following Hippocrates' departure, and of the reputation of the physicians of Kos, in particular through epigraphy of Hellenistic and Roman times. All the same, we know little about the development of the school of Kos, especially when the ancient city of Astypalaia, on the west side of the island, was replaced with a new Hellenistic city on the east side.

However that may be, the school of Kos lost its leadership as the smaller cities made way for the larger Hellenistic realms, with their capitals, Alexandria and Pergamum. The two great physicians of the Hellenistic period, Herophilus and Erasistratus, were not natives of Kos, and they practiced at Alexandria, which had become the great medical center. By this time the physicians of Kos enjoyed privileged ties only with Alexandria, no longer with Macedonia. Praxagoras of Kos was the master of Herophilus; but Herophilus was the master of Philinus of Kos. This reversal perfectly symbolizes the passage from the medicine of Kos to the medicine of Alexandria. History had turned a page, but Hippocrates remained a presence, with the Hippocratic collection, which the scholars of the Library of Alexandria strove to assemble and annotate.

The Hippocratic Question and the Composition of the Hippocratic Collection

Under the authorship of Hippocrates, tradition has handed down some sixty medical texts in the Ionian language, which we can peruse in the monumental ten-volume edition edited by Emile Littré (Greek text with French translation).[35]

Between the life of Hippocrates and the vast body of work that bears his name lies a broad moat of obscurity that modern scholarship will probably never succeed in filling. The body of treatises—despite an undeniable unity consisting chiefly of a spirit of medicine freed of all reliance on magic—cannot possibly have been written by just one man. Many different reasons militate against the idea of a single author. A close examination of the contents of the Hippocratic collection reveals a number of differences in vocabulary, as well as contradictory doctrines. Moreover, the few ancient documents that we possess concerning the question of the author prove that certain of the treatises were not written by the master. In his *Historia animalium*, Aristotle quotes from a lengthy description of the blood vessels and attributes it to Polybus.[36] Actually, this description is taken from a Hippocratic treatise entitled *De natura hominis*.[37] This work, therefore, should be attributed to Polybus, the disciple and son-in-law of Hippocrates, and not to Hippocrates himself. This treatise sets forth the famous theory of the four humors (blood, phlegm, yellow bile, and black bile), which has been considered—throughout Western thought, beginning with Galen—as the cornerstone of Hippocratic doctrine. The creation of the disciple, then, has been attributed to the master. In the same passage of his *Historia animalium*, Aristotle also quotes from a brief description of the blood vessels, attributing it to Syennesis of Cyprus;[38] this description, too, can be found in the Hippocratic collection.[39] Syennesis, as already mentioned, was also a disciple of Hippocrates. Thus, the only two passages of the Hippocratic collection that we can reliably attribute to a known author, through an ancient and trustworthy source, come not from Hippocrates himself but from two of his students.

If, however, we must disencumber ourselves of the illusion that everything traditionally attributed to Hippocrates was in fact written by him, it would be equally wrong to slip into the wholesale skepticism now so fashionable, consisting in the belief that these writings are the work of various physicians, assembled by pure happenstance. A core of major treatises is doubtless the work of Hippocrates or his circle, that is, what was traditionally called the school of Kos. To this original nucleus, however, other treatises were added later, from sources other than the school.

Originating from various sources, these treatises were also written in different periods. Certainly, many of them were written during Hippocrates' lifetime; others date from the time of Aristotle, or even later. The heterogeneity of this collection also derives from the purpose of the writings and their contents. Some of the treatises seem to have been lectures, meant primarily to be addressed to a large audience, made up of specialists and laymen. Other treatises were written for publication, and clearly speak to a public of specialists. Lastly, certain writings are notes or memorandums originally meant for internal use of the physician or the physicians of a school, while yet others are mere compilations taken from other treatises (some of which survive while others have been lost) and serve as manuals. As for the topics covered, they are all the more varied in that Greek physicians were general practitioners and had not become specialists, as was the case in Egyptian medicine.[40] This does not mean, however, that in this period there were no specialized treatises. Two major groups of the Hippocratic collection consisted of surgical treatises and gynecological treatises.

The composite nature of this collection was later accentuated by the vicissitudes of textual transmission, beginning from Hellenistic times, and continuing all the way down to the medieval manuscripts that formed the basis for modern editions. Works that originally composed a whole, or at least a set, were broken down into separate treatises, such as the *Epidemiae*. But certain treatises that were originally separate have been assembled into a whole or a series such as the four books of *De morbis*.

In an effort to organize this set of works, scholars have attempted to separate the wheat from the chaff. As early as Hellenistic and Roman times, and even now, a primary concern of Hippocratic scholars has been determining which works were actually written by Hippocrates himself. There exists a Hippocratic question, just as there is a Homeric question.[41] The trusting optimism of ancient times, when most treatises attributed to Hippocrates were thought to have been written by his own hand, is now opposed by the critical skepticism of modern times. Erotian, a physician who lived at the same time as Nero, and who wrote a *Vocum Hippocraticarum collectio*, was the first author to compile a list of the treatises attributed to Hippocrates. In his lifetime, the treatises considered to be authentic amounted to at least two-thirds of our contemporary list.[42] In the nineteenth century, the trend was the opposite. Littré attributed only eleven treatises to Hippocrates: *De prisca medicina, Prognosticon, Epidemiae I* and *III, De diaeta acutorum, De aere, aquis, locis, De articulis, De fracturis, Mochlikon, Iusiurandum [Oath]*, and *Lex*. Twentieth-century scholarship is even more skeptical. The discovery of Anonymus Londinensis (in 1890) offered new indications on the theories of Hippocrates. These trace back, in the final analysis, to the Aristotelian school, once again bringing up the problem of authorship and casting the spotlight on a work rejected by Littré, *De flatibus*.[43] The oldest source, Plato's *Phaedo*—which Littré used to attribute the treatise *De prisca medicina* to Hippocrates—provides no reliable criterion, in view of the identification of the authentic treatises. If we limit ourselves to the other ancient documents, which are less ambiguous than Plato, concerning the treatises that are potentially attributable to Hippocrates (Ctesias of Cnidus for *De articulis*,[44] Diocles of Carystos for *Epidemiae I*,[45] and Herophilus for *Prognosticon*),[46] we still encounter obstacles. The problem is that analysis of the terminology employed seems to show that the three treatises could not possibly have been the work of the same author, unless we accept that there were major changes in the style of Hippocrates. It becomes easy to understand, therefore, why the Hippocratic question has come to an impasse, and why scholars have tended to stop thinking in terms of a single author and have preferred to talk about a collection of treatises.[47] Research based on groups of treatises—assembled according to relatively objective criteria and in accordance, where possible, with the information provided by ancient sources concerning the medical centers of Kos and Cnidus—has in turn been subjected to criticism. Nowadays, as a result, we use two critical models that are, in theory at least, contradictory. In fact, however, they are complementary. The first model attempts to sharpen the criteria of pertinence for the treatises that could come from the Hippocratic circle or else reflect the Cnidian production; the other model, which considers ancient sources to be inadequate, studies the Hippocratic treatises in and of themselves, with no consideration of their origin.[48]

A summary of the contents of the Hippocratic collection must begin with the set of treatises traditionally attributed to the school of Hippocrates.[49] To this set, first of all, belongs the clearly defined group of surgical treatises. Perfectly organized, these treatises masterfully illustrate the various wounds of the head, caused by missiles and projectiles, and their treatment. They also offer a precise description of trepanning *(De capitis vulneribus)*, as well as the various methods for reducing and treating dislocations or fractures, while respecting the natural configuration of the limbs, and eschewing needlessly spectacular procedures (*De fracturis* and *De articulis*). Alongside these works, intended for publication, a number of extremely concise treatises must have been meant as memorandums: *De officina medici* sets forth the general rules concerning operations or medications in the medical clinic; *Mochlikon* (the title is taken from the Greek name for a surgical instrument designed to reduce dislocations, the "lever") is a compendium, with some rewriting, of the treatises *De fracturis* and *De articulis*.

A second, consistent group attributed to the so-called school of Kos is *Epidemiae*. As we have seen, these treatises should be linked with the activity of Hippocrates and his disciples during the Thessalian period. They are broken down into three subgroups (the first and third; the second, fourth, and sixth; and the fifth and seventh); this division is universally accepted. These subgroups were completed at different times in a period that runs from the last decade of the fifth century to the middle of the fourth century B.C.[50] They are the product of the experiences of physicians who traveled and practiced in a number of different cities, staying for one or more years. In their original form, particularly well preserved in *Epidemiae I* and *III*, these treatises describe, year by year, in connection with the climatic constitution, the diseases that prevail, season by season, in a given place. In certain cases, they add general propositions that sprang from these observations, and clinical descriptions of certain patients. The progress of the disease in those cases is scrupulously noted. To the group *Epidemiae*, certain other treatises are linked, in particular *De liquidorum usu.*[51]

The treatise *De aere, aquis, locis*, expressly written for a physician who takes up residence in a city with which he is unfamiliar, also concerns the work of a traveling physician. A first section sets forth the various external factors that a physician should observe to understand, foresee, and treat diseases successfully: first, the way that places are oriented with respect to the winds; next, the waters used by the inhabitants; finally, the climate. This medical part is followed by an ethnographic section, in which the author applies his medical method to the study of peoples, with a well-known comparison between Europeans and Asiatics. Physical and moral differences are explained, beginning essentially with the nature of the climate and places, and secondarily with the political regime and the various customs; moreover, in rejecting any reference to divine intervention, the author establishes a rational ethnography. The importance placed on climate and, above all, the rejection of explanations based on divine intervention, reappear in the brief but noteworthy treatise *De morbo sacro*, quite likely by the same author. This treatise begins by denouncing, with a lively polemic, those physicians who attribute the various forms of the "sacred disease," epilepsy, to various deities and who claim to treat it with magical procedures (interdictions, purifications, and incantations). The author demonstrates that this disease is no more sacred than others and can be attributed to natural causes: the crisis is triggered by changes in the winds.

Whatever the importance of climatic factors for a traveling physician, the fact remains that a practitioner, summoned to the bedside of a sick patient, must be able to interpret the symptoms so as to understand the nature of the disease and prognosticate its progress, in order better to treat it. This is the argument of the renowned treatise *Prognosticon*, which discusses the favorable or unfavorable symptoms to be observed in acute diseases. It is this treatise that contains the classic description of the face of the patient, altered by disease, foretelling imminent death (the so-called *facies hippocratica*). The therapy of acute diseases is the subject of the treatise entitled *De diaeta acutorum*. Its author offers a lengthy presentation of the use of a decoction of barley, or barley water, also known as ptisane. This explains why the treatise, in ancient times, was known as *De ptisana*.[52] It ends with a discussion of the proper use of beverages and baths. Throughout the treatise, the physician warns against sudden changes of regimen.

The set of treatises of Kos are linked, lastly, with those works whose aphoristic form assured Hippocrates' works a widespread diffusion. The *Aphorismi*, which begin with the best-known maxim of the entire collection ("Life is short, the Art long"), present—in unsystematic order—a lavish harvest of propositions concerning various aspects of the medical art, prognosis, the influence of seasons and ages, and therapy (evacuation, regimen). This was by far the most widely read, published, and commented on of all the Hippocratic treatises. The more recent *Praenotiones Coacae* are a sort of descriptive encyclopedia of Hippocratic prognosis.

Alongside the treatises by Hippocrates and his circle we find a body of work that, in all likelihood, came from the school of Cnidus. In the introduction to *De diaeta acutorum*, we learn, for the first time, of a Cnidian work written and revised by a collective of physicians: the *Cnidian Maxims*. The Hippocratic author of *De diaeta acutorum*—whether Hippocrates himself, as Galen believed, or some other physician—criticizes the Cnidian work on many points. Among those points are insufficient observation of symptoms to establish a true prognosis; an excessively precise enumeration of diseases; and a summary therapy that emphasizes treatment based on evacuants, milk, or whey, while overlooking diet. In addition, many of the treatises of the Hippocratic collection—whose parallel structures indicate that they are derived, in part or entirely, from a common model—show a number of affinities with what *De diaeta acutorum* and other sources tell us about the *Cnidian Maxims* and Cnidian medicine.[53] It is therefore reasonable to consider them to be Cnidian treatises, or of Cnidian derivation. These are nosological treatises, such as *De morbis II*, *De morbis III*, and *De affectionibus interioribus*.[54] As for the Cnidian subdivision of diseases, about which Galen offers specific information, it corresponds with what we find in the treatise *De affectionibus interioribus:* its author distinguishes, exactly as the Cnidians did, four jaundices, four diseases of the kidneys, three cases of tetanus, and three forms of phthisis.[55] This group of nosological treatises are linked to the gynecological treatises, which, like them, present parallel structures: *De natura muliebri*, the complex set of *De mulierum affectibus (I, II)*, and the treatise *De virginum morbis*.[56]

The bonds linking these treatises can especially be seen in the expository structure. For the most part, if not entirely, they consist of a succession of files on different diseases or varieties of disease. These files are put together in accordance with a fairly regular outline involving three fundamental parts: a description of the symptoms, the prognosis, and the therapy. Some of these treatises also contain lists of remedies. Not all the nosological treatises date necessarily from the same period: given the parallel structures, it is possible to single out innovations over time from one treatise to another, especially in the area of the etiology of the diseases.[57] All the same, this group contains on the whole a fairly closed medical tradition, not guided by the experience of traveling physicians, as is, instead, the case with *Epidemiae*. The authors here are less interested in the individual patients and much more interested in the diseases themselves, which they codify and subdivide into subtle varieties. These diseases are, moreover, described as entities that are on the whole independent of the place, the time, and, in many cases, the nature of the patient. Unlike the treatises of the school of Kos, the treatises in question do not even contain any general thoughts about method and the medical art.[58] Their authors seem not to have been affected by the intense critical thought of the sophists about the arts. The description of symptoms is quite minute, however, and we find here for the first time a mention of direct auscultation. This group of treatises represents, on the whole, a more traditional medicine than that of the treatises attributed to the school of Kos.

Lastly, treatises independent of both the school of Kos and the school of Cnidus were added to the Hippocratic collection. For the most part, these writings are absent from Erotian's list. The most important among them are medical treatises with a philosophical bent. They assert that medicine requires a preliminary awareness of the basic elements of human nature. These primary elements are mingled with those of the universe. The two great treatises of a philosophical bent not mentioned in Erotian's list are *De carnibus* and *De diaeta [Regimen]*, both dating from the lifetime of Hippocrates. Of later date, though the subject of some debate, is the treatise *De hebdomadibus [De septimanis]*.[59] Two treatises, known to Erotian and dating from the lifetime of Hippocrates, contain vigorous reactions against this medicine with a philosophical bent. One of these, *De natura hominis*, certainly belonged to the school of Kos; it was written, as already noted, by Polybus. The other, entitled *De prisca medicina*, is not directly linked to the group of treatises traditionally attributed to the school of Kos, although it does present links with *De diaeta acutorum.*[60]

Among the treatises not mentioned by Erotian but present in medieval manuscripts, a number certainly date from later than Hippocrates. The treatise *De corde* shows anatomical knowledge much broader than that of the time of Hippocrates. The precision of the description of the heart found in this treatise is unrivaled until the sixteenth century.[61] Three treatises on ethics, *De habitu decenti, Praeceptiones,* and *De medico,* may be recent in character, but they preach a medical ethics that derives directly from the Hippocratic ideal: a horror of charlatans and respect for the patient. "For where there is love of man, there is also love of the art," one of them says.[62]

The Hippocratic collection is so vast and so varied that any classification we might attempt is necessarily inadequate. A classification into these three major sets is certainly the least objectionable, because it corresponds as far as possible to what we can observe in the history of the formation of the collection, the earliest nucleus of which was the work of Hippocrates and his disciples. By its very nature, the last set is heterogeneous, while the first two, comprising respectively the writings of Kos and Cnidus, are more homogeneous.

In any case, aside from the conflicts, the contradictions, and the differences that may exist among the medical writings gathered in this collection, it is easy to detect a certain degree of unity, both in the medical practice and in the rational approach to diseases and their treatment. Thus, without any wish to overlook differences or contradictions, which are real and so remain, it is possible to speak of a Hippocratic physician in a broader sense, or, for ease of reference, of Hippocrates, without therefore taking a definite position upon the Hippocratic question. In fact, "Hippocrates" means two things. He was a historical figure, but he was also a handy name to denote the body of work that has survived under his name. The ambiguous use has remained constant throughout the course of history, in the reading of this collection of medical writings. It is difficult to avoid it. The important thing is to be aware of it.

Hippocratic Rationalism and the Sacred

When we speak of Greek rationalism in the age of Pericles, we naturally think of the historian Thucydides, who refused—in contrast with Herodotus—to explain the progression of historical events through the intervention of deities in human affairs. A kindred approach can be found in the Hippocratic collection. One can find, here and there in the vocabulary of these medical treatises, the heritage of archaic thought, which viewed disease as a demoniacal force that penetrated the patient from without, to possess him, and which considered proper therapy to be the expulsion from the body of the disease through the use of *pharmakon,* or an evacuant, in the same way that the *pharmakos,* meaning expiatory victim or scapegoat, made it possible to expel evil from a city. But on the whole Hippocratic thought ignored or rejected any intervention of a particular deity in the progress of a disease, as well as any magical therapy involving prayers, incantations, or purifications.[63]

From this point of view, the exemplary treatise is *De morbo sacro.* Epilepsy, which produces sudden and terrifying crises in the epileptic, was traditionally attributed to the intervention of a deity, prior to Hippocrates, and was hence commonly called the "sacred disease." Now, in the first section of the treatise entitled *De morbo sacro,* the Hippocratic author harshly attacks those responsible for considering the disease sacred; the author then sets forth what he believes to be the natural causes that explain the disease. The first, polemical section is a document of great importance to the history of ideas, since it is the earliest known text in which a rational medicine is opposed to a religious and magical medicine. Through a detailed description of the practitioners of this religious medicine, who attributed the cause of epilepsy to various deities in accordance with the differences among symptoms, and who treated the disease through interdicts of more or less magical nature, as well as with incantations and purifications, we seem to see a crowd of strolling charlatans return to life, as we already have in the pages of Plato, and we understand just how important the religious conception of disease remained in the popular mentality during the century of Pericles. In the face of this popular conception, the Hippocratic author categorically rejects any possibility of intervention in the production of diseases by an anthropomorphic deity and, as a result, rules out all therapy directed toward the placation of the divine wrath or the purification of the sufferer. The author claims the existence of natural causes, that is, of a flow of cold humors caused by changes in the winds, and suggests a natural treatment with the opposite means.

The so-called sacred disease is not the only ailment in the Hippocratic collection to prompt criticism of a belief in the divine origin of a disease. An entire chapter of the treatise *De aere, aquis, locis* is devoted to a confutation of the belief that the impotence of certain Scythians, known as Anarei, was caused by a deity.[64] The polemic here is less marked than in *De morbo sacro*, since the author is not attacking a belief voiced by certain physicians or self-described physicians (thus potential competitors of the author), but is rather attacking a belief held by a people that live outside the area in which the Hippocratic physicians practiced their art. The confutation takes the form of an initial acceptance of the hypothesis of divine explanation, only to demonstrate that this leads to consequences that conflict with reality. If the disease were more sacred than others—the author declares—then it should strike chiefly those who offer the fewest sacrifices and offerings to the gods, namely, the poor. Instead, the disease chiefly strikes the wealthy. The hypothesis of a personal intervention on the part of a deity is therefore not acceptable.

Given the diversity of authors found in the Hippocratic collection, however, we should not expect total consistency in the attitudes of Hippocratic physicians concerning the divine. For example, the treatise *De diaeta* [*Regimen*] goes so far as to recommend that patients offer prayers to the gods, above and beyond a rational therapy.[65] This is an exceptional case, however. In *Prognosticon,* the physician is advised, when establishing his prognosis, not to fail to determine whether there might be a divine factor present in a disease. Unfortunately, it is impossible for us to determine with any certainty just what is meant by this expression.[66]

The rational conception of disease and treatment, which is one of the principal characteristics of Hippocratic medicine, is all the more noteworthy in that it was at the exact time in which the Hippocratics were practicing medicine that a religious medicine, characterized by miracle cures, enjoyed an unprecedented development in the temples of Aesculapius at Corinth, Athens, Epidaurus, and Kos. The earliest major literary documentation of these miracle cures can be found in Aristophanes' last comedy, entitled *Plutus* (388 B.C.), in which the deity Wealth, stricken blind, is healed in the temple of Aesculapius.[67] This type of healing, however, is chiefly documented through epigraphic finds: four large stelae uncovered at Epidaurus, dating from the fourth century B.C.[68] The accounts of miraculous healing that can be found on them are in clear contrast with Hippocratic medicine. The patients fall asleep in the sanctuary, see the god in a dream, and awaken the next day miraculously cured. It was therefore the personal intervention of the deity, appearing in a dream, that caused healing in the medicine of the priests of Aesculapius, while any intervention of a personal deity is ruled out in the medicine of the descendants of Aesculapius. The difference between these two contemporary forms of medicine, one miraculous, the other rational, is so evident that we cannot accept the tradition, attested to by the geographer Strabo,[69] according to which Hippocrates made use of treatments inscribed on the votive offerings of the sanctuary of Aesculapius at Kos. The rational medicine of the Asclepiads does not derive from the temples of Aesculapius.

All the same, the rationalism of the Hippocratic authors is cautious not to enter into open conflict with this medicine of the sanctuaries, and stops short of rejecting as a whole the category of the divine. The author of *De morbo sacro* has steered safely clear of accusations of atheism, which were a genuine danger to enlightened thinkers in the century of Pericles. On the one hand, with all the ability of a sophist, he has overturned the position of his adversaries by accusing them of atheism, setting up against them a purer conception of the divine; on the other hand, he has maintained in his own explanation the concept of the divine, assimilating it into the concept of nature. The sacred disease is no more divine than other diseases, but all diseases are at the same time natural and divine.[70] We find the same conception of the divine in the treatise *De aere, aquis, locis*,[71] expressed in such similar terms that it is generally deduced, in a very plausible manner, that the two treatises were written by the same author. This adaptation of the divine to the natural derives from the assumption by the author of *De morbo sacro* that natural phenomena, such as climatic conditions and the winds, are divine.[72] In this way, while rejecting the intervention of a specific deity, which would only upset natural causation, the two treatises preserve the concept of a divine factor that manifests itself in the very regularity of natural laws. Nevertheless, this recovery of the divine as a factor is accepted solely on the condition that the concept be emptied of any anthropomorphic contents.

Medicine and the Birth of the Sciences of Man

The fifth century can be seen as the time of the birth of humanism, as well as rationalism, as long as we attribute to the term "humanism" the broad meaning of man's thought concerning himself and his condition. Man became aware of his place in the universe that surrounds him and, at the same time, of his history. This transition from nature to culture depended on the resources of inventiveness found in his reason.

A New Vision of Man in His Environment:
From Meteorological Medicine to Ethnography

Hippocratic medical literature contributed greatly to the redefinition of humanity in the century of Pericles. Beginning with the Homeric epic, moving on through lyric poetry, and culminating in tragic poetry, man chiefly found his identity through his relations with the gods. The values of piety and justice were the focus of his concerns. If there was a single common denominator that allows us to capture the unity of humanity, this was the contrast between gods and men. Poets compare the power and knowledge of the gods with the weakness and heedlessness of men. This traditional conception was still current in the theater of the classical period. Hippocratic medicine, for its part, offered a different vision of man, one in which man measures himself no longer against the gods but through his ties to the universe that surrounds him. Man, according to Hippocratic physicians, cannot be considered a whole unless one takes into account as well the external environment in which he lives. For instance, according to the treatise *De natura hominis,*[73] man—despite the basic stability of his natural constitution, made up of the four humors—regularly experiences rises and drops in his humors, in accordance with the seasons: phlegm, cold and moist, prevails in winter; blood, warm and moist, in spring; yellow bile, warm and dry, in summer; and black bile, cold and dry, in autumn.[74] Thus, for a Hippocratic physician, human affairs no longer come about in time with caprice and the will of the gods; rather, it is to the pace of the seasons that the humors in the body rise and fall, in accordance with a law of nature.

This new vision of man contextualized in his environment is typified in the treatise *De aere, aquis, locis,* which is considered both the first treatise on medical climatology and the earliest piece of anthropological research known.[75] Written for the use of a wandering physician who arrives in an unfamiliar city, it presents, in its first section, all of the factors that a physician should observe to make a prognosis and determine treatment of the general and specific diseases that may come about over the course of a year. Health and disease are not solely products of the way men live, but also result from a series of natural factors. First, there are local factors, such as the particular orientation of a city with respect to winds and the rising sun, the quality of water used, and the type of soil. Another general factor comes into play, valid in any city: the climatic makeup of the year. All of these factors exert a major influence on individuals, who are affected and react each according to their nature, gender, and age. This relationship between man and environment is not limited to the physical aspect but covers also character and intelligence. Man is defined, therefore, in his totality, through a network of multiform, complex factors that the physician must take into account, considering them as a whole. This medicine, described as "meteorological," inasmuch as it takes into account the influence that "the phenomena on high" (in Greek, *meteora*) exert on health and disease, is based on the idea that man is an integral part of the geographic and climatic setting in which he lives. He enjoys the best health when the external influences that affect him, whether local or general, are balanced and moderate. The idea of moderation, traditionally applied by the Greeks to human behavior, was transferred by the physician to the natural environment of man. This transposition entails a number of accompanying shifts in meaning. In the field of morals, the opposite in behavior of moderation *(metriotes)* is excess *(hybris)*. The new medical outlook replaced excess with change *(metabole)*. And it is, in fact, change that particularly marks unfavorable local or climatic conditions.[76]

One of the most intriguing aspects of this treatise is that, in the second part, which is devoted to a comparison between European and Asiatic peoples, the author extends the etiological method that he has learned from his medical experience to the study of peoples. Medicine thus develops into ethnography. In extending to healthy populations his narrower method of analysis of diseased individuals, the author adds a new dimension to ethnographic research, which, in this context, becomes more explanatory than descriptive. The diversity of the physical or moral features of different peoples can be explained using the same rational principles of explication. Peoples are, first of all, shaped by the climate in which they live: the major moral or physical differences between European and Asiatic peoples are primarily a product of the climate, in accordance with a theory that foreshadows the one Montesquieu developed in *De l'esprit des lois*. This determinism, which places man in a natural environment, is later compounded, or corrected, by a cultural factor, the so-called *nomoi*, which is to say, customs and laws. This two-fold causality is especially notable in the field of morality.[77] The Asiatics' lack of courage, which is weighed against the courage of the Europeans, can be explained primarily through climate, which is homogeneous in Asia and variable in Europe. Moreover, the political regime, usually despotic in Asia and democratic in Europe, reinforces this opposition. In effect, a despotic regime aggravates a lack of courage, since men are fighting on behalf of their lord; whereas a democratic regime reinforces courage, since men are fighting on their own behalf. It may happen that a political regime counteracts the effects of the climate: suffice it to think of those peoples living in Asia under a democratic regime—and here the author is referring primarily, though not exclusively, to the Greek cities in the Ionian area—who are more courageous than others. It is for this reason that man, while subjugated to some extent by the natural environment in which he lives, can elude nature through culture.

It may seem surprising that the author of the treatise *De aere, aquis, locis* should have ventured no further than the traditional division of the world into two continents, arbitrarily separated by the Meotite Swamp (the Azov Sea).[78] The factors that he singled out to explain the physical and moral differences among peoples might well have led him to question this division of the world, or at least to ignore it. We may also be surprised at a certain wavering in the explanations: now the physician feels that climate explains the earth and humans, and later he feels that it is climate and earth that explain humans. We should not expect total rigor from a still-embryonic science. Rather, we should note the unprecedented effort expended by Hippocratic physicians in thinking about man, as an individual or a people, in the context of rational factors that can be applied to one and all without distinction. In this sense the author surpasses the point of view of Hellenocentrism, thus appearing in our eyes as the true founder of a science of humanity.

A New Vision of the History of Man: The Birth of the Art of Medicine

Hippocratic physicians not only defined the place of man in his own environment in the process of thinking about the causes of disease. They further reconstructed the history of man in the context of their thinking about the art of medicine. The treatise *De prisca medicina*, in fact, presents a reconstruction of the birth of medicine, in this way helping to clear up a crucial transition in the history of mankind, the moment in which humanity passed from a state of savagery to a state of civilization through the discovery of this *techne*. The author adopts the conception of historical process typical of modern minds during the age of Pericles.

In contrast to the Hesiodian conception of human history, that of a steady decline following the golden age, in the fifth century B.C. the history of man was considered to be one of progress, both by the tragic authors and by the historian Thucydides.[79] This progress begins with man in a state of savagery, clearly the opposite of the golden age, and continues up to the stage of civilization, brought about through the appearance of the various arts. And among those arts that have led to the birth of civilization, a prominent place is enjoyed by medicine, which saves men from disease and death.[80]

It is therefore only logical that the treatise *De prisca medicina* should offer a reconstruction of the birth and progress of the medical art in a historical narrative that features many similarities with the great texts of the fifth century celebrating the progress brought to humanity by the arts.[81] The twofold discovery of cooking and medicine—to use a term that was not used by the author, who does not mention cooking, but rather speaks of the diet of people in good health—constituted, for humanity, a point of departure, marking a transition from life in a state of unhappy savagery, in which man ate like the animals, to a civilized life. The first of the two discoveries, that of cooking, which consists of mixing and heating, put an end to cannibalism and took man out of the condition of the animals.[82] We might say, then, that humanism was born with cooking. The second discovery, that of the regimen of the sick—that is, medicine proper—is simply an extension and improvement of the other. The second discovery extends the first, inasmuch as it is based on the same reasoning and has the same ultimate goal, which is to say, the adaptation of a nutritional diet for man. It improves upon the first discovery because it is more complex. While there is only one diet for those in good health, it was necessary to invent a number of diets for the sick, because their degree of weakness varies in accordance with the strength of their disease: a solid diet for the least ill, a liquid diet for the most serious cases, and a diet of soups for the intermediate cases. Medicine, therefore, is a sort of personalized cooking. The existence of medicine is the sign of a higher level of humanism, to which not all men have access. Incidentally, but significantly, the author of *De prisca medicina* notes that barbarians are not familiar with medicine.[83] If cooking is a sign of general humanism, found equally among Greeks and barbarians, medicine is a sign of its more highly developed form, Hellenism. Despite his efforts to think of humanity in general, the Hippocratic physician could not quite free himself from the viewpoint of Hellenocentrism.

What chiefly characterizes this reconstruction of the development of mankind is the way it links a realistic vision of man's physical weakness with an enthusiastic faith in the power of man's reason. On the one hand, the author of *De prisca medicina* insists on the role played by necessity and need in research and discovery: it is because the diet of savages, far from being useful to the earliest men, caused suffering, disease, and death, that man sought and discovered the diet of persons in a state of good health. Moreover, it was because the diet of a healthy person was not suited for the sick that men were forced to seek and find the various diets suited to various degrees of sickness. Paradoxically, the weakness of man helped drive him to greatness. On the other hand, it was by virtue of his reason, and not by chance, that man emerged from a profound state of ignorance, making discoveries that the author considers worthy of admiration.[84] These discoveries, accomplished through reason, continue in the present and extend into the future, through the efforts of the trainers of athletes, as far as the diet of men in a state of good health is concerned, and through the efforts of physicians, in a narrower sense, concerning the sick. Such a conception of open-ended progress is evident to a modern mind, but it should be underscored as highly original to a fifth-century mind. Other Hippocratic physicians declared, somewhat rashly, that all of medicine had already been discovered.[85]

Efforts have been made to find the sources of this history of humanity, outlined by the author of *De prisca medicina* in various thinkers of the fifth century, either sophists or pre-Socratics. Among the sophists, the earliest of these, Protagoras, has long been mentioned, and among the pre-Socratics, Democritus has been cited.[86] Actually, our knowledge of these philosophers is far too indirect and spotty to allow us to make any definitive judgments as to their specific influence on this Hippocratic treatise. The resemblances are evidence of a common knowledge upon which anyone could draw and adapt to their own needs. In any case, the theory of *De prisca medicina* is the only fifth-century theory concerning the development of humanity to have survived in its entirety. For this reason, it constitutes a major piece of documentation for any history of human thought concerning its own origins and the birth of civilization.

The Birth of Epistemology: The Criteria of the Art

In the view of all the thinkers of the fifth century B.C., the transition from primitive barbarianism to civilization was the result of the birth of the arts, whether they attributed that birth to the gift of a god or to a human discovery, and whatever the arts to which they might refer.[87] Simultaneous with the birth of the arts came discussions—exceedingly lively at times— concerning the existence of those arts and the methods to be employed in practicing them. The Hippocratic collection offers the best image of these debates on the concept of art, because it is the only collection of texts of the fifth century to have preserved in their entirety examples of those treatises that were called *technai*.

A paradox of this period of intellectual ferment was that the existence of the arts was already being radically debated at the very moment when specialists were attempting to establish the rules of those arts. The Hippocratic treatise entitled *De arte* is quite illuminating on this subject.[88] The author opens with this striking statement: "Some there are who have made an art of vilifying the arts"; and the entire purpose of his exposition is the demonstration that an art of medicine exists, in response to the numerous objections of detractors. According to these detractors, there is no such thing as medicine, since some patients get well without relying on physicians, while other patients die despite all the efforts of physicians.

One merit of the treatise *De arte* is that it clearly shows how this lively debate was able to offer a positive contribution, by encouraging and deepening the thinking of physicians about their own art. Indeed, the treatise gives some idea of the earliest discussions of science, at a time when science was becoming aware of its own development and when it was first establishing itself against its external enemies. It is not excessive to speak of the first epistemological considerations, since this confutation of outside enemies involved an initial defense of all the arts.[89] This surprisingly refined discussion of general epistemology required, on the part of the physician, a solid familiarity with contemporary discussions of ontology and with the philosophy of language. The arguments developed here are of great importance to the history of ideas, not only because this is the earliest known documentation of epistemology as a discourse concerning science, but chiefly because this document was written by a scientist and not by a philosopher. We know that epistemology was long to remain the domain of philosophers; we know that its founder was traditionally considered to have been Plato. Actually, however, this body of epistemological thought should be traced back to the time prior to Plato, when it was not reserved to sophists and philosophers alone, but also involved men of science.

When the author of *De arte* narrows his analysis to medicine proper, he begins to deal with problems that are closer to what we might expect from a discussion of knowledge and the criteria of science. The criteria of art can be defined by examining art's antonym, chance. This antithesis between art and chance or, if we prefer, between science and fortune, established the structure from the fifth century onward for all discussions of the various activities that aspired to the status of art. We find it in the classical theater as well. Euripides, in his *Alcestis*, put it nicely and vividly: "The outcome of our fortune is hid from our eyes, and it lies beyond the scope of any teaching or craft."[90] It is in the technical writing of physicians, however, that this antithesis can most frequently be found, prior to Plato and Aristotle.[91]

Chance, already in *De prisca medicina*, is evoked by the Hippocratic physician to reject the absurd hypothesis according to which there is no medical art: "If an art of medicine did not exist at all . . . the treatment of the sick would be in all respects haphazard."[92] And when the same author boasts of the discoveries of medicine, he points out that these discoveries were "the work, not of chance, but of inquiry rightly and correctly conducted."[93] This antithesis plays a major role as well in the treatise *De arte*, specifically in the response offered to adversaries who claim that "those who escape do so through luck and not through the art."[94]

Since it is the antonym of undifferentiated chance, art is defined primarily by the possibility of establishing prescriptive distinctions. Knowledge implies being able to discriminate between that which is correct and that which is not.[95] This theoretical distinction marks the difference between good physicians and poor physicians, a difference that is spotlighted especially in the cases of the most dangerous diseases, when poor physicians are unmasked just as poor helmsmen in a tempest are.[96] Thus, while chance is the realm of the undifferentiated, art manifests itself through distinctions among values and a hierarchy of all those abilities that are revealed in critical moments. The realm of art is the realm of differences: "For a leech is of the worth of many other men," we read in the *Iliad*.[97] This traditional idea of the superiority of a man of science is inherent to the very definition of the art, ever since its birth in the fifth century B.C. Science, inasmuch as it is not equally shared among citizens, will not appear as a political virtue. This is the meaning of the end of the myth of Protagoras recounted by Plato, in which the phase of the discovery of the arts, the phase of difference, is completed by the phase of the acquisition of political virtues, the phase of equal sharing among men.[98]

The world of science is not only the world of differentiation of values and men, but also a world of perception of the consistency of things. Whereas chance is synonymous with disorder and apparent spontaneity, science discovers the regularity of the natural order of things. One of the greatest merits of the Hippocratic physicians is that they articulated, in its most universal form, what was later to be called the principle of determinism. Everything that happens has a cause. The most theoretical articulation appears in *De arte:*

> Indeed, under a close examination spontaneity disappears; for everything that occurs will be found to do so through something [*dia ti*], and this "through something" [*dia ti*] shows that spontaneity is a mere name, and has no reality. Medicine, however, because it acts "through something" [*dia ti*], and because its results may be forecasted, has reality, as is manifest now and will be manifest forever.[99]

Probably, this physician was not the first in classical Greece to have formulated the idea of the necessary concatenation of events. Leucippus, the master of Democritus and the founder of atomism, already had written in his treatise *On the Mind:* "Nothing is produced in an absurd manner, rather all things are produced according to a reason and a necessity."[100] The physician's text, however, foreshadows even more closely, in its formulation, Aristotle's belief that art is defined by its knowledge of a "through something."[101] And that is not all: the concept of causality—and this is the most important new idea of the Hippocratic text—is already linked to that of prediction. If a knowledge of causes seemed indispensable to the physicians of the Hippocratic collection, it is not only for the prediction of diseases, but also so as to combat them with a correct and natural treatment. The author of *De arte* puts it in his own way: "If indeed they understood their diseases they would never have fallen into them, for the same intelligence is required to know the causes of diseases as to understand how to treat them with all the treatment that prevents illnesses from growing worse."[102]

Similarly, the author of *De flatibus* begins his discourse with a number of general considerations that all lead in the same direction: "For knowledge of the cause of a disease will enable one to administer to the body what things are advantageous. Indeed, this sort of medicine is quite natural . . . To sum up in a single sentence, opposites are cures for opposites."[103]

According to this last passage, it is clear that the causal method is the condition *sine qua non* of a full-fledged medical art. The treatise *De prisca medicina*, moreover, insists on the need for men of science to go beyond the limits of mere descriptive or prescriptive statement, and to venture on to the stage of the interpretive postulate, by taking into consideration the causes, as well. This passage is well known. After defining the task of the physician, who must study the influence of foods and the entire regimen on men, the author takes the example of cheese: "It is not sufficient to learn simply that cheese is a bad food, as it gives a pain to one who eats a surfeit of it; we must know what the pain is, the reasons for it, and which constituent of man is harmfully affected."[104]

In other words, science is causal or it is not. And physicians are able to further refine the analysis by distinguishing triggering causes from deep causes, by virtue of a technical vocabulary still in the course of formation.[105] We can thus see the emergence, even in the earliest epistemological texts of ancient Greece—beginning with a remarkably lucid reflection on the art of medicine—of a number of key concepts that were to guide the development of science for centuries to come. Certainly, there is quite a difference between theoretical declarations and practical applications. For example, the author of *De prisca medicina,* despite his admirable declarations concerning the need for causal understanding, fails to proceed to any experimental investigation to further implement his own program.[106] A certain conceptual architecture, in any case, had already been created. In particular, the field of science, which establishes distinctions, unifications, and predictions, excludes the field of chance, where the indistinct, the unexplained, and the unpredictable all hold sway. In this manner, the cognitive paradigm of order, with the exclusion of disorder, was inaugurated. It was to be the foundation of the deterministic conception of science.

Relations between Medicine and Philosophy

Against the attacks from without, all physicians were obliged to close ranks, presenting a united front in defense of their art. But when it was time to discuss the methods of the medical art, rather than the basic issue of its existence, specialists began to take sides. The fundamental methodological problem, which was widely debated within the ranks of physicians, concerned the relations between medicine and philosophy.[107] There were those in favor of philosophical medicine, just as others were opposed. While the external enemies, those rejecting the medical art entirely, are known to us only indirectly through the depiction of their standpoint offered by a Hippocratic physician, the debate between medicine and philosophy is found in the heart of the Hippocratic collection. Because of its variety, the collection preserves works representative of both positions, offering a direct documentation of a "crisis" of medicine, that is, a decisive moment in which the medical art began to establish its independence from philosophy.

Let us go straight to the heart of the debate. According to the partisans of philosophical medicine, it is not possible to understand medicine without having a prior understanding of human nature and the various elements of which man is composed.[108] In this context, the constituent elements of man are dependent on the elements that make up the universe. The art of medicine is based, therefore, on principles extraneous to the art itself, deriving from cosmology. If, however, in all proponents of philosophical medicine the method never varies, it should be noted that at least the conceptions of man and the universe do differ sharply. One treatise hearkens back to monism: the author of De flatibus believed that air was the only cause of all disease.[109] Another adopts a dualistic solution: according to the author of De diaeta [Regimen], man is composed of two opposite and complementary elements: fire, which is dry and warm; and water, which is cold and moist.[110] One remarkable aspect of this treatise is that it presents the most ancient formulation surviving in Greek literature of the micro- and macrocosmic theory. Man—it says—is "made in the image of Everything."[111] A third treatise, entitled De carnibus, is based on a three-element cosmology: fire, earth, and air;[112] this work is unique in its field, in that it precisely responds to the program of the "investigation of the nature" of philosophers, mentioned by Plato in Phaedo.[113] This dialogue comprises an explanation of the initial formation of the various parts of the human body, beginning with the mixture and transformation of the primary elements of the universe, as well as an explanation of thought and the senses. Lastly, the author of De hebdomadibus [De septimanis], who established, as did the author of De diaeta [Regimen], a correspondence between man-microcosm and universe-macrocosm, is noteworthy for his attempt to explain everything—both man and the universe—with the number seven.[114] The variety of solutions adopted in the many treatises considered reflects the diversity of cosmological systems found among the pre-Socratics, even if we cannot establish exact correspondences between theories of physicians and theories of philosophers. In any case, it is possible to draw a link between the monism of the author of De flatibus and the ancient theory of Anaximenes of Miletus, a sixth-century (B.C.) philosopher who believed that air was the only substance in the universe; this theory was proposed once again in the fifth century by Diogenes of Apollonia. It is likely that Aristophanes, in The Clouds, was poking fun at this latter philosopher, through the figure of Socrates.[115] The osmosis between this medicine with a philosophical bent and pre-Socratic philosophy is such that some have spoken of an influence of philosophy on medicine, as well as an influence of medicine on philosophy. Although it may seem a bit much to postulate a direct influence of Hippocratic medicine on pre-Socratic philosophy,[116] it is clear that the philosophers of the fifth century, closely interested in the development of medicine, placed far greater importance on thinking about living creatures than their sixth-century predecessors had done, once cosmology had been enriched with an anthropology.

Faced with this medicine with a philosophical bent, the authors of two treatises reacted vigorously, affirming the medical art's autonomy from philosophy. The first, *De prisca medicina*, had the considerable merit of setting forth the problem of method with great clarity. We have already seen how this treatise reconstructed the "archaeology" of the medical art. The occasion for this apologetic history of medicine was furnished by a polemic against certain innovators, whose ambition had been to found a new medicine that, to explain diseases, began from such simple postulates as heat, cold, dryness, and moisture. These innovators were probably reacting against what they saw as the excessive empiricism of the medical art; they wished to refound medicine on one or two clear and simple principles, precisely as had the philosophers who proposed to explain the diversity of reality by starting off from a small number of fundamental elements.[117] In the eyes of the author of *De prisca medicina*, these basic postulates were simplistic and did not correspond to reality. The polemic spread later to cover the entire current of philosophical medicine; and it was here that the author presented the position of his adversaries properly, while contrasting his own method with lucidity. Whereas the physicians who supported philosophical medicine believed that, to practice medicine properly, it was necessary to begin with a prior understanding of human nature, the author of *De prisca medicina* declared that it was a knowledge of medicine, as properly defined, that best served as the source of an understanding of human nature. Through a simple reversal of terms, the author brought about a full-fledged revolution. Physicians were no longer obliged to attempt to recreate man, beginning from a few first elements, the way a painter who depicts man begins with a few primary colors. The physician's task, then, was to observe the various reactions of the human body to the different actions of a regimen (food, drink, exercise). Through the causal study of these actions and the corresponding reactions, a physician could determine the different categories of human nature. In this way, the physician had replaced the general concept of human nature, which comes from a body of knowledge shaped by philosophical thought (*physis*, in the singular), with the different categories of human nature obtained through reasoned observation (*physeis*, in the plural). From this point on, medicine acquired a new standing: it was no longer driven by philosophical anthropology, but rather became itself a science of man.

The second attack against philosophical medicine came at the beginning of the treatise *De natura hominis*. From the very first sentence, Polybus attacks those who, in treating of human nature, go beyond that part of human nature that pertains to medicine. At first, the set of problems is quite similar, therefore, to that of *De prisca medicina*. Later, however, the critique follows different paths: Polybus denounces the ideas of philosophers who believe that man is composed of, variously, air, fire, water, or earth. He rejected these beliefs for two reasons. First, they went beyond what the physician can observe in man;[118] the basic principles of the universe, such as air, fire, water, and earth, cannot be observed, as the humors blood, phlegm, and bile can be. Second, these conceptions evinced monism. Monism permits no explanation of pain, nor of the diversity of diseases and remedies, nor of conception and birth.[119] And for the same reason, Polybus disapproved of physicians who believe that man is composed of a single principle, whether blood, phlegm, or bile. According to the author of the treatise *De natura hominis*, human nature is composed of four humors (blood, phlegm, yellow bile, and black bile); in a state of health, they are mingled and balanced.

The mistrust expressed in these two treatises toward philosophy, though it did not result in identical conclusions concerning human nature, manifested itself in a direct denunciation of two pre-Socratic philosophers mentioned by name: the author of *De prisca medicina* cited Empedocles as an exemplar of philosophical medicine,[120] while the author of the treatise *De natura hominis* named Melissus of Samos, probably a pupil of Parmenides of Elea,[121] in his polemic against monist philosophers. These citations are all the more remarkable in that the use of proper names in a polemical context was not a custom typical of the fifth century.

From the Observation of the Visible to the Reconstruction of the Invisible

Despite the internal debates that might pit certain Hippocratic authors against one another, there remained a shared foundation of thought, the unity of attitude of physicians toward the sick and toward disease. And it is this common approach that we can describe as Hippocratism. Among the chief characteristics of this Hippocratism, aside from the rationalism that we have already explored, there was a remarkable faculty of observation and of recording one's observations in the greatest detail.[122]

Clinical Observation

Everything that could be perceived concerning the manifestations of a disease was noted and recorded, for the slightest detail might well have the value of a sign. Prognosis, like diagnosis, could result only from a set of signs. Certain texts provide advice to physicians concerning the best way of making observations: "Take the body of the patient as a subject under examination: sight, hearing, smell, touch, taste, reason."[123] Physicians were not satisfied with merely observing; they knew that there existed an art of observation. The observation of a patient by a physician should be performed through the concerted use of all the senses, and with intelligence.

If sight is mentioned first in this text, that is not only because sight is the sense that allows the greatest array of observations; it is also because sight is naturally the first sense to be stimulated when the physician first approaches the patient. It may even happen that a physician will formulate an initial prognosis at some distance from the patient, performing his preliminary examination strictly through visual observation.[124] In any case, the first signs that a physician will observe upon reaching the bedside of a sick patient are those perceptible through sight: the patient's face, the way in which the patient is lying, and the movement of the patient's hands. The author of the *Prognosticon* made observations of astonishing accuracy on all these aspects; his visual description of the alterations of the facial features during the onset of death remains celebrated, under the name *facies hippocratica*.[125] It goes without saying that visual observation can go no further than that which can be seen with the naked eye. The well-trained eye of a Hippocratic physician, however, saw details that a modern physician can no longer see, chiefly because a modern physician no longer needs to see them. Modern analytical instruments render those observations superfluous. All the same, certain visual observations made by Hippocratic physicians remain an established part of modern science and still constitute significant symptoms, such as carphology, or floccillation, and the Hippocratic, or clubbed, finger.[126]

Observation through listening led certain physicians of the Hippocratic collection to practice direct auscultation in cases of pneumopathy; this meant placing one's ear directly against the patient's chest and listening to the noises within ("it seethes inside like vinegar," "a sound like new leather"). Physicians did not stop with passive auscultation; they went on to cause sounds of internal surging by shaking the patient before listening, so as to establish the site on which to make an incision for the drainage of water or pus. This procedure of direct auscultation, whether or not it was accompanied by succussion of the patient, was long forgotten or ignored. It was not until the turn of the nineteenth century that this procedure was given renewed consideration, by René Laennec.[127]

In the programmatic passages, in which the physicians give advice as to the best way to perform an examination of a patient, the enumeration of the senses is completed by a mention of either intelligence *(gnome)* or reason, that is, the faculty of calculation *(logismos).*[128] The physicians never explicitly explain in these passages the role played by this faculty, mentioned on the same level as the other senses. Still, it is clear (at least from the point of view of the author of the *Prognosticon,* certainly a paragon of Hippocratism) that they are talking about the faculty of calculating *(logizesthai)* the value of the entire set of signs observed, balancing those favorable against those unfavorable, comparing them with one another to form an accurate appreciation of the state of the patient, and thus formulate a sound prognosis.[129]

This attention to the minutest of details led these physicians to compile remarkably precise records, or files, on their patients. As mentioned earlier, for the first time in the history of medicine, we find these sorts of observations made on the case histories of individual invalids. What was found prior to this—even prior to Greek medicine—were individual records, or files, on each disease. In Egypt, texts on medicine were made up of a series of short annotations on diseases, arrayed *a capite ad calcem,* from head to foot. The files consisted of three major sections: description of the symptoms, prognosis, and therapy. We find the same form of presentation in certain nosological treatises in the Hippocratic collection, traditionally attributed to the Asclepiads of Cnidus, though we do not know with any certainty whether this is due to the influence of Egyptian medicine. What is clear is that unlike the Egyptian texts, the Greek nosological treatises do not prescribe magical or religious procedures, such as prayer or spells. These treatises betray a notable spirit of observation in the description of symptoms of disease.

We first find records of individual patients in the writings of the school of Hippocrates, following his departure from Kos for Thessaly. They are preserved in the body of the treatises entitled *Epidemiae*. To give some idea of the number of files, let us consider the earliest group, comprising the first and third volumes and including the files of forty-two patients. Galen counted fifty individual case histories in *Epidemiae V.*[130] If we assemble all the case histories contained in all of *Epidemiae*, we would have a tragedy in one hundred acts. These files note the patient's symptoms day by day, from the onset of the illness to the resolution (usually fatal) of the case; there is every indication that these records are impromptu and made on the spot. All the same, this apparent spontaneity should not hide the fact that in forming their descriptions, physicians applied a preexisting body of knowledge, a precise familiarity with the array of points to be examined and with the intrinsic value of each of the signs.

The clinical descriptions made by Hippocratic physicians thus attained an unquestioned level of perfection, making use to the greatest possible degree of all that can be perceived through the senses, and painstakingly determining from that evidence—through intelligence—its prognostic value. This art of external observation, however, was considerably limited by those physicians' ignorance of the invisible world inside the body.

The Reconstruction of an Invisible World

The Hippocratic physicians did not practice dissection on human beings. They were obliged to reconstruct the internal structures of the human body, either by working from what they saw or felt through an external examination or else by making use of what they observed in dissections of animals.[131]

We should not therefore be surprised if their understanding of this internal world, which remained fairly obscure to them, was partial, erroneous, or even quite fanciful. Translators of the works of the physicians of antiquity commonly stumble into anachronisms, making use of terms that imply a level of knowledge which they did not possess. Even such simple words as "organs," "nerves," "veins," and "arteries" can give rise to anachronisms. Of course, the Hippocratic physicians were familiar with the principal organs, such as the brain, the heart, the lungs, the liver, the kidneys, the spleen, and the bladder, all arranged in two large cavities, upper and lower, which were separated by the diaphragm. They did not yet describe them as "organs," however: the concept of "organ" is Aristotelian.[132] The modern-day term "nerve," although it does derive from the Greek word *neura,* used commonly by Hippocratic physicians, no longer corresponds to the ancient meaning. They confused tendons with nerves, and they were not aware of what we now describe as the nervous system. To their minds, these were simply ligaments, required to hold together the whole body or to cause movement through increases or decreases of tension. Although they were aware of muscles, the Hippocratic physicians knew nothing of their property of contraction. Certainly, they were familiar with the fibrous tubes that transport blood, but they called them *phlebes* (hence the term "phlebitis"); moreover, on the whole, they made no distinctions between veins and arteries.[133] The word "artery" was used to designate what we now call the trachea, which is actually an abbreviation of "trachea-artery."[134] The arterial pulse had not yet been discovered, and was not used for diagnosis prior to the Hellenistic age.[135] The pounding in the temples, in particular, had been observed, but only as a pathological perturbation.[136] It is therefore better, in speaking of the Hippocratic age, to use the term "vessels": it was believed that these vessels transported not only blood but also air and perhaps other humors as well.[137] The arrangement of vessels within the body was pretty much left to the imagination. Each of the major descriptions contained in the Hippocratic collection offered its own general system.[138] In particular, the point of origin of the various systems diverged. Hippocratic physicians, evidently, had no idea of the circulation of the blood, which was discovered only in the seventeenth century. One physician thought the point of origin was the head; another thought it was the liver; a third, the heart. Paradoxically, from Aristotle onward, the best-known description was also the most fanciful. To show that his predecessors had traced the vessels back to the head, and that he himself was the first to have understood clearly that they began at the heart, Aristotle quotes as an example a lengthy description written by Polybus, which is also preserved in the treatise *De natura hominis.* This illustrious disciple of Hippocrates spoke of four pairs of vessels running down from the head, all the way to the feet, with ramifications in the arms, without once mentioning the heart!

It was probably in connection with the female genitalia that physicians most relied on their imaginations. The uterus, correctly identified as the source of certain feminine diseases,[139] was thought to roam on odd voyages throughout the body. That the uterus is subject to deviations or many sorts of prolapse is accurate. But that it could drop as far as the legs, provoking convulsions in the big toe, or that it could venture as far as the liver, hip, loins, or ribs, or that it could rise up to the heart or even the head—these ideas are truly astonishing in the context of a medical art that had freed itself from the errors of magic.[140] In certain cases, the uterus seems to be endowed with a life of its own. We see it, dehydrated, and "running" madly toward moisture, lunging at the liver, which is gurgling with humor,[141] thus causing the sudden suffocation of the woman. Or, suffering from excessive heat, we see it "leap" toward the external coolness;[142] this was an explanation for a certain type of prolapse.

In the description of the internal world, not everything was left quite so much to the imagination. The arrangement and the shape of the bones were easier to discover than those of the vessels and the uterus. Surgical treatises reveal a solid understanding of the human skeleton and above all a clear awareness of the need for complete knowledge of the shapes of bones and ligaments to make diagnoses and to treat properly dislocations or fractures. The author of *De articulis*, for instance, accurately described the spinal column,[143] and then proceeded with an angry denunciation of certain of his colleagues who confused a fracture (benign) of the spinous apophysis of a vertebra with a forward dislocation (grave) of the entire vertebra.[144]

When we move from anatomy to physiology, the gaps in understanding are even more serious and the free play allowed the imagination far greater. Such vital functions as respiration and digestion lacked any adequate explanation. There is a sharp contrast between the precision with which certain physicians observed respiratory disturbances in order to single out certain prognostic signs[145] and the explanations offered by others for the role played by respiration. Just as certain Hippocratic authors were able to describe the system of vessels without involving the heart, so other authors—of no lesser standing—described the path of air through the body without mentioning the lungs in any significant role.[146] The phenomenon of digestion is treated in purely vague and metaphorical terms. Physicians used an imprecise term, such as "cavity" *(koilie)*, to refer to the "stomach" even when discussing digestion.[147] Among the viscera, the stomach was not considered to be particularly important.[148] Digestion was conceived of as a sort of wrestling match between man and his food, normally ending in the triumph of the former over the latter. It was also compared to cooking in a pot, or to a sort of fermentation in a vat. The three explanatory models could even be combined.[149] For Aristotle, digestion was still seen as a form of cooking.[150]

Hippocratic Humoralism

The field of humors in Hippocratic physiology was one in which physicians relied on their imaginations to produce a perfectly clear system explaining an entirely dark interior world. Certainly, the observation of the various fluids secreted by the body when in a state of health, and especially when wounded or during the course of various diseases, allowed the imagination to depict an internal environment in which these fluids must have "flowed" *(rhein)* through the body, given that they emerged into the outside world in the form of a flow (spit, urine, stools, discharges from the eyes and the ears). "First we have the more obvious symptoms, which all of us experience and will continue to do so," to borrow the terms in which one of the physicians expressed himself, referring to "those of us who suffer from cold in the head, with discharge from the nostrils."[151] What, then, could be more natural than to imagine that such a flow should proceed as from a spring, from some higher point, and hence from the head and from the brain? This conception still survives in modern French, in which a cold is called *rhume* (from the Greek *rheuma*) or *rhume de cerveau.* We can say with certainty that the Hippocratic physicians must have had to perform a remarkable feat of the imagination to construct, from this point, an exceedingly elaborate system of humors that rise and descend within the body. It was usually beginning from the brain that the humors would flow into various parts of the body; but if the brain could generate such a flow of humors, it was because the brain had attracted them from the rest of the body. One curious passage from *De prisca medicina*, in which the author describes what we call the organs (which he calls the "structures"), shows clearly the role that physicians assigned to the various organs in this model. The shape and the makeup of the organs determines their functions. The piriform and hollow organs in particular attract the humors: the head, the bladder, and the uterus. The spongy and porous organs are those most capable of absorbing the humors upon contact: here we find mention of the spleen, the lungs, and the breasts. A number of Hippocratic physicians systematically reconstructed the path of the humors, which, having flowed to the head from the belly, flowed out into the various parts of the body in which they fastened themselves and caused various diseases. An arithmancy served at times as a support for this type of reconstruction: the humors flow by chance from the brain, but chance then works with considerable precision, given that the destinations of that flow are seven.[152]

The number of the humors, as well as their internal paths, was reconstructed. Humors such as blood and bile were easily observable in everyday experience (wounds, sacrificial offerings), and were therefore well known prior to Hippocrates' time. Greater imagination was required for the reconstruction of the other humors, such as phlegm, which had originally been conceived as the inflammatory humor and later, following a development about which we know little, was considered the coldest humor in the body; or for the distinction between yellow bile and black bile. Hippocratic physicians, for that matter, did not all agree on the same theory of the humors. In many treatises, it was bile and phlegm that played essential roles in the explanation of diseases.[153] The theory that remained linked to the name of Hippocrates, however, was that of the four humors (blood, phlegm, yellow bile, and black bile), even though it was actually the work of his pupil Polybus. Health prevails when the four humors are balanced and mixed. Sickness prevails when one of the humors is isolated and begins to flow, causing a twofold pain in the point from which it flows and in the point to which it flows, attaching itself.[154] At the time, this was only one more theory among many. Its spread, through Galen, can be explained by virtue of the clarity with which it is presented and, above all, by its consistency as a system that links the four humors with the four elementary qualities (warm, cold, dry, and moist) and the four seasons (winter, spring, summer, and autumn).

The Analogic Method and the Interpretive Method: The Visible as Model or Sign of the Reconstruction of the Invisible

Physicians, frequently aware of the difficulties involved in penetrating this world of the invisible that lies within the body, attempted to guide and to justify their reconstruction of invisible internal phenomena by analogy with visible phenomena on the exterior of the body. To understand the properties of the "structures" (the organs) on the interior of the body, "One should learn this thoroughly from unenclosed objects that can be seen," wrote the author of *De prisca medicina*.[155] The method was not peculiar to physicians. The pre-Socratics, who were as interested in the human body as physicians were, found themselves faced with the same difficulties and employed the same analogic method. The visible thus became a criterion of the invisible. This method was linked permanently to the name of Anaxagoras, who is quoted as the source of one particularly effective

formulation, cited approvingly by Democritus, in time becoming prover-
bial: "The visible is the eye of the invisible."[156] Coining an effective slogan,
however, does not mean inventing a procedure. Empedocles, who—
though younger than Anaxagoras—wrote his works first, had already applied the method in question in a celebrated passage of his poem "On
Nature," in which he explained the workings of respiration through analogy with the behavior of air or water in a clepsydra.[157] Hippocratic physicians, more or less consciously, made use of this reasoning by analogy
when they attempted to reconstruct their own physiology or their own
pathology. One of them distinguished himself by his constant use of this
form of reasoning with reference to everyday reality. This is the author of
the treatises *De genitura* [*De semine*], *De natura pueri*, and *De morbis IV*, a
true specialist in analogy.[158] Greek physicians drew visible facts from
which to deduce by analogy the internal functioning of the human body
from quite disparate fields: plants, animals, arts, and so on. Cooking, in its
wider meaning, was the favorite field: a pot of water boiling over the fire
was, implicitly or explicitly, one of the preferred models for explaining the
internal functions of the body, beginning with the physiology of digestion
(seen, as noted, as a form of cooking) and encompassing the pathology of
fevers, in which it is used to explain the vaporization of humors and the
condensation of sweat.[159] The manufacture of butter or cheese helped in
visualizing the coagulation and separation of the humors inside the
body.[160]

Utilizing this analogic method, physicians limited themselves to observing carefully, on the whole without intervening in any way, the "external reality." In certain cases, they went further, organizing rudimentary
experiments, and thus acting upon the external reality in order to understand more clearly the internal reality. The author of *De morbis IV*, for
example, recreated externally—using a wineskin filled with earth, sand,
and lead shavings, into which he blew through a tube—what he believed
to be the conditions of the embryo, in order to explain the differentiation
of the parts, in accordance with the rule that similar entities attract each
other reciprocally.

More elaborate than the analogic method is what we could call the
interpretive method. Rather than reconstructing the invisible through
analogic transposition of the visible, this method deciphers the invisible
through the interpretation of visible signs. According to the author of *De
arte*, for instance, the interior of the body, although it is invisible, allows a
number of signs to escape, such as "clearness or roughness of the voice,

rapidity or slowness of respiration, and for the customary discharges the ways through which they severally pass, sometimes smell, sometimes colour, sometimes thinness or thickness."[161] The physician will take these signs as criteria in evaluating the points affected and the diseases suffered. He is even capable of producing these signs artificially when nature does not reveal them. For instance, to prompt the respiration to reveal what he wishes it to reveal, he will have a patient climb a hill, or he will set him running, so that the patient's breathing may reveal what it ought. The art of medicine, therefore, may go so far as to constrain nature, when the signs that it provides on its own are not sufficient for diagnosis and prognosis: "When this information is not afforded, and nature herself will yield nothing of her own accord, medicine has found means of compulsion, whereby nature is constrained, without being harmed, to give up her secrets; when these are given up she makes clear, to those who know about the art, what course ought to be pursued."[162]

The same idea was adopted by Francis Bacon: "Nature, irritated and tormented by art, shows itself more clearly than when it is left to itself."[163] The Hippocratic physician added an important consideration: it is fundamental that this forcing of nature by art should cause no harm to nature. The violence of the physician does not resemble the violence of disease; it can only be a gentle violence. The ultimate goal of medicine, the welfare of the patient, is never lost sight of.

The Hippocratic Ethic

In the Greek city in which he was practicing, the physician would care for men, women, citizens, strangers, freedmen, slaves, Greeks, and barbarians. He accepted payment but made no apparent distinctions among his patients. The physician considered that he had, first and foremost, a human being before him. Even the terminology used was tangible evidence of this humanism: the Greek word *anthropos*, which designates "the human being," recurs quite frequently in the writings of Hippocratic physicians in referring to the sick. Other distinctions—such as gender, social standing, or racial origin—are secondary, and that what counts most is the invalid whose health must be restored. The goal of medicine becomes crystal clear in a maxim that has remained famous: "You should have two things in mind in treating sickness: to be useful, or at least to do no harm."[164] The Hippocratic physician here states, well before Plato or Aristotle, that the goal of medicine is not the success of the physician but the health of the invalid. Yet the essential point of view of the practicing physician renders nuanced a position that was to become far more dogmatic among the philosophers. "To be useful" is an ideal that a medical practitioner cannot always achieve; thus "do no harm" is added. If a physician cannot be useful, at least he should not worsen the condition of the patient by intervening in an untimely manner. This provides the justification for refusing to accept certain patients, whose illness escapes the theoretical knowledge of modern science.[165] Of greater concern to our subject is the recommendation to avoid all spectacular treatment and to eschew any pursuit of innovations more for the sake of the doctor's reputation than for the patient's well-being;[166] another interesting point is the probity of the physician who admits his own errors so that others may not repeat them.[167]

In their reflections on their own work, Hippocratic physicians succeeded in grasping the fundamental elements that constitute medicine, as well as in analyzing the relations between those elements. The medical art, according to a Hippocratic physician, includes three terms: disease, the physician, and the patient. And he defines the relations among those three terms in the following manner: "the physician is the servant of the art; the patient must cooperate with the physician in combatting the disease."[168] The relationship between patient and disease is thus conceived in terms of a struggle: the disease must be combatted. The struggle against the disease is waged by the patient. The physician, in turn, is the patient's ally, helping him to combat the disease. Here, the reader will note the physician's modesty and profound humanity. This human dimension, in the relations between the physician and the patient, constitutes one of the great original contributions of Hippocratism. The physician knows that the drama is that of the patient fallen prey to disease, and that he, the physician, can provide nothing more than help. How will he provide that help? Without doubt, through his knowledge, but also through his devotion and selflessness,[169] with his sense of dialogue and give-and-take,[170] and with his understanding approach to the invalid (sweetness, courtesy).[171]

The reflection of the Hippocratic physician on his own art, then, opens the path to a discussion of professional ethics that still serves as a model; these ethics constitute the deathless gem of the second portion of the oath, the founding text of professional ethics and medical secrecy:

> I will use treatment to help the sick according to my ability and judgment, but never with a view to injury and wrong-doing. Neither will I administer a poison to anybody when asked to do so, nor

will I suggest such a course. Similarly I will not give to a woman a pessary to cause abortion. But I will keep pure and holy both my life and my art. I will not use the knife, not even, verily, on sufferers from stone, but I will give place to such as are craftsmen therein. Into whatsoever houses I enter, I will enter to help the sick, and I will abstain from all intentional wrong-doing and harm, especially from abusing the bodies of man or woman, bond or free. And whatsoever I shall see or hear in the course of my profession, as well as outside my profession in my intercourse with men, if it be what should not be published abroad, I will never divulge, holding such things to be holy secrets.[172]

The Presence of Medicine and Medical Thought in the Literature of the Classical Era

At the time when the earliest medical literature known to us was being written, there was as yet no clear distinction between technical literature and a more general literature of artistic value. The Hippocratic physician could write for the public at large, composing a medical treatise in an artful prose,[173] just as the philosopher Empedocles was able to write a philosophical treatise in verse. The spread of medical knowledge to the public at large had not yet encountered the barrier of technical language.

Medicine and Tragedy

Despite the inevitable differences between something of a technical nature written in prose and a text written in verse and destined to be performed on stage, there is a natural affinity between the point of view of a tragic poet and that of a physician.[174] To quote a celebrated phrase by a Hippocratic author, the physician "sees terrible sights."[175] The tragic poet, by contrast, portrays terrible sights, so much so that fear, according to Aristotle, is one of the driving forces of tragedy.[176] The spectacle of human suffering links physicians and tragic poets.

Of course, there is a considerable gap between the rational conception of disease in Hippocrates and the archaic conception of disease in tragic poets, whether we are talking about disease in general or specific diseases. One may take as an example the "pestilence" *(loimos)* as discussed by Hippocrates *(De flatibus, De natura hominis)* and by Sophocles *(Oedipus Tyrannus)*. There is clearly a sharp distinction in the conception of cause, because although both authors make use of the same Greek term, *miasma*, they give it two different meanings: a religious meaning for Sophocles (the stain of spilt blood), and a rational meaning for Hippocrates (miasma suspended in the air). There is an equally sharp distinction between the means employed to end the pestilence: in *Oedipus Tyrannus*, no one bothers to consult a doctor to combat the scourge; appeals are made to the gods, oracles, and soothsayers. For the Hippocratic physician, the precaution that should be adopted is that of breathing miasmatic air as seldom and as little as possible.[177]

Tragedians could hardly remain unaware of or indifferent to medical progress and to the blossoming of medical literature. Since ancient times, mention has been made of the similarities between tragic verse and passages from the Hippocratic collection. Clement of Alexandria, for instance, compared Hippocrates and Euripides: "The physician Hippocrates first wrote: 'it is thus necessary to examine the season, the region, the age, and the diseases,' and Euripides says in an observation in hexameters: 'All those who wish to heal correctly must take into consideration the way of life of the inhabitants of the city and the territory, when they examine diseases.'"[178]

The rational conception of Hippocratic pathology, which established ties between diseases and the physical environment and with the diet and way of life of the inhabitants, therefore, was familiar to the tragic poet who expressed the greatest curiosity concerning intellectual developments of his time. In more general terms, tragic authors made direct use of medical information, both in terminology (*phagedaina, leichen,* and so on), and in the description or depiction on the stage of pathological cases (Io, Orestes, Ajax, Hercules, Philoctetes, Agave, and others). For some time now, mention has been made of similarities between medical descriptions of epileptic seizures *(De morbo sacro, De flatibus)* and the descriptions of fits found in Greek tragedy when the hero falls prey to an excess of grief or madness (such symptoms as rolling and diverging eyes, foaming at the mouth, trembling hands). This opens the issue of what links there might have been between Hippocrates and the Greek tragedians. We should refrain from attempting to provide a complete answer. The idea of any direct influence of the Hippocratic treatises on the work of Aeschylus can be ruled out immediately for reasons of chronology; this does not mean, however, that the earliest tragic poet might not have been familiar with some nosological treatises that have not survived. Moreover, the idea that the oldest treatises in the Hippocratic collection may have had some influence on the later work of Euripides, or even of Sophocles, is plausible. The realism of the two scenes in which we witness a crisis of an invalid on stage (Philoctetes, in Sophocles' work of 409 B.C.; and Orestes, in Euripides' play of 408 B.C.) corresponds to the realism of the clinical descriptions offered by Hippocratic medicines. Finally, the thoughts of tragic authors concerning medicine may link up with the observations made by the physicians. In particular, Euripides reflects some of the problems dealt with in medical writings by having his characters make general observations. For instance, Phaedra's wet nurse, in lamenting her condition as a nurse, declares, somewhat paradoxically: "It is better to be sick than to care for the sick" (v. 186). This idea certainly reflects the observation made in the treatise *De flatibus*, which was famous throughout late antiquity, concerning the hard life of the physician who "sees terrible sights, touches unpleasant things, and the misfortunes of others bring a harvest of sorrows that are peculiarly his; but the sick by means of the art rid themselves of the worst of evils, disease, suffering, pain and death."[179]

Medicine and History

Historians may find themselves having to describe some of the pestilences that strike humanity. In works of history, one may compare the description of diseases and the explanations of them with those offered by physicians.[180]

There are some remarkable and striking resemblances between explanations of diseases given by Herodotus and those found in the Hippocratic collection. Explaining why the Egyptians are, after the Libyans, the healthiest people on earth, Herodotus states: "The reason of which to my thinking is that the climate in all seasons is the same; for change is the great cause of men's falling sick, more especially changes of seasons."[181] Now, the idea that major changes in the seasons are the main cause of diseases is a fundamental concept in *De aere, aquis, locis* and can be found in other treatises, notably in *Aphorismi*, where the statement is made, in terms remarkably similar to those used by Herodotus, that "it is chiefly the changes of the seasons which produce diseases."[182] Unlike physicians, however, Herodotus did not possess a coherent system of etiology regarding pathological events. For, having said of a southern people that climate is an important factor in health and disease, Herodotus makes no more reference to climate when he speaks of a disease afflicting a northern people—the impotence of the Scythians. Instead, at this point, Herodotus accepts a religious explanation, which the Scythians themselves credited, that of a curse placed on them by the goddess Artemis; in contrast, the Hippocratic author of *De aere, aquis, locis* examines each religious explanation encountered, offering a rational account in its place. Herodotus, therefore, offers explanations ad hoc, attributing diseases to the climate here, and to deities there.

This is no longer the case by the time we get to Thucydides, who was as consistently rational as the Hippocratic physicians. Like Herodotus, he was aware of the importance of changes in the production of disease;[183] but unlike Herodotus or Sophocles, he refused to accept the intervention of a deity as an explanation of the scourges that strike mankind; indeed, Thucydides made an even clearer distinction between nature and the divine than did the Hippocratic authors. He provides a masterly description of the "pestilence" that ravaged Athens at the beginning of the Peloponnesian War, taking his distance from the traditional explanation in divine terms and favoring a more medically oriented approach.[184] In effect, on the one hand, Thucydides points out the total inefficacy of all religious means of recourse against the disease, such as supplicating the gods and consulting oracles. His descriptions clearly show that religious desecrations, such as the presence of corpses in holy shrines, far from being the cause of the outbreak, were a consequence of it. On the other hand, he reflects the influence of medical literature in two areas. He describes with considerable accuracy the symptoms of the disease, making use of a technical vocabulary similar to that used by physicians; his analysis of the pathological aspects is as purely rational as that of the Hippocratic texts. Still, we should not overemphasize Thucydides' reliance on the physicians. The historian makes it clear, as a preliminary to his description of the pestilence, that his experience was personal: he personally suffered from the disease and witnessed the sickness of many others. He was therefore eminently capable of describing the disease as a well-placed observer, from without and from within, without depending on the words of others. What truly sets Thucydides apart from the physicians of the Hippocratic collection, however, is his refusal to identify a cause; for a Hippocratic physician, it was absolutely necessary to know the cause of a disease, for the therapy must be based thereon. Thucydides, by contrast, rejects equally the arguments of supporters of a rational medicine and those of adherents of religious medicine. He underscores with parallel eloquence the inadequacies of both approaches.[185] One surprising result of this refusal to speculate as to a cause is that the historian was more clear-eyed than the physicians, his contemporaries. Since he was not wearing the conceptual blinders that prevented specialists from crediting the idea of contagion through contact, Thucydides was able to note clearly the chain of infection,[186] and observe that physicians, through their close dealings with the sick, were those most greatly exposed to the disease.

Though Thucydides inaugurated in this description of the pestilence a new skeptical positivism, describing facts and events while refusing to venture an opinion on their specific medical causes, he certainly attempted to give historical explanations of events, such as the war between Athens and Sparta, which lay at the heart of his work. Indeed, his analysis of causes delved profoundly into the distinction between apparent causes and real causes, employing a vocabulary clearly related to that found in the Hippocratic treatises. In particular, Thucydides used the term *prophasis*— not in the usual sense of "pretext," but rather in the technical sense of "cause," just as it is used in medical literature.[187] Other similarities have been noted between the historical method of Thucydides and the method of the Hippocratic physicians, especially concerning the importance of the concept of "human nature" in explaining the behavior of individuals and nations, with a view to forecasting that behavior in some future application.[188] We should also note references to medicine in the speeches that Thucydides attributed to various politicians, showing how the medical paradigm and the Hippocratic ethic ("be useful, or at least do no harm") could be used in political thought to define good policy.[189] And this is a first sketch of what was later to become, in the work of Plato, both a didactic and a heuristic method: the transposition of the medical model from the realm of the body to that of the soul. Of course, Plato had not been the first thinker to make use of this analogy. The sophist Gorgias, in his work *Encomium of Helen,* had already formulated quite clearly the parallels between the powerful effects of discourse upon the soul and those of medications upon the body.[190] This analogy, however, was not used by the sophist to establish a full-fledged *techne* of rhetoric.

Plato

Among the arts *(technai)* that served as models for the thought of Socrates and Plato, medicine occupied a considerable position, alongside the art of the helmsman. These two arts are analogous inasmuch as they belong to the category of the arts of well-being. A helmsman must ensure the well-being of his passengers as he conveys them through raging storms to bring them safe and sound into harbor; likewise, a physician must allow an invalid to pass through the tempest of disease, so as to escape death and recover his health. This comparison, which had already been presented in the writings of a Hippocratic physician (*De prisca medicina*, 9), became quite familiar in the realm of Socratic thought. These two arts, both directed toward the preservation of physical well-being, served as paradigms for the definition of those arts directed toward the well-being of the soul. Even more than the art of the helmsman, the art of the physician was well suited to this transposition, since it operates directly on the body, just as an orator or a politician acts directly on the soul. Plato made continual reference to the medical model in his work; he does so first in his early dialogues, particularly the *Gorgias*, and continues to do so in *Phaedrus* and up to the last dialogues, particularly the *Laws*.[191] Such confidence in the worth of the medical art is that much more remarkable if we consider that its very existence had been questioned among the sophists of the fifth century.

In the *Gorgias*, medicine is the authentic art that corrects the body. It promotes the well-being of the body and operates with an awareness of cause, precisely as did the medical art in *De prisca medicina;* whereas, however, the Hippocratic treatise states that the discovery of medicine was simply an extension of the discovery of cooking, Plato makes a distinction between the basic nature of medicine, which is a true art, and cooking, which he defines as a luxury for the body's pleasure and an empirical method, operating on chance.

This reorganization of knowledge derives from Plato's distinction, unknown to the Hippocratic physicians, between science and empirical method. After defining these two models for activities acting on the human body, Plato transposes them to those activities that act on the soul: rhetoric and politics. Sophists, such as Gorgias, and the illustrious political figures of Athenian democracy, such as Themistocles or Pericles, were nothing more than political cooks; the only physician of politics was Socrates. Plato characterizes this Socratic medicine in the *Gorgias* as consisting of a strict diet, bitter medicine, or painful operations.[192] Painful therapy seems, in the *Gorgias*, to ensure the authenticity of the art, so sharp is the distinction between pleasure and well-being.

Plato returns, in *Phaedrus*, to the definition of rhetoric as a "psychagogy,"[193] making renewed use of the medical model. And it is here that we find an allusion to the Hippocratic method, in a passage whose interpretation has been the subject of great controversy.[194] As in the *Gorgias*, medicine is a model because a physician does not operate by chance and seeks out causes. In the later work, Plato's analysis delves to greater depth and the medical model is broader and richer. For the physician in *Phaedrus*, unlike the one in the *Gorgias*, employs different regimens and different remedies, according to the different physical constitutions, to restore bodily health. The true orator is one who can distinguish among the different sorts of souls, knowing which discourse should be employed to persuade different categories of the public. The goal of the art remains the same, but the means employed—remedy or discourse—is diversified in accordance with the various categories, of body or soul.

Finally, in the *Laws*, the physician is still a prime example, along with the helmsman and the general, for establishing a definition of the legislator; the medical model, however, has developed further. Plato envisages at this point a medicine in which the bitterness of the useful remedies is tempered by pleasant foods,[195] somewhat reminiscent of the courtesies of the Hippocratic physicians. Above all, in the renowned composition in which he compares and contrasts the scientific medicine practiced by free physicians with the empirical medicine practiced by assistant physicians, who were generally slaves, Platonic medicine gained a new dimension, in the relationship between physician and patient;[196] the importance of this relationship had already been glimpsed in Hippocratic ethics. A Platonic lawgiver would be, like an authentic physician, not only a man of the art but also a master of persuasion. It is quite possible that Plato's encounters with Hippocratic medicine—toward which he recognized his debt as early as *Phaedrus*—helped to enrich his conception of the medical art in the *Laws*, over against that of the *Gorgias*. Plato thus discovered, in the very core of medical activity, not only a rational method to borrow but also a type of human relation to imitate.

Plato, once he had transposed medical thought into rhetoric, politics, and ethics, was still not done. He further set forth his medical ideas in *Timaeus*. Here, however, despite his admiration for Hippocrates, Plato describes a philosophical medicine that has little in common with what posterity has generally considered to be the Hippocratic spirit: specifically, clinical observation and opposition to philosophy. The micro- and macrocosmic conception of *Timaeus* presents certain precise analogies with the Hippocratic treatise *De diaeta* [*Regimen*]."[197] Moreover, *Timaeus* also reveals, as does the *Laws*, a development of Plato's thought regarding a medicine that links up with another feature of Hippocratism: the importance of regimen. Although a celebrated passage of the *Republic* comes out in favor of the pharmacological medicine of the ancients over the dietetic medicine of Plato's contemporaries,[198] *Timaeus* warns against the dangers of remedies that may make diseases more virulent, preaching the benefits of a natural and dietetic medicine.[199] The various readings made, from antiquity onward, of the Hippocratic collection differ so widely that diametrically opposed judgments have been offered of the relations between Hippocrates and philosophy in general and Plato in particular. While Celsus, in the first century A.D., considered Hippocrates the founder of medicine by breaking it away from philosophy,[200] Galen saw in Hippocrates the very model of a philosopher-physician, and tried to show the resemblances between Hippocrates and Plato, who both believed that the activity of thought occurred in the brain.[201]

Hippocrates was to exert an influence on medical thought, over the course of more than twenty centuries, roughly comparable with the influence of Aristotle on philosophical thought. At times hotly debated, often admired, and, more often still, misread by those in search of support for their own conceptual agendas, the Hippocratic opus was to be a constant model of reference for Western medicine from antiquity up to the turn of the twentieth century. Although the work handed down under the name of Hippocrates is now scientifically obsolete, the human aspects of the work remain a model for physicians. In any case, the body of work endures as one of the greatest monuments to the awakening of the scientific spirit in Greece and in the Western world.

~ 3 ~

Between Knowledge and Practice: Hellenistic Medicine

MARIO VEGETTI

Very few eras in the history of medicine—modern or ancient—have seen as sharp an acceleration in development, as far-reaching a structural transformation, as the first half of the third century B.C. During this period, not only was there a remarkable increase in medical knowledge, there was also a veritable epistemological revolution (although that revolution was left in part incomplete, as we shall see). It is likewise rare that innovations of this sort can be attributed to the work of a limited and well-defined group of individuals, who in the case at hand are also clearly identified. We are referring to four remarkable physicians, two masters and their respective disciples. The first pair consisted of Praxagoras of Kos (whose acme should be dated at about 300 B.C.) and his pupil Herophilus of Chalcedon, who lived between 330 or 320 B.C. and 260 or 250 B.C., and who worked chiefly in Alexandria. The second pair consisted of Chrysippus of Cnidus (dates uncertain) and his pupil Erasistratus of Ceos, who also lived from 330 to 250 B.C., and who worked in Antioch, the Seleucid capital, as well as—in all likelihood—in Ptolemaic Alexandria.[1]

These geographic parameters alone allow us to delineate with considerable precision the geopolitical setting in which the great transformation occurred, as well as the quite remarkable relations between tradition and innovation that emerged as a result. The masters had roots in major centers—Kos and Cnidus—of the great medical tradition of the fifth and fourth centuries B.C. The texts that survive from this tradition were incorporated in the great collection that is known as the Hippocratic collection. The disciples, in contrast, gravitated toward the capitals of the new Hellenistic monarchies, and especially to Alexandria under the Ptolemies, a city that ruled over the entire Aegean, including Kos and Cnidus, at the turn of the third century.

An Incomplete Epistemological Revolution

The Hippocratic tradition handed down, both to masters and disciples, an image, a theory, and a practice of medicine that revolved entirely around the problem of disease. In that tradition, the figure of the physician was that of a professional wholly dedicated to the pressing demands of clinical practice, and therefore first and foremost to prognosis and therapy. The human body—not yet explored by anatomical investigation—was perceived as a sort of "black box." Inside the unexplored body the processes of humoral physiopathology were believed to take place, based solely on the knowledge of the materials taken in (the air breathed, the food and drink ingested) and expelled (excrement, hemorrhages, sweat).[2] Even in this narrow epistemological context, however, an unparalleled clinical experience had been accumulated. The factors that made up this clinical experience were careful observation of individual patients; remarkable semeiotic skill; and relatively efficacious therapeutic knowledge, especially in terms of pharmacology, surgery, and—above all—diet (which grew to include the patient's entire regimen of life).

The innovative daring of masters such as Praxagoras and Chrysippus, and especially of their disciples, Herophilus and Erasistratus, can be understood only if we consider that they triggered, as it were, the demolition of this immense traditional heritage, which constituted the sole model of medicine then known in the Greek world. Commensurately vast and—understandably enough—largely unsolved were the problems that emerged as a consequence of their subversion of the medical tradition in which they had themselves developed.

The overall direction of the transformation can be identified with considerable precision. It involved, in the first place, a reconsideration of the nature of medical knowledge. Included in this reconsideration—indeed, central to it—was the problem of understanding the natural, normal state of human bodies, and hence, *health*, in contrast to the overwhelming attention that had hitherto been focused on disease. The new dimension of medicine coincided with the scientific, rational, and

73

epistemic aspects of that discipline. The rest of medicine, however necessary (clinical medicine, therapy), was relegated to the epistemological shadows of guesswork and trial and error. Thus, Herophilus distinguished among three parts of medical knowledge: that having to do with health (also described as *logikon,* or "rational"), that concerned with disease, and that described as "neutral" (meaning surgery and pharmacology).[3] Erasistratus distinguished a "scientific" part *(epistemonikon)* of medicine, which was concerned with etiology and anatomophysiology, from the "stochastic" part, concerned with therapy and semeiotics.[4] Erasistratus's greatest work concentrated on anatomophysiology, and hence on the first part (the *General Discourses*); his writings on pathology, fevers, and paralysis focused partly on the second area.

The emergence of this new, epistemic dimension of medicine found its justification and at the same time exhausted itself in the establishment of an equally radical new body of knowledge, without precedents in the "Hippocratic" tradition: the anatomical investigation of the structures of human and animal bodies, achieved through the practice of dissection. By this point, the practice had become systematic and allowed physicians successfully to open and examine the contents of the corporeal black box. The knowledge thus obtained about the solid organs—beginning with the brain, heart, and liver and the vascular, nervous, and muscular systems— also immediately led to a rethinking of the Hippocratic physiology of humoral fluids, in favor of new, anatomically based explanations. What thus developed, occupying and defining the new epistemic field of medicine, was an anatomophysiological body of knowledge, engendered by dissection and previously unknown, at least to the medical profession.

These innovations—both in the epistemological structure of medicine and in the content of medical knowledge—were so drastic with respect to certain basic and inescapable therapeutic problems of medicine, that they produced a lasting and, over time, critical state of tension between the two polar extremes of the medical art, epistemic on the one hand and clinical on the other. I shall return to the effects of this development, but for now consider the observations of someone who was attentive both to this innovative process and to its problematic effects. The historian Polybius (second century B.C.) was close, both chronologically and intellectually, to this great turning point in thought. He wrote that, in the medicine that had developed at Alexandria, and especially through the work of Herophilus, the "theoretical" part *(logikon)* became much more important than dietetics, surgery, and pharmacology; that the physicians who possessed theory acquired both an air of distinction and a reputation that overshadowed those of other practitioners; but that their problems began when they were faced with a single patient instead of a crowded audience for one of their lectures. Faced with a patient, they often came off looking like a helmsman who was trying "to sail a ship from what he had read in a book."[5]

The Aristotelian Foundation of a Science of Life

Before taking a closer look at the epistemological forms and the contents of the knowledge that characterized the great rupture produced by Hellenistic medicine, with all the resulting tensions, we should devote some discussion to the array of factors, both intellectual and institutional, that made that rupture possible.

Between the old Hippocratic tradition and the new masters of the late fourth century B.C. lies the colossal intellectual event that was the work of Aristotle. Toward the end of the fifth century, it was still possible to conceive of conflict between the *physiologia* of philosophers and that of medicine for supremacy in the overall field of knowledge of nature. The Hippocratic author of *De prisca medicina* had been able to write sarcastically that *physiologia* as practiced by Empedocles more closely resembled "painting than medicine," adding, "I also hold that clear knowledge about natural science can be acquired from medicine and from no other source, and that one can attain this knowledge when medicine itself has been properly comprehended, but till then it is quite impossible."[6]

But the new role of the *physikos* delineated in the work of Aristotle put an end to this rivalry. The philosopher of nature now possessed a general theory of natural processes (physics), as well as a doctrine of elements (air, water, earth, fire) and qualities (hot/cold, solid/fluid) as primary components of both inorganic *(De generatione et corruptione)* and organic bodies *(De partibus animalium,* 2).[7] He possessed, moreover, a well-structured theory of the major processes of animal life (nourishment, perception, reproduction, and movement). As a result of all this, scientific knowledge concerning nature appeared clearly to be the domain of the *physikos* philosopher. The physician, far removed from Hippocratic ambitions, was relegated to a secondary—though not insignificant—status as one versed in a specific *techne,* concerning the general realm of disease. In the context of this fundamental hierarchical transformation, Aristotle still recognized a linkage between natural philosophy and medical knowledge:

75

"It is further the duty of the natural philosopher to study the first princi-ples of disease and health; for neither health nor disease can be properties of things deprived of life. Hence one may say that most natural philoso-phers, and those physicians who take a scientific interest in their art, have this in common: the former end by studying medicine, and the latter base their medical theories on the principles of natural science."[8]

Although medicine remained locked in a hierarchical relationship, Aristotle here indicated the possibility of an epistemological reevaluation of medicine, so as to make it a knowledge as much of health as of disease, enjoying ties with the basic role of natural philosophy. This was a possibil-ity that Hellenistic medicine was to seize upon to a considerable degree.

It was not only in epistemological terms, however, that Aristotle's work came to constitute a watershed between old and new medicine. There was also, and indeed especially, the incursion of anatomy into the science of life and living things.[9] With the widespread and methodically regulated practice of animal dissection, Aristotle had begun the systematic process of opening up the body. Upon this foundation, he had constructed an imposing edifice of comparative anatomophysiology. On the one hand, no school of medicine that aspired to an elevated level of scientific legiti-macy could forego a knowledge of that structure. On the other hand, faced with the devastating superiority of Aristotelian anatomical knowledge, the old medicine saw a definitive check to its claim of privileged standing in terms of knowledge of the body and its processes.

The Aristotelian edifice thus came to embody a challenge, and a fundamental point of reference, for the new medicine. In fact, that medi-cine was largely to be anatomical in subject but would work to overcome its empirical limitations. Constituted as it was by a compact interweaving of elements of knowledge, theoretical presuppositions, and ideological prejudices, the Aristotelian edifice in question would—henceforth—represent to medicine a mass of problems to be solved, as well as preju-dices and presuppositions to be accepted or rejected.

First of all, there was the primary theoretical underpinning of that intellectual structure, the teleological approach. Aristotelian teleology pos-sessed practically none of the cosmic providentialism that was later to distinguish Stoic teleology and that was to be so broadly incorporated in the work of Galen. Rather, it constituted the great founding axiom of anatomophysiology: the presupposition of the existence of a rational rela-tionship between the structure of an organ and its function, with its logical corollaries (there are no useless organs; it is best for each organ to perform

76

only a single function).[10] In these terms, Aristotelian teleology could be usefully accepted in the field of medicine. Indeed, it was so accepted, both by Herophilus and by Erasistratus. It was not, however, without its problems. In general, it was a theory of the normal functioning of the organism, and as such it could act as an "epistemological obstacle" to a scientific understanding of pathological dysfunctions, which despite all else continued to be one of the central problems of medicine. In particular, it was to greatly influence the anatomophysiology of the vascular system, with problematic results.

Then there was the entire cluster of problems inherent in what Aristotle saw, believed he saw, or refused or was unable to see in his exploration of the body's internal organs. Some of Aristotle's "errors" of observation were rectified fairly quickly and easily. An instance of this was his failure to distinguish between veins and arteries, or between tendons and nerves. Far more complex, however, proved the set of problems that sprang from his emphasis on a thermic-cardiocentric paradigm as the foundation of his entire physiology.[11] For example, Aristotle linked the sensory organs to the heart rather than to the brain and reduced the brain, along with the lungs, to organs for cooling the heat of the heart; he also supposed the existence of an innate heat, located in the cardiac "hearth," responsible for the most important physiological processes; these processes he considered as successive levels of "coction" of foods (transformed into blood for nutrition, and then from blood into seed for reproduction, though only in males).[12] Lastly, Aristotle accorded a growing emphasis to a "pneuma," likewise innate to the heart, with no relationship to the air taken in during respiration.

The problem of the pneuma unquestionably constituted the most ambiguous aspect of the heritage that Aristotle bestowed on medical posterity. The pneuma—a semimaterial organic substance, innate air that was thus different from the external air, heated with a similarly innate heat that was not the same as fire, a mysterious cardiac "vapor"—was a concept that was progressively tested by Aristotle in the function of "hypothetic agent allowing the solution of problems,"[13] that is, as an unobservable somatic substrate that was needed to explain the superior psychic functions found in the interface between body and soul. In full-fledged Aristotelian biology, the pneuma was variously called upon to explain the transmission of perception from the sensory organs to the heart, via "conduits full of innate pneuma";[14] to translate into terms other than metaphorical the formation and transmission to the muscles of impulses to voluntary motion, following the arousal of such psychic states as desire;[15] and to explain the transmission of the soul-shape from the seed of the father to the embryonic material provided by the mother.[16] In the latter manifestation, the pneuma was defined by Aristotle as analogous to the ether, the quasi-divine material of heavenly bodies. The more the pneuma was found to be unobservable, the more it was felt to reveal a "nearly miraculous potential"[17] in the explanation of the most complex and secret of psychophysical processes. In this guise, pneuma was to constitute one of the most important (and burdensome) bequests of Aristotelian natural philosophy. On the one hand, due to the linkage that pneuma suggested between the world of life and the sphere of the divine cosmos, it was to play a central role in what can in fact be defined as Stoical "cosmobiology."[18] On the other hand, because of its unprecedented capacity to explain psychophysical processes, it became a crucial heritage for post-Aristotelian medicine. In the second half of the fourth century, as C. R. S. Harris has observed,[19] it became a given, commonly accepted by all physicians, cardiocentrists or encephalocentrists though they might be.

Ties between the Aristotelian School and Hellenistic Medicine

There are many links, both direct and indirect, between the Aristotelian school and Hellenistic medicine.[20]

The first of them may in all likelihood be identified in the work of Diocles of Carystos, whose acme can be dated around the middle of the fourth century:[21] he was traditionally described as the "second Hippocrates," showing that the innovative nature of his medical thought had been understood. Diocles may have taken his inspiration from the epistemological hierarchy established by Aristotle, when he denied that it was appropriate or useful to medicine to search for the "first causes of all nature,"[22] clearly a search that belonged to the pursuit of philosophy. According to tradition, moreover, Diocles wrote a treatise entitled *Anathomia*, which should be considered a first effort to transpose this body of knowledge from the zoological context proper to Aristotle to a more specifically medical area. Similarly Aristotelian were his failure to distinguish between veins and arteries and his interpretation of respiration as a means of cooling the innate heat. Most strongly linked to Aristotle, however, was the cardiocentrism that we find in Diocles; he placed both innate pneuma and heat in the heart's left ventricle. Since the right ventricle was considered to be the source of the blood, and the heart was considered to be the origin of the vascular system, it followed—according to Diocles—that both blood and pneuma were present in all vessels.[23] The Aristotelian influence in Diocles was certainly perceived as well in the traditional centers of medicine, as we learn from Praxagoras at Kos and Chrysippus at Cnidus.

Praxagoras was a complex and contradictory figure, in whom both innovation and tradition were closely intertwined. Influenced by Aristotle and Diocles, he introduced cardiocentrism into what had long been the stronghold of Hippocratic encephalocentrism. Praxagoras believed that the heart was the center of thought and of all psychic functions.[24] Unlike his two masters, Aristotle and Diocles, Praxagoras was capable of distinguishing between the veins and the arteries (he may thus have been the first to do so). He did so less on an anatomical basis (through the difference in thickness of the respective membranes or tunics) than on the basis of the fluids that the two vessels contained. The veins contained blood, while the arteries contained only pneuma, as did the heart's left ventricle, from which the arteries led.[25] This was "really one of the tragical mistakes in the history of Greek medicine," as Harris puts it,[26] and a mistake freighted with consequences. Still, it was a mistake with a foundation in observation, since in effect when a cadaver was dissected, both the left ventricle and the arteries proved to be almost empty of blood.

Once Praxagoras had established the pneumatic fluid as the centerpiece of his physiological system, he was obliged to explain its formation and functions; in this he was faithful to the Hippocratic tradition (suffice it to mention *De morbo sacro*), and indeed he did not accept the Aristotelian hypothesis of an innate pneuma. Less mysteriously, he linked the pneuma to the external air obtained through respiration.[27] From the lungs, the pneuma was then sent to the heart through the pulmonary artery; once in the heart, through the effect of the cardiac heat (likewise not innate, produced most likely through the digestion of food), the air was transformed into a humid and vaporous fluid *(atmodes)*[28] and channeled into the arteries. And indeed the presence of pneuma in the arteries explained the phenomenon of the pulse.

Still, Praxagoras—probably influenced by *De motu animalium*—attributed another important function to pneuma, using it to explain the dynamics of voluntary movement. In this idea he was encouraged by another error, less "tragical" if for no other reason than that it was easier to correct. Praxagoras not only failed to distinguish between tendons and nerves, but believed that the system of nerves and tendons originated in the narrow, tough, terminal portion of the arteries. Thus, the expansion of pneuma in the arteries could immediately produce traction of the limbs. Although much remained unclear, in this way there was direct communication between the heart (seat of the psychic principle), arteries, tendons-nerves, and muscles, through the medium of the pneuma. Thus, a basis was established for an elasticofluid explanation of a major psychophysical process such as voluntary movement.

In clinical and pathological terms, Praxagoras remained entirely faithful to the Hippocratic tradition. He developed that tradition into a complex humoral physiopathology, involving no fewer than ten principal humors, including blood. He attributed all diseases to imbalances in these humors.[29] His therapy was the fruit of an extreme refinement of Hippocratism. Aside from diet, a crucial role was played in the therapy by an almost obsessive concern with the evacuation of excess—and therefore pathogenic—humors. Among other therapies was a systematic reliance on phlebotomy, or bloodletting. It also appears that Praxagoras tended to use medicines of considerable complexity.[30]

It must have been quite an undertaking for Herophilus to sort out the exceedingly complex and often contradictory teachings of his master. In effect, as we shall see, he was to make radical corrections in many areas (cardiocentrism primarily). At the same time, however, he accepted many other equally problematic ideas, such as humoral pathology. Praxagoras, for that matter, was cited extensively by the Stoic Chrysippus, supplying the precious figure of medical authority for Chrysippus's cardiocentrism, after—and in the face of—the work of Herophilus and Erasistratus.

We possess far less information concerning the second of the two masters, Chrysippus of Cnidus. The one thing we do know is that tradition tells of his sharp departure from the old Hippocratic medicine, a departure that found expression, for instance, in his refusal to make use of phlebotomy.[31] This may have been an indicator of his overall rejection of humoral pathology, a line in which Erasistratus was to follow him.

It was not through their masters alone, however, that Herophilus and Erasistratus entered into contact with Aristotelianism. It is not impossible that Herophilus visited Athens before going to Alexandria. As for Erasistratus, we have solid documentation concerning his apprenticeship at the Peripatetic school, where he was supposedly a student of Theophrastus and perhaps of Strato.[32]

Although the relationship between Erasistratus and Aristotelian thought has probably been given undue emphasis by the Peripatetic tradition (this point was indeed challenged repeatedly by Galen in his polemic against Erasistratus), and while our estimation of Strato's influence should doubtless be revised downward,[33] there can be no doubt that Erasistratus was thoroughly familiar with the heritage of Aristotelian biology.

A New Professional Setting for the Physician

Any discussion of the conditions that made possible the break with the past and the innovation produced by Hellenistic medicine cannot be limited to the array of intellectual events that, in the second half of the fourth century B.C., made the theoretical universe of medical tradition obsolete, at least in part. There were also radical institutional transformations, which modified the old professional standing of the physician. The physician had always been an itinerant professional, without ties to any institutional structure, whose survival and reputation depended on winning patients and performing therapy successfully. This was the reason for the interest, to the nearly total exclusion of all else, in problems of immediate clinical application: the Hippocratic physician had neither time nor space—in the twofold sense of the Aristotelian term, *schole,* meaning both leisure and school—to engage in theoretical research that was relatively detached from therapy. Not only did the "schools" of medicine commemorated by tradition (such as those of Kos and Cnidus) never actually serve as regular centers of development and transmission of medical knowledge (a form of institutionalization that was in fact unknown to ancient medicine). Those schools cannot be compared even to so informal an organization as that of Aristotle's Lyceum. The Lyceum may not have had any state sanction, but it did possess a library, rooms for lessons and research, and permanent teaching courses. The medical schools of the fifth and fourth century B.C. were probably never anything more than centers for the training of practitioners, formed through family dynasties or apprenticeships. These schools were also (in the case of such remarkable individuals as Hippocrates of Kos, or respected manuals such as the *Cnidian Maxims*) points of reference for doctrinal orientations, however elastic.

Here too there was a sharp break that came with the experience of Aristotle's Lyceum, and especially with its export (probably at the suggestion of authoritative members of the Peripatetic school, such as Demetrius of Phaleron and Strato) to the Alexandrian circle. In Alexandria the model of the Lyceum finally acquired recognition from the state, in the form of the patronage accorded by the Ptolemaic kings to the library and the museum. These new institutions provided, respectively, a place in which to meet, work, and "live in common," for scientists and researchers in every field and of all origins, throughout the Hellenistic world; and a place in which to collect, transcribe, and catalog the entire body of writing that had thus far been created by Greek culture. Although there are regrettable gaps in our understanding of the structure and operation of these institutions,[34] it would be difficult to overstate their revolutionary importance in the transformation of the conditions in which intellectuals, particularly scientists, worked.

Still, we must clarify a few points—both positive and negative—concerning the specific standing of physicians in the context of the museum. It is not known with certainty whether Herophilus was a member of the museum, entitled to a royal "pension." We can, moreover, determine that neither he, nor any of the other physicians connected with the museum, performed the functions of a court physician (this position was filled by professionals recruited in the traditional centers of Kos, Cnidus, and Carystos). Finally, we can reject the idea that Herophilus held regular courses in the museum: tradition describes his disciples and successors as "those from the House of Herophilus," clearly alluding to a still-private, almost family-style transmission of medical knowledge.

None of this, however, should in any way be seen as diminishing the role played by the institutions of Alexandria in the intellectual watershed of Hellenistic medicine. First and foremost, there was what Heinrich Von Staden has described as a climate of "scientific and literary frontiersmanship."[35] There was a general encouragement of research, openness, and innovation, generated by the context of a "new Greece," wealthier and more cosmopolitan, on Egyptian territory. This situation was further promoted by the new dynasty of the Ptolemies, who were both ambitious and in need of prestige and intellectual legitimation. All this added up to facilities, leisure time, and tools—predominantly books—made available for the work and cooperation of scholars. Scholars were thus allowed a certain, at least partial, relief (with or without other direct financial incentives) from the immediate demands of their professional activity. They were afforded, in short, the *schole* needed for theoretical research. Of more direct concern to the physicians, then, was the fact that the new atmosphere and the state support that embodied it together produced a further decisive contribution to this research. The new climate allowed physicians to venture to shatter an age-old taboo, tacit but daunting: anatomical intrusion into human cadavers. This step was necessary if they were to overcome the limitations of observation inherent in the dissections of animals practiced by Aristotle. It was especially fundamental to the in-auguration of anatomopathological research. And state support had an even more sensational effect: according to the unquestionable assertion of Celsus, Herophilus and Erasistratus were allowed to practice human vivi-section upon criminals who had been sentenced to death and who were delivered into their hands for this purpose by the royal authorities.[36] The valuable knowledge and understanding acquired through this practice—as cruel as it may have appeared to both pagan and Christian posterity—also formed part of the heritage of Aristotelian epistemology, in a certain sense. Aristotle, in fact, had pointed out that "now a corpse has the same shape and fashion as a living body; and yet it is not a man," while "none of its parts remains the same, except only in shape," and that these parts had the same names as the organs of a living body, but nothing else in common.[37] It was therefore necessary to dare to go further than Aristotle, by moving from the dissection of animal cadavers to human dissection and, to satisfy Aristotle's own theoretical demands, by progressing from human dissec-tion to vivisection. Had it not been for the practice of vivisection, many of the anatomophysiological advances of Herophilus and Erasistratus would have been impossible.

Dissection of the human body, whether living or dead, was possible even in Alexandria for only about fifty years. After the middle of the third century, with the exhaustion of the "frontiersmanship" of earliest Ptole-maic Alexandria, human dissection once again became unthinkable, and so remained throughout the rest of the history of the ancient world. Even Galen was forced to rely on animal dissection and vivisection. To his students, he recommended fairly furtive procedures for the observation of human cadavers (going perhaps so far as to break into graves in the cemetery), as well as pilgrimages to Alexandria, where it was still possible to observe at least human skeletons.[38]

It would be appropriate here to clear up one fairly common misun-derstanding: it is widely believed that the Egyptian practice of mummi-fication provided anatomists with access to the human body. As has been shown, nothing could be further from the truth. Those who actually did the mummification were shunned as being tainted and were social out-casts. It may well be, therefore, that the renewed influence of the native traditions in the Alexandrian court, after the middle of the third century, had precisely the opposite effect, that is, they reestablished religious taboos against the manipulation of the human body, whether dead or alive. For that matter, and in more general terms, it is astonishing to see the amply documented gap between traditional Egyptian medicine—with its static and timeless repetitiousness and its unrelenting blend of clinical experience with magical practice—and Hellenistic medicine. The latter may have developed in the Alexandrian circle, but there clearly was no intellectual or social contact with the Egyptian tradition.[39]

The dichotomy between Greek medicine and native medicine was hardly the most important effect of the new institutions of Alexandria. These new institutions, in effect, redesigned the entire field of medicine. Following the turn of the third century B.C., the sources no longer employ the term "Asclepiads." This religious and semicorporative emblem—to which all physicians belonging to the prior tradition had made reference, and which had endowed those physicians with both a social and cultural identity and a form of divine protection against possible suspicions of contamination (not to mention suspicions of bad faith or incompetence)—was now gone. In place of the relatively homogenous world of the Asclepiads, the medical profession experienced a sharp division. On one side were physicians belonging to the groups of high-level research, like those tied to the museum and more generally to the elevated circles of the Hellenistic monarchies, who tended to come from considerable social stock and enjoy respectable cultural levels.[40] On the other side was the common, scattered multitude of practicing and itinerant physicians, cut off from access to both theoretical research and the production of the treatises which expressed that research. Thus, the unity of *techne*, so proper to the Hippocratic tradition, expressed in a diffuse and anonymous writing, was broken up. And as a result, the teaching and texts of such great scientists as Herophilus and Erasistratus, and those of their students, recognized by their affiliations with this or that school, contrasted with the anonymous obscurity of the marginal and secondary practitioners, who no longer even recognized a shared membership in the "family" of the Asclepiads.

In any case, the revolutionary rupture and the innovations in medical knowledge produced by Hellenistic medicine could not possibly have come about had it not been for the array of intellectual and institutional factors that we have thus far explored. Let us now take a closer look at their epistemological setting and their contents in terms of medical theory and practice.

Herophilus and His School

The work of Herophilus[41] provides an exemplary demonstration of the tensions and contradictions between innovation and tradition that marked the epistemological revolution of Hellenistic medicine; these conflicts prevented that revolution from attaining fulfillment. Let us begin with the innovation: it was epistemologically based. As we have seen, Herophilus established in medicine a new theoretical aspect, concerned with the normal conditions of a healthy body, alien to the Hippocratic tradition. It is interesting to consider the language that Herophilus used to describe this new dimension of medical knowledge: "relating to health are all things that equip [*kataskeuazonton*] the parts in man to be such that, if they are harmoniously fitted to each other [*hermosmenon*], the state of being healthy is constituted as a result [*synistatai*]."[42] The language clearly refers to what has been described as the "constructive paradigm" of Greek technology,[43] the earliest and most respected of such paradigms, whose application ranged from architecture to the construction of such artifacts as ships. Herophilus, therefore, abandoned—on this level, anyway—the description of the body as a container of fluids, in the older tradition of humoral physiology. He replaced this description with that of an assembly of solid parts, perfectly suited one to another.

Herophilus adhered to the model of Aristotelian anatomophysiology. In delineating the epistemological outlines of medical knowledge, however, he dissociated himself from natural philosophy, in the direction indicated by Diocles. He did so with an axiomatic declaration: "Let these things be first even if they are not primary."[44] Galen, who quoted these words, considered them proof that Herophilus was only a half-dogmatic, who had stopped midway along the path of rationalization of medicine,[45] as was further demonstrated by Herophilus's skepticism concerning the possibility of ascertaining in this context the "first causes."[46] What we have here is not so much a case of incomplete rationalism, or even—as has recently been put forward—the influence of skeptical philosophy on Herophilus.[47] What Herophilus fundamentally rejected was the necessity of incorporating into medicine, at its very foundation, the philosophical theory of elements or qualities over which medicine could not possibly exert any control. In effect, the things that are "first even if they are not primary," upon which medicine should be based, according to Herophilus, were the *phainomena*, to be precise, the phenomena brought to light through anatomical dissection, consisting, of course, of the organic parts and the vascular systems.[48] In denying that it was either possible or useful for medicine to make reliance on the theory of elements, and in asserting that anatomical evidence was the proper foundation for medicine, Herophilus remained faithful, at the same time, to the Aristotelian division between natural philosophy and scientific medicine, as outlined in *De sensu*. In another area, Herophilus was thus establishing an epistemological protection of medicine's independence from philosophy.[49] He thus fended off the danger that medicine might find itself entangled in the debate between rival schools over the elements (Aristotelian qualities versus Epicurean atoms).

This approach, moreover, established immediately innovative results in Herophilus's work, even beyond the narrow bounds of the epistemological context. Abandoning the theory of the elements and replacing it with an emphasis on anatomy tended to undermine the foundations of the great thermic paradigm, upon which Aristotelian physiology had been based and, with it, Aristotelian cardiocentrism. This dislodged the postulate of heat as the active principle of natural processes. Thus, the hypothesis of an innate heat in the heart became unnecessary, as did the parallel hypothesis of an innate cardiac pneuma, that is, a pneuma unconnected with respiration. And in this manner, supported by anatomic discoveries, Herophilus was already hacking away at the central buttresses of Aristotelian vitalism. What remained intact was Aristotle's finalism. The presupposition of a nonredundant relationship between organs and functions led Herophilus to begin constructing a new paradigm. The three great diffuse systems that anatomy had uncovered (nerves, arteries, and veins) necessarily served different functions, and this discovery led to the hypothesis that they constituted vessels for equally differentiated fluids. The paradigm "three vessels, three fluids" was to play a central role in the physiology of both Herophilus and Erasistratus.[50]

The remarkable innovations that Herophilus brought to this field, with respect to the Aristotelian model (not to mention traditional medicine), were largely the product of the cultural and institutional setting in which Herophilus worked. This setting not only offered a scientist the *schole* required for theoretical work, but also eliminated the taboo against anatomical study of the human body. There is no doubt that Herophilus practiced dissection of human cadavers,[51] and there is likewise no reason to question Celsus's statements concerning human vivisection. "They laid open men whilst alive . . . and whilst these were still breathing, observed parts which beforehand nature had concealed, their position, colour, shape, size . . . Nor is it, as most people say, cruel that in the execution of criminals, and but a few of them, we should seek remedies for innocent people of all future ages."[52]

One can only observe that Herophilus's vivisection did far more to advance "pure" theory than it did to increase knowledge of therapeutic remedies, though Celsus adduces the latter in moral justification.[53]

Nevertheless, Herophilus's contributions to the progress of theory were truly astounding.[54] His greatest achievement lay in his identification of the nervous system, clearly distinguished for the first time from both the tendons and the arterial endings. Herophilus believed that the nervous system originated in the cerebellum and the adjoining spinal cord.[55] He further classified the nerves into two categories: the nerves responsible for voluntary movement, which he called "decisional nerves" (using, significantly, the Aristotelian term *proairetika*), and the sensory nerves *(aisthetika)*. In anatomophysiological terms, the differences between the two categories were noteworthy. The motor nerves were classified, along with the tendons and ligaments, in a "hard" and elastic system, the *neurodes genos*, or the family of nerves and tendons.[56] The body of these nerves was solid, and movement was thought to be transmitted through that nerve body directly, without its being a vessel for any fluid. Galen later criticized Herophilus for this idea, but we know that the transmission of voluntary movement from the brain to the muscles was a problem that sorely tried Galen, too.[57] The sensory nerves, by contrast—especially the optic nerve, which connects the eye and the brain—were described as soft conduits, hollow and filled with pneuma, which presumably served as the medium through which the perceptual message was transmitted.[58] On the whole, therefore, Herophilus transferred to the *neurodes genos* the functions that Praxagoras had attributed to the arteries regarding voluntary movement. Likewise, he attributed to the system of nerves, pneuma, and brain the perceptual functions that Aristotle had ascribed to the system of veins, blood, and heart. In terms of theory, this marked the end of cardiocentrism (though that system continued to flourish at length as a tradition; its special benefactors were the Stoics, who continued to rely on Aristotle and Praxagoras).

It was at this point that the first problems with Herophilus's anatomophysiology began to arise. Why did pneuma play no role in voluntary movement? What was the source of the sensory pneuma that appeared to be located in the fourth cerebral ventricle? We have no answer to these questions, either because our sources are incomplete or because Herophilus himself failed to complete the system.

His description of the second major system appears more thorough. That system connects heart, veins, and arteries (distinguished for the first time, at least in part on an anatomical basis, through the differences in thickness of the respective membranes or tunics). The veins, naturally enough, were blood vessels, distributing nutrition throughout the body. The arteries instead contained pneuma, in accordance with the teachings of Praxagoras. It may be—though we cannot be sure—that Herophilus conceded that there was a certain amount of blood present in the arteries as well, to nourish the membranes or tunics.[59] Here he differed from Erasistratus and came closer to the beliefs set forth by Galen.[60] The pneuma found in the arteries originated in the heart and not in the brain, as did the sensory pneuma. (Here we begin to see the distinction, which later became standard, between psychic pneuma and vital pneuma. This distinction was made necessary by the quasi-axiomatic requirement that different vessels be assigned different fluids, as is the case with the sensory nerves and the arteries.)

It is worth noting that Herophilus believed not that the heart pumped pneuma into the arteries but rather that the arteries attracted the pneuma by expansion.[61] Here we see another fairly primitive technological model, that of the bellows. The pneuma, for that matter, was attracted not only by the heart but also directly by the external air, through the pores of the skin. Arteries and pneuma were also responsible for involuntary movement, in particular for the heartbeat, caused by arterial systole and diastole.

Herophilus's theory of respiration is interesting for more than one reason. First, it once again stated that organic pneuma derived from the external air, in accordance with Praxagoras but differing with Aristotle, and rejected any significant role for the heart in the respiratory process. Second, Herophilus made further use in this context of the technological model of the bellows. The external air, in fact, was inhaled following the expansion of lungs and chest. This was the beginning of the distribution of pneuma—through a mechanism that is not clear to us—to the nerves and arteries. Excess pneuma was exhaled through the contraction of the lungs.[62] Herophilus's deep-seated opposition to Aristotle led him to ignore any function of cooling organic heat in the respiratory process, and he especially rejected the cooling of cardiac heat. Respiration, therefore, served solely to supply the organism with pneuma.

Thus far, we have delineated the central features of Herophilus's anatomophysiology. The transitional element between that system and the clinical context was his theory of the pulse. Herophilus was the founder of this theory, as well as a genuine virtuoso of the pulse, so to speak. With respect to this innovative tool of medical semeiotics, Herophilus displayed a taxonomic sensitivity that was almost musical in nature. He may have been inspired by Aristoxenus. The typology of the pulse was categorized according to the age of the patient, but also by rhythm, frequency, magnitude, and so on. Herophilus had detected a link between the pulse and states of fever, and consequently made use of one of the most advanced pieces of Hellenistic technology, the water clock. It served as a replacement *ante litteram* for an instrument that antiquity was never to develop, the thermometer. Herophilus actually had a portable water clock built and calibrated it according to age. He used it to measure the fevers of his patients.[63] We also have documentation that Herophilus used the pulse rate in his prognoses.[64] This was a radical innovation—based on his anatomophysiological knowledge—of the old Hippocratic semeiotics.

But this work marked the boundary of Herophilus's innovations, a measure of his unfulfilled epistemological revolution in medicine. We are left with a distinct gap, which Peter Marshall Fraser describes as a "surprising contrast,"[65] between the profound anatomophysiological renewal of medical knowledge brought about by Herophilus and his persistent traditionalism in the clinical field. The gap and contrast—despite the effort made by Erasistratus—were to have a lasting effect on the progress of ancient medicine right up to Galen himself. They derived from a deep-seated contradiction, between anatomophysiology as a theory of the normal state of the organism and clinical medicine as knowledge concerning the organism's pathological alterations, where the ancient experience of Hippocratism continued to be viewed as indispensable and unrivaled.

In reality, it may be that Herophilus tried, at least partially, to bridge this gap. He may have made anatomophysiological efforts to diagnose the cause of death of a cadaver.[66] In substance, however, he was unable to venture far from the humoral pathology of his master, Praxagoras, and so he returned to the canonic doctrine of the four humors, sustained in *De natura hominis*. Disease was always caused by an imbalance between organic humors. They were the dominant fluids, in place of pneuma and blood.[67]

The therapy that Herophilus practiced, as a result, was just as traditionally Hippocratic. The hygiene was based, as always, on a nutritious diet and vigorous exercise (meant to assist in a correct coction of the foods, so as to establish humoral equilibrium). Phlebotomy, of course, was used to rid the patient of excess sanguinary humor, and simple and compound medicines, primarily of vegetal origin, figured prominently. Herophilus so valued these medicines that he referred to them as the "hands of the gods."[68] What is most striking is the absolute lack of mention in the sources of any surgery practiced by Herophilus. If, indeed, this silence corresponds to an absence, it only widens the gap that separated his anatomical knowledge from any clinical and therapeutic practice. What is certain, at any rate, is that Herophilus's inability to draw solid and systematic links between the theoretical dimension of medicine—which he was the first to develop—and the hygienic, etiological, and therapeutic aspects of medicine lay at the basis of the radical new direction taken by his school, in various forms, as early as the first generation of disciples.

Philinus of Kos broke away from the circle and initiated the empirical school. This move may not have been entirely unfaithful to Herophilus, if it is true, as the pseudo-Galenic *Introductio sive medicus* informs us that he had received "the impulse for doing so" from his master.[69] Philinus's place of origin, for that matter, may already be considered in a certain sense an indicator of what was to remain one of the basic qualities of empirical medicine. That quality can be identified as a return—leaving aside the anatomical revolution—to the tradition of Hippocratism, and hence an opting, within the work of Herophilus, for the more conservative aspects (humoral pathology) as opposed to the more innovative aspects.

Within the bounds of the school Baccheius had begun an intellectual process that was to continue up to the end of antiquity. The process in question was the commentary of Hippocratic texts, which also marked a return to that tradition. At the same time, the school was gradually shedding anatomical practice and concentrating on the clinical aspects of the art (sphygmological prognosis, pharmacological therapy, surgery). Hippocratic commentary and surgical technique were to meet and be joined particularly in the first century B.C., in the work of Apollonius of Citium.

Of course, both of these directions—Hippocratic commentary and the abandonment of anatomy—in part resulted from social and cultural trends independent of the school itself. The crisis of the Ptolemaic dynasty—which culminated, as far as we are concerned, with the expulsion from Alexandria of the intellectuals, ordered by Ptolemy III Euergetes in the middle of the third century B.C.[70]—along with the return to influence of the native Egyptian element and Greek religious conformism, certainly brought about the death of that climate of intellectual frontiersmanship that had so strongly marked the rule of the earliest Ptolemies. With the loss of that remarkable intellectual climate, the institutional and cultural conditions that had allowed the astonishing development of anatomy in the first half of the third century B.C. were likewise lost. As for the practice of commentary, it should surely be set in the context of philological and antiquarian interests so heartily promoted—in and about the museum—by such prestigious men of letters as Aristophanes of Byzantium, who was carrying on the tradition of Callimachus. Exegesis, philology, and the lexicographic study of classical texts probably emerged—for physicians as much as for everyone else—as a form of intellectual distinction, and even a social requirement, to the point that Apollonius declared that he had composed his commentary on the Hippocratic *De articulis* "by order of the king."

All this, however, is not sufficient to explain the evolution (or, in a certain sense, the involution) of the Herophilean school, any more than the attacks made by empirical medicine suffices to explain it. The empirical school certainly adopted a set of critical tools taken from the skeptics, but there is no denying that the original impulse came directly from Herophilus. And this is not to say that Herophilus was in any sense already a skeptic, but rather to single out the theoretical impasse that Herophilus had already encountered in his effort to build an epistemic and rational system of medicine based on anatomy. Precisely this impasse was singled out for attack in the two chief arguments of the Empirics. The first of these held that anatomy was useless to the therapeutic and clinical practice of medicine, as had been shown by Herophilus's acceptance of humoral pathology, despite his best efforts. The second argument held that, consequently, it was not practicable for medicine (as useless as it was epistemologically unsound) to try to find causal explanations that involve inferences from the visible to the invisible, from the known to the unknown, from clinical experience to an anatomophysiological theory of the normal state of the organism.

The Herophileans were unable to find in the teachings of the founder of their school arguments sufficiently powerful to withstand this attack. The ensuing abandonment of anatomical research and return to commentary upon Hippocratic texts are indicators of precisely this surrender and, with it, of the inability to find reasons sufficient to justify the continuing independent existence of the school. In the Hippocratic texts, precisely that heritage of clinical experience was stored up that once again began to appear fundamental to medicine. The Empirics themselves considered it to be a level of *historia* necessary to the integration of direct observation. The final episode in the history of the school of Herophilus was the *didaskaleion* founded by Zeuxis—part Herophilean and part empiric—in Laodicea in Phrygia in the middle of the first century B.C. After that point, we find no further documentation of an organized Herophilean school. It took Galen to rediscover in Herophilus the great and unrivaled master of anatomical knowledge (and to reproduce, in more sophisticated forms, Herophilus's unresolved dichotomy between the epistemic and anatomophysiological aspects of medicine and the clinicotherapeutic aspects, once again "temperamental" and humoral). But from Zeuxis's time to Galen's, Herophilus was seen as boxed in, along with Erasistratus and others, in a dogmatic and rationalist "sect," largely a historiographic construct produced by empirical polemics. This sect described an intellectual attitude (a holdover from the epistemological revolution attempted by Hellenistic medicine) more than it did a homogeneous school of medicine with its own precise doctrinal boundaries.[71]

The Systematic Reorganization of Medical Knowledge: Erasistratus

Were we not fairly well informed on the chronology, we would be tempted, and justifiably so, to consider Erasistratus as a successor to Herophilus, rather than his contemporary. In terms of anatomical knowledge, Erasistratus was perfectly aware of Herophilus's innovations concerning the brain and the nervous system, while he appears markedly ahead of Herophilus in his knowledge of the heart and the cardiac valves. If we may look at indicators from outside the sphere of medicine, Erasistratus's references to mechanics and pneumatics also seem to allude to a more modern and sophisticated technical context than that known to Herophilus. Above all, Erasistratus gives us the distinct impression of having made a systematic effort to resolve the epistemological problems inherent in an overall reorganization of medical knowledge, problems that developed in the heart of the "Hellenistic revolution," problems that Herophilus had left unsolved.[72] Since, however, it is clear that the two masters were contemporaries, we are forced to conclude that Erasistratus was simply more consistent, and perhaps more ambitious, in his approach to the problems raised by the revolution in question.

Not only did he reaffirm the split between a theoretical and a clinical dimension of medicine, but he attributed a different epistemic weight to each of the two. Anatomophysiology, which was now accompanied, significantly, by etiology (a theoretical commitment that Erasistratus attempted to respect), was assigned a full epistemic status *(epistemonikon);*

clinical medicine (semeiotics, therapy), by contrast, was recognized only as having a character of probabilistic approximation *(stochastikon).*[73] This was a basic difference that, on the one hand, helped to lower the standing of the Hippocratic tradition, while, on the other, was destined to leave a profound mark in the self-awareness of physicians, as well as in the different degree of dignity accorded the medical professions of "theoretician" and practicing clinician.

Thus far, Erasistratus had continued to adhere to well-known Aristotelian indications, while striving for greater precision. Of greater complexity, however, was his relationship with Aristotle's teleology. According to Galen, Erasistratus professed a teleological persuasion, describing nature—with language that was more Stoic than Aristotelian, at least in appearance—as the "providential author" of the living *(technike, pronoetikè).*[74] Nonetheless, Erasistratus was to further undermine Aristotelian teleology by admitting the nonteleological nature of many organs.[75] Indeed, he was to wind up giving an excessively literal value to the "technical character" of nature, maintaining that "animals grow like a seine, a rope, a sack, or a basket, in which the incrementation takes place by braiding onto the extremity of each other material, similar to that of which they are initially made up."[76] Galen certainly had an interest in contesting the legitimacy of the Peripatetic influence to which the Erasistrateans of his time laid claim, on the basis of the clearly established ties of Erasistratus himself with Theophrastus and Strato.

Nonetheless, Galen's polemic hit its target, at least in part. There is no question, as we shall see below, that the model of the twisted cord played an important part in the anatomophysiology of Erasistratus. And it is equally certain that Erasistratus rejected the salient points of Aristotelian vitalism, such as innate heat, innate pneuma, and the thermocardiocentric paradigm. Thus, the art of nature was in the end limited to providing a good initial building plan for a living organism, while its providentialism consisted of nothing more than supplying that organism with the materials and energy needed for it to function.

One sign of this approach can perhaps be found in Erasistratus's memorable belief in a relationship between the development of human intelligence and the greater complexity of the convolutions of the human brain compared with those of other animals. This relationship implied no causal precedence of the psychological datum over the anatomical datum.[77]

It was chiefly in the effort to "axiomatize" medicine that Erasistratus's epistemology proved more deep-seated and more demanding than He-rophilus's, even as Erasistratus continued to respect the limits of Aristotle's partition between natural philosophy and medical knowledge. The language that Erasistratus used in identifying the first and fundamental "principles" and "elements" of this knowledge was clearly inspired by Aristotle's logic, from which he derived such terms as "suppose" and "presume" (*hypotithesthai* and *katalambanein*).[78] Alongside these terms, however, we find an innovative epistemological concept specific to Erasistratus, the concept of "theoretical observability" *(logoi theoreton)*.[79] The meaning of this apparently paradoxical concept lay in the necessity of assuming the existence of structures and entities that were invisible to anatomical observation and that were nonetheless required for the completion and perfection of the system. The observability of these invisible data can be interpreted in two convergent senses: that, in any case, these are physical entities, and hence observable in principle if not in fact; and that said observability is possible indirectly, if not directly, through quasi-models or metaphorical references.

The system of postulates that was required, according to Erasistratus, included two "primary and fundamental matters [*hylai*], by which the animal is governed."[80] One of these was food, a nourishing material that, when transformed into blood, maintained the organism's integrity by replacing those parts of it which were consumed during the vital processes. The other was pneuma: "collaborative [*synergos*] in natural activities [*energeiai*]."

To these two "matters" should be added, in the role of "principle [*arche*] and element [*stoicheion*]," a "principal structure," whose theoretical observability must be assumed.[81] This is the *triplokia*, or invisible interweaving of equally invisible nerves, arteries, and veins (though theoretically observable), which supposedly made up the walls of the anatomically visible nerves, arteries, and veins.[82] Concerning this complex and trying hypothesis of Erasistratus's, we must wonder what factor made it necessary, and in what manner it can be considered "observable."

The hypothesis of the *triplokia*, first of all, was necessary to explain nutrition, that is, the adduction of blood to the membranes or tunics of nerves and arteries. In Erasistratus's view the nerves and arteries themselves had to be scrupulously free of blood, given the distinction of the three systems and the fluids they carried. This adduction of blood was assured by the invisible vein interwoven in the *triplokia*—if there is no blood *inside* the arteries and nerves, there must be blood in their walls.[83]

The invisible nerve served, in turn, to explain the existence of feeling in the three great systems.[84] The function of the artery in the *triplokia* was less clear. It can be supposed that, with its vital pneuma, it assured the energy principle required for the systems to function.

This twisted cord made up the three major elasticofluid systems that in turn constituted the load-bearing structure of the organism. The "soft" organs, such as the brain, the marrow, the liver, the spleen, and the lungs, were, in contrast, made up of deposits *(parenchyma)* of sanguinary nutrition.[85]

As for the theoretical observability of the *triplokia*, the much-repeated Galenic comparison of an elastic cord made of three plaited leather straps[86] allows us to think that Erasistratus had in mind the model of a torsion spring, made up of hairs and then of plaited tendons, which constituted the power and propulsive element of the artillery developed by Hellenistic technology. Based on this model, the theoretical observability derived from a metaphoric transposition of an actual observation.[87]

In the axiomatic set posited by Erasistratus there appeared—alongside the primary materials and the principal structure in which these materials were contained—a general principle of a physiological, or rather "biophysical," nature.[88] This principle was formulated as the *pros to kenoumenon akolouthia*, literally, "the filling of that which has been emptied" by contiguous material (known later, with some slight inaccuracy, as the principle of the *horror vacui*).[89] In its more generally accepted form, this principle held that whenever there was a loss of material in the organism (whether through physiological consumption or for pathological reasons), nature immediately tended to replace it with other, spatially adjacent material, which may be of the same type, in normal cases, or of a different type, in pathological cases.

It may be—though this is far from certain—that Erasistratus's hypothesis had some connection with Strato's theory of the vacuum, to which we find reference in Hero. In any case, we can rule out the possibility that either Strato or Erasistratus had anything to do with the atomistic doctrine of the vacuum.[90] Assuredly, the principle of the filling of a vacuum played a central part in the pathology and the physiology of Erasistratus. It replaced wholesale the family of physiological concepts that derived from both the Hippocratic tradition, such as that of coction, and Aristotelian physiology, such as the thermic paradigm.

In connection with this assumption of Erasistratus's, Galenic testimonies provide clear indications of its technological provenance: no longer mechanical, but dictated rather by the functioning of pneumatic devices. "In the case of reeds or tubes immersed in the water, it is safe to say that when the air is removed from them, in their interior either there will be an entirely empty area or there will be an inflow of the contiguous fluid."[91] Here the model to which reference is made is that of the siphon, while elsewhere pumps are indicated[92] or compressed-air or compressed-steam devices.[93]

The set of principles assumed by Erasistratus made it possible to think of the organism as an elasticofluid system, that is, as a device driven by fluids under pressure, contained in expandable and contractible vessels. The living organism therefore represented a synthesis, or a functioning assembly, of the two models offered by Alexandrian technology—torsion-spring artillery and pneumatic devices—although that technology never succeeded in combining them, despite occasional sporadic efforts in this direction.[94]

On this foundation, at any rate, Erasistratus was able to produce with consistency both an anatomophysiological system and a pathology, and was finally able to present them as conceptually unified—the first to do so. In terms of direct observation, Erasistratus's anatomy was based on human dissection and vivisection, as was Herophilus's. In addition, Erasistratus certainly conducted experiments of animal vivisection (upon oxen and kid goats); these experiments were intended to verify critical points of his theory.[95]

An exposition of Erasistratus's anatomophysiological system can well begin with the processes through which the organic mechanism is nourished with the two fundamental materials, pneuma and food. Respiratory dilation of the thorax and lungs produces a vacuum that is immediately filled by outside air. This air serves no cooling function whatsoever. Rather, it supplies the pneuma required in physiological processes, replacing the pneuma that has been consumed or lost through visible transpiration via the epidermal pores. From this point forward, the pneuma circulates through the body as it would in an almost perfectly sealed pneumatic machine (save only for the transpiration of the skin).[96] The diastole of the heart's left ventricle recalls the pneuma from the lungs to the heart; the heart then distributes it successively to the other organs, where it is specialized as psychic pneuma and "animal," or vital, pneuma.[97] The pneuma reaches the heart from the lungs through the pulmonary artery (nowadays considered a vein, but its connection with pneuma and the left ventricle obliged Erasistratus to see it as an artery, though an anomalous one).

As for the food consumed, it undergoes an initial processing in the stomach: significantly, this is not coction but a grinding performed by stomach muscles activated, in this involuntary movement, by the swelling of the arteries with "animal" pneuma. This is an entirely mechanical process, therefore, in which the stomach acts as a pestle.[98] The liver completes the transformation of the food thus far processed into blood; from the liver the food is recalled to the heart, through the vena cava, by virtue of the diastole of the right ventricle.

The heart plays a central role in the processes of distribution of both principal organic materials. And if the strategic step in Herophilus's anatomy was that of identifying the link between the brain and the nervous system, for Erasistratus this strategic move was, without a doubt, his discovery of the cardiac valves, which allowed him to form a precise conception of the heart as a double pump equipped with unidirectional valves. This pump was the fulcrum of all the major organic processes.[99]

The systole of the right ventricle, in fact, pumped blood into the veins, through which it was distributed throughout the body. Here the blood served to rebuild tissues, filling the gaps left by the consumption of organic material, in compliance with the principle of the filling of a vacuum. For its part, the systole of the left ventricle pumped pneuma into the arteries (it should be noted that the pulse represented the arterial diastole that followed the cardiac systole). From there the pneuma was divided in two. Most of the pneuma was conveyed through the arteries to the muscle cavities, constituting the energy principle of all ensuing movement—as in the case of digestion—through the swelling of muscles by virtue of the pneuma.[100] Another portion of the pneuma was conveyed, likewise through the arteries, to the meninges and the cerebral ventricles, where it was transformed into psychic pneuma.[101]

As for the brain and its connections with the nerves, Erasistratus by and large followed the findings of Herophilus—though with a few significant variations. The nerves were divided into the customary two groups, which Erasistratus identified as sensory *(aisthetika)* and motor *(kinetika)* nerves. The former originated in the meninx, while the latter came from the brain and the cerebellum.[102] All of the nerves were necessarily hollow in order to accommodate the psychic pneuma that, presumably, was pumped there by the systole of the cerebral ventricles.[103]

While the adduction of perception to the brain via the pneuma contained in the sensory nerves did not seem to pose any particular problems for Erasistratus, the dynamics of voluntary movement did. It appears that his two models—the former being elasticomechanical, the latter being fluidopneumatic—overlapped.[104] In the first of these two models, the fact that Erasistratus treated nerves and tendons as relatively indistinct, identifying them together as something not unlike the cord of a sling or a bowstring, was the prime influence:[105] this model supplied an energy-based explanation of voluntary movement, leaving unclear—as had Herophilus—the function played in all this by the psychic pneuma. In the second of these two models, the idea of the perforation of the nerve for the flow of pneuma arose. The pneuma was adduced to the muscle cavities, setting them into motion by expansion, as in the case of involuntary movement caused by the vital pneuma contained in the arteries. It is likely in any case that, here as elsewhere, Erasistratus's physiology was directed toward producing a combination of both models.

Erasistratus found himself facing two formidable problems. The first was posed by an observation that constituted a true epistemological brain-teaser: the undeniable presence of blood in the arteries whenever they were perforated, during dissections and in the case of wounds. The imperative of distinction between systems and respective fluids required—at the risk of the entire system's collapse—that arteries be vessels only for the "animal" pneuma, just as the nerves were for the psychic pneuma and the veins were for the blood. The phenomenon of blood in the arteries thus needed to be explained or, better, explained away.

The second major problem lay in the need to overcome the gap—which Herophilus had simply left yawning—between the new anatomo-physiology, the epistemic foundation of medicine, and the old humoral pathology of the Hippocratic tradition. Erasistratus did not intend to accept so feeble an epistemological compromise, and he had therefore ambitiously included etiology as part of the rationally "strong" section of medicine. For this reason, it was necessary to produce a general model for the explication of diseases, based directly on the anatomophysiological system.

Erasistratus overcame both problems with a single solution of remarkable scientific efficacy. He simply introduced a new, theoretically observable structure, an invisible synastomosis, equipped with valves, between the capillary endings of veins and arteries (thus "inventing," rather than discovering, the vascular capillaries).[106]

On this basis, Erasistratus was able to deal with the obstacles. In the case of the perforation of the arterial membrane or tunic, no matter how minimal, there was an ensuing (invisible) leakage of all of the pneuma contained in the artery. The vacuum thus created was immediately filled by a flow of blood that (by the principle of *horror vacui*) forced its way past the valve of the synastomosis, overflowing from the vein into the artery.[107] The presence of blood in the open artery did not call the system into question. Rather, it confirmed it. (We are quite familiar with the determination with which Galen worked to demolish this "explanation" of Erasistratus's.)

Erasistratus succeeded in finding in his system itself a clear basis for his theory of health and, consequently, for his theory of pathology. Health consisted of the hermetic seal between the three elasticofluid systems. This meant that the three "materials" (blood, psychic pneuma, and animal pneuma) should remain in their respective vessels. His definition led to a sharp narrowing of the concept of "cause" of disease: there might be potentially pathogenic factors, such as heat or cold, dietary excess or strains, but these are not truly causes. A cause is solely that which directly and necessarily determines the onset of the disease. In these terms, Erasistratus was able to drastically reduce his etiology to a single pathogenic condition: plethora, an excess of materials entering the organism, especially the excess of blood that ensued.[108] If there was more blood in the veins than they could contain, that blood would tend to overflow into the other linked systems. This phenomenon, called *paremptosis,* was the first and, one might say, the sole cause of all diseases.[109]

On the basis of so audaciously simplified an etiology, which was directly derived from the anatomophysiological system, Erasistratus was thus able to reduce all diseases to two major groups. The first was that of inflammations and fevers. This group was caused by the passage of excess blood from the veins to the arteries, forcing its way past the valves located in the synastomosis and resulting in a blockage of the free flow of animal pneuma in the arteries themselves.[110] The second group of diseases were those of "paralysis," which affected the nervous system controlling sensation and voluntary movement. These diseases were a consequence of the passage of blood into the nerves, thus blocking the flow of psychic pneuma. Since there was no natural synastomosis between nerves and veins, we must suppose that this passage took place through the *triplokia,* filtering from the invisible vein to the invisible nerve.[111]

It thus became possible to formulate, with equal clarity, in a quasi-deductive manner, the general principle of any therapy: it was necessary to return the material (the excess blood) to its natural location (the veins), by reducing its quantity, which was the cause of *paremptosis.*[112] Erasistratus pursued this end with fairly bland means of therapy: through diets that were capable of progressively reducing the nourishment that reached the organism; to a lesser degree, he made use of purgatives.[113] One may be surprised to learn that Erasistratus rejected the use of phlebotomy, as had his master, Chrysippus.[114] This therapy might seem to offer the quickest and most efficacious means for reducing an excess of blood, and indeed the Erasistrateans who lived in Galen's time had begun to make use of it again. But we must suppose that Erasistratus's chief concern was to avoid damaging in any manner the hermetic seal between the organic vessels, which ensured health, and that he would therefore be afraid of compromising it in any way by cutting the veins.

Overall, Erasistratus seems to have crossed the barrier between anatomy and surgery, a barrier that Herophilus had failed to overcome. Tradition tells us, for example, of a daring liver operation performed by Erasistratus.[115]

The Fate of the Erasistratean System

Erasistratus had therefore completed the anatomically based epistemological revolution that Herophilus had undertaken but failed to complete. Above all, he had succeeded in incorporating into his system the clinical dimension of medicine, from etiology to therapy. The price he had paid for this achievement, however, was high, perhaps too high. If the thought of Herophilus had been too weak, and his school had ebbed back into the streambed of Hippocratic tradition, the thought of Erasistratus appeared to be too strong, leaving itself open to criticisms and lending itself to uses that proved equally fatal.

There was a paradoxical contradiction at the system's heart. A conception of medicine that claimed to be based on the anatomical observability of the organic structure was, in fact, forced to rely on entities and structures that were impossible to observe by their nature. These veritable theoretical constructs appeared precisely at critical points in the construction of the system: the pneuma itself, the *triplokia*, and the synastomoses. At the same time, the system found itself denying the value of such easily observable phenomena as the normal, nonpathological presence of blood in the arteries.

From this point of view, Erasistratus was vulnerable to the attacks of the Empirics, who handily decried him as an intemperate rationalist and a hyperdogmatic. His success in completing the system could be interpreted, paradoxically, as further proof of the inability of anatomy to serve as a positive foundation for clinical medicine. On the one hand, in fact, the transition from anatomy to clinical medicine demanded reliance on the invisible and indemonstrable. On the other hand, this transition impoverished, to an unacceptable degree, etiology, diagnosis, prognosis, and therapy. Indeed, what became of seasonal and environmental factors, factors of age and diet in the etiology of Erasistratus? What became of the observation of individual clinical cases, of semeiotic competence, of the theory of the crisis—abandoned along with the idea of coction—and of the complex and learned therapeutic virtuosity that had been accumulated by traditional medicine?

All of this, from the standpoint of empirical criticism, simply confirmed the uselessness or, worse, the harm done by founding the medical art on anatomy. It consequently appeared necessary to adhere rigorously to the observable links between symptomatic patterns and therapeutic interventions of proven efficacy.

Even those who seemed in some way to be making use of Erasistratus's rationalism were in fact dealing devastating blows to his system. Consider the Stoics (with their unquestionable influence upon pneumatic medicine).[116] The central role they attributed to pneuma in psychophysiological processes, their interest in the energy-oriented dimension of the organism, and their reliance—in the explanation of psychic dynamics—on mechanical and pneumatic models taken from Hellenistic technology (quite evident, for instance, in the concept of the *tonos* of the soul),[117] all brought the Stoics closer to the Erasistratean framework of physiological thought. But the Stoics were entirely uninterested in the anatomical foundation of that thought, for practical and theoretical reasons. Chrysippus was satisfied with making reference to the archaic anatomy of Praxagoras.[118] He sought to serve the requirements of his own system by reconciling a theory of pneuma with the supremacy of the heart (cardiocentrism). Reference to the connection between nerves and brain, the foundation of the anatomy and physiology of Herophilus and Erasistratus, would have thrown cardiocentrism into crisis. In theoretical terms, the anatomy and physiology of the three systems of conduits were useless, even damaging for the Stoics: pneuma did not require specific vascular receptacles (because of the Stoic doctrine of the presence of pneuma in the organism as a whole). The rationalism of the Stoics could thus derive from Erasistratean thought ideas connected with energy and pneumatics; at the same time, that thought reinforced the opinion that the whole of the

Erasistratean anatomophysiological structure had been a useless hypothesis. For that matter, Erasistratus offered no psychophysiological theory of the emotional states, such as passions, which lay at the heart of Stoic philosophy.

Among physicians, we find a few echoes of the ideas of Erasistratus—although they are quite ambiguous—in the "dogmatism" of Asclepiades of Bithynia (at the end of the second century B.C.). This physician was building a new system, based on the idea of entities and structures that were theoretically observable, but two suppositions were sufficient to allow him to explicate all physiological and pathological phenomena: those of the *onchoi*, small material masses that made up the body, and the *poroi*, vascular conduits through which the *onchoi* moved from place to place. This meant a drastic epistemological reduction of the postulates, in comparison with the Erasistratean system.[119] The detailed and complex knowledge of anatomy as the foundation of medicine was eliminated as a requirement. Asclepiades began a process of reduction that was carried further by Roman methodic medicine.

The dogmatism of Asclepiades and the methodic sect—much like the dogmatism of the Stoics—took its inspiration in a certain sense from the Erasistratean model; in contrast to the Empirics, it shared Erasistratus's fundamental systematic approach. This contributed all the same to the collapse of the model, in that the approach deprived the model of its foundation and raison d'être: the reconstruction of medicine based on the anatomical revolution.

Nevertheless, the Erasistratean school—in contrast with the Herophilean school—was not destined to vanish entirely. Erasistrateans existed during the lifetime of Galen. To defend themselves from Galen's critical pressure, they tended to reduce the originality and specific nature of the thinking of their master. In effect, in theoretical terms, they insisted on his bonds with the finalism of Aristotle and the Peripatetics; in clinical terms, they returned to the bloodletting that Erasistratus had rejected during his lifetime. All this was not enough to shelter the teachings of Erasistratus and his supporters from the twofold attack of Galen. On the one hand, they were portrayed as hyperdogmatics, because they persisted in refusing to recognize an observable fact (the presence of blood in the arteries), for the sake of maintaining intact their system. On the other hand, they were depicted as representatives of an incomplete rationalism, for they refused to venture past the level of anatomophysiology into the theory of the elements. The Erasistrateans believed that this incompleteness was the price they had to pay to assure the epistemological autonomy of medicine with respect to natural philosophy. The acceptance of the Aristotelian doctrine of elements and qualities, proposed by Galen, led back to the thermic paradigm, putting the focus on coction—and this was entirely incompatible with the original thought of Erasistratus.

Galen himself was not proof against the problems for which he criticized Erasistratus. He wanted to reconcile the Aristotelian philosophy of nature, the anatomophysiology of Alexandrian origin, and the clinical medicine of Hippocratic inspiration. The system would not hold together: Hippocratic clinical medicine was compatible with the doctrine of elements and qualities (through the theory of humors and temperaments) but irreconcilable with Hellenistic anatomophysiology. For that matter, this latter school of thought—a magnificent instrument for obtaining an understanding of the normal functioning of the healthy organism (hence the foundation for a providentialistic view of nature)—was at the same time wholly inadequate in terms of diagnosis, prognosis, and therapy. Galen was thus obliged—despite his program of unification and epistemological reorganization of medicine—to allow the two models and two descriptions to coexist. The first, the "high," finalistic, and providentialistic model, was based on anatomophysiology. The second, the "low" model, situated at an epistemologically inferior level, established a sort of short circuit between the theory of elements and qualities and Hippocratic clinical medicine.[120] This dualism was the last symptom of the incompleteness of the epistemological revolution undertaken by Hellenistic medicine. And this incompleteness was to continue in Galen's work, despite all his efforts; Galen continued to uphold that medicine, although he was its greatest critic.

~ 4 ~

The Paths of Knowledge:
Medicine in the Roman World

DANIELLE GOUREVITCH

For many centuries, most of those physicians who were not simply charlatans were "rationalists," "Dogmatics," or "logicists," without even realizing it, in much the same way that Jourdain, the central character of Molière's play *Le Bourgeois Gentilhomme*, wrote prose. All physicians had adopted the same method for acquiring knowledge, believing, with Hippocrates, that medicine is a science of hidden things *(episteme)*, on the basis of which one could reason in therapeutic terms.

Medical Sects

The idea of a medical sect first appeared in Alexandria during the third century B.C., in one of the cradles of ancient medicine, then at the height of its glory.[1] The idea developed and was adopted throughout the Roman world.

It seems that it all began with Herophilus, a great innovator and charismatic figure. He attracted a solid group of brilliant pupils; these disciples admired Herophilus's anatomical discoveries and, like him, believed in the need for dissection of human cadavers.[2] Among these students were Philinus of Kos and Baccheius of Tanagra, who played leading roles in the years that followed. Philinus soon parted ways with his teacher. Although he remained in Alexandria, he imparted teachings that were diametrically opposed to those of Herophilus and his followers. Philinus founded the empirical sect and attacked Baccheius, who was still faithful to Herophilus, in a six-book treatise. Philinus's successor at the head of the empirical sect, Serapion of Alexandria, wrote a book entitled *Ad sectas*,[3] in which he apparently attacked not only the school of Herophilus but all other physicians of differing schools. That started things rolling; the medicine of the sects had come into being, and "heretical" medical literature began to flourish.

Why do we now speak of "heretical" literature? Why do we speak of "sects" or "factions"? These are words that are decidedly pejorative nowadays. What terms were used to describe these developments in the languages spoken in those days, freely coexisting in this field, namely Latin and Greek?[4] A sect was a group that accepted leadership *(agoge)* and followed a set of teachings *(didaskaleion)*; it was a school *(schole)*. In metaphorical terms, a sect was a chorus, with its *choragi*, or leaders of the chorus, as in a tragedy; a sect was an army of loyal soldiers. The terms that were properly used to designate a sect were, however, in ancient Greek *hairesis*, and in Latin *secta*. The Greek term described a group that had made a set of choices, while the Latin term indicated a group that followed a master or a set of principles (in ancient Greek, a verb with the same Indo-European root, *hepomai*, was employed to indicate that a certain physician followed the opinions of some other physician). With the growing influence of Christian thought, both of these words began to acquire—from the second century A.D. onward—a pejorative meaning, the same as that of the word *factio*, used by Pliny to denigrate the empirical sect.

Any given group had a founding father, a master thinker, a guarantor of authority. A group might or might not have, at a specific time, a leader or a chief member. Members of the group frequented the master, either listening directly to his words or learning indirectly from his teachings.

The cohesiveness of a group was expressed through such formularies of obedience as "it is the general opinion that"; other terms included "to follow," "to believe," "to place reliance on," and "consider oneself among the followers of . . ." Internal solidarity could be strengthened by attacks from other sects, the publication of polemical books, and a specific form of oral teaching called debate *(agon)*, which was invariably directed against others. This harsh form of confrontation was often conducted with considerable verve, wit, and linguistic creativity. The controversy *(antilogia)* frequently became rough, the opponent's position being discounted as mere error *(hamartema)*. Differing points of view resulted in separation of the schools *(diaphora)* and failure of their voices to harmonize *(diaphonia)*. More important, each of the physicians-authors of each of the sects had no qualms about expressing reservations or even aggressively criticizing their forerunners or even their masters. The members of a sect rarely agreed, and only under quite exceptional circumstances would they all concur on a point. Still, following the initial dissidence that underlay the sect's foundation, true dissidence was uncommon. Much the same case prevailed, in all likelihood, among humble practitioners, who wrote no books yet felt strongly about inscribing upon their tombstone a proclamation of their membership in a given sect.

Disagreements among the members of the methodic sect were so sharp that their *diaphonia* became the subject of much mockery. Despite this discord, there was mutual recognition among them as to their membership in the sect; the same was true of the Empirics. Indeed, the mind of an ancient physician seemed incapable of entertaining doubts as to the membership in the sect of a given colleague. It is unquestionably difficult for us clearly to grasp the ideas that made such doubt untenable, as we are strongly influenced by the later events that occurred at the beginning of the Christian era: a major effort was made to resystematize these sects, leading to the canonical classification into three sects, which persisted throughout the Middle Ages. This threefold partition was certainly useful, but it was quite simplistic. This tripartite classification, however, serves nicely to delineate the crucial problem in question here, that of the acquisition of knowledge.

The distinct presentation given the three different sects in the preface of Celsus's *De Medicina* is the earliest surviving example of this.[5] A considerably greater abundance of information can be found in the works of the Galenic corpus: *Subfiguratio empirica,* which survives in the translation into medieval Latin by Nicola da Reggio; *De experientia medica,* preserved in Arabic; *De sectis ad introducendos (De sectis ad eos qui introducuntur),* which survives in Greek.[6] In *Definitiones medicae,* the logical scheme is presented to the reader in even simpler terms,[7] and we shall allow ourselves to be guided by it:

> The logical sect is the science that has to do with hidden things and
> the actions that derive therefrom in the art of healing. The empiri-
> cal sect is the science of what is observed most of the time, in the
> same way, and in more or less the same manner. The methodic sect
> is a knowledge of the apparent communities, which are in accord-
> ance with the goal of the medical art and are necessary to it.[8]

In other words, the true issue was not the choice of therapy, which was debatable but never worth fighting over; the question was rather the method by which medical knowledge was acquired, the nature of this knowledge, its origin, and its final purpose. How should a physician, in such or another case, determine the appropriate treatment for a given illness? And how could the physician conclude that this was the right treatment?

Dogmatic Medicine

In chronological terms, the first sect to be recognized as such was that of the Empirics; this sect developed as a response to what was then seen as the outmoded rationalist medicine, given new life by the discoveries of anatomistic medicine. For a complete understanding of these matters, we must take a step backward and attempt to grasp the medicine that the Empirics were to describe as dogmatic, logical, analogistic, or rationalist. This was the earliest school, based as it was upon the rationalist postulate that provided the very foundation of the birth of the medical art. With a slightly embarrassed insistence, the pseudo-Galenic author of the *Introductio* wrote: "Hippocrates of Kos was the founder of the logical sect. After him came Diocles of Carystus, Praxagoras of Kos, Herophilus of Chalcedonia, Erasistratus of Ceos, Mnesitheus of Athens, Asclepiades of Bithynia, also known as Asclepiades of Prusa, Athenaeus of Attalia, in Pamphylia."[9]

This dogmatism, ineluctably subordinated to reasoning, older and yet not well organized, was sufficiently confident of victory to trigger the development of a skeptical movement, the empirical sect. Faced with this new development, the dogmatic sect found itself forced to define itself more firmly and to undergo transformation. At that time, all physicians who considered speculation to play a role in medical discovery were classed as Dogmatics. In the eyes of the Dogmatics themselves, however, there really was no dogmatic sect—rather, there was a certain state of mind that was shared by numerous groups. Those groups were named by referring not to a method but to their founding father. There were thus physicians who relied on the work of Hippocrates, Erasistratus, Herophilus, or even Asclepiades, Diocles of Carystus, or Praxagoras. A certain Tiberius Claudius Menecrates, who was an official physician to the emperors, and who lived in the first century A.D., claimed to have invented a special dogmatic system, which he described in 156 books. He boasted of it in his epitaph.[10] No physician belonging to this school could write *pro secta sua*, in defense of dogmatism, as the Empirics did in defense of empiricism.

These believers in *rationalis medicina*, to use the expression of Celsus,[11] believed that the medical art—by reconciling recent discoveries with the older, Hippocratic clinical tradition—could discover the most recondite things, through the systematic application of certain principles, and thus attain a state of perfection. They also agreed upon the following main points:

1. There are obscure causes of disease that escape the immediate notice of the senses but that the physician can discover, enabling him to construct a true etiology of diseases. According to Celsus's view, these causes lie in the state of the body's component elements, which are accessible only to the mind.

2. These hidden causes are opposed to the more evident causes, which are instead perceived directly by the senses; these more evident causes immediately precede or even trigger the disease. Among them are heat or cold, hunger or overeating, and other such causes. They must be taken into consideration.

3. Reasoning, based upon experimentation and the dissection of cadavers (the matter of vivisection is of minor importance in the history of ideas, and has been somewhat blown out of proportion),[12] can solve even the most difficult problems of anatomophysiology, nosology, and therapy.

4. Treatment is essentially discovered by conjecture, following the discovery of the hidden cause, which serves as an indicator by its nature. Experience can play a role, however, as can experimentation, to a lesser degree.

Upon this overall landscape, the two most important logical sects stood out—the sect of the Herophileans and the sect of the Erasistrateans: "Both these schools flourished after Herophilus's death."[13]

In the persuasive chronology suggested by Von Staden, the Herophileans consisted of Andreas of Carystus, physician of Ptolemy IV Philopator, one of Herophilus's earliest disciples; Callianax, who was remembered for his coarseness toward his patients; Callimachus, considered to be one of the founders of the sect by the historian Polybius, who placed him on a level with Herophilus himself (second half of the third century B.C.); Baccheius of Tanagra, who looms large in the medical tradition for his

Lexeis, a lexicographical work concerning certain uncommon or difficult words used by Hippocrates; Demetrius of Apamea; Mantias, whose fame was chiefly based on his pharmacological expertise; Zeuxis, founder of a Herophilean school near Laodicea in Phrygia; Apollonius Mys, an Alexandrian Herophilean (second half of the first century B.C.); Aristoxenus, student of Alexander Philalethes (first half of the first century A.D.), whose book *De Herophili secta* was doubtless known to Galen; Gaius, who may have been a Roman; and Demosthenes Philalethes, head of the sect at Laodicea, the last known Herophilean (first half of the first century A.D.).

The chief of the rival rationalists was Erasistratus of Ceos, who took up residence in Alexandria. Among the Erasistrateans were, first and foremost, his direct disciples, such as Strato. It is in this medical context that Plutarch's works are steeped, especially the discussions of the *Quaestiones conviviales.* During Galen's time, there was a major group of Erasistrateans in Rome. Then they disappeared, leaving no followers. Perhaps their about-face on the matter of bloodletting led to their decline in repute.[14]

Empirical Medicine

Let us return, then, to the source of so much trouble, the Empirics.[15] "At the head of the empiric sect was Philinus of Kos, who was the first to divide it and separate it from the logical sect; he had received the necessary encouragement from Herophilus, of whom he had been a direct pupil."[16] The first to proclaim its existence as a sect, the first to appoint a chief, and the first to establish a set of principles and a name, this sect was for many years confined strictly to Alexandria. The Empirics, under the influence of skeptical philosophy, did not consider medicine to be a full-fledged science. According to Sextus Empiricus, they even ventured further than the skeptics, in a certain sense. They declared that what the senses could not apprehend was incomprehensible in nature, which is more than the skeptics would ever have dared to claim. The Empirics believed that medicine was simply an accumulation of knowledge, attained through what were essentially fortuitous observations.[17] And it was from this stance that they derived their name: "se empiricos ab experientia nominant,"[18] or else "alia factio, se ab experimentis cognominans empiricam."[19] In this fundamentally negative context, no doctrine could really develop, properly speaking.

Particularly sensitive to the differences of opinion among the Dogmatists, the Empirics were, furthermore, certain that nature was incomprehensible and that only that which could be observed was real. It was therefore pointless and superfluous to insist on seeking out the invisible; the study of physiology and anatomy—and to an even greater degree, vivisection itself, which had been practiced for some time in Alexandria— were not advisable. Since that which is hidden is secret, and since there are no reliable signs, it was perfectly useless to engage in reasoning based solely on some likelihood or other; this meant relying on opinions, and what is more, opinions that diverged one from another and that had no real effect on the choice of therapy. A disease was entirely composed of its symptoms; the causes of disease were evident: hunger, thirst, chills, heat, lack of sleep, fatigue, and so on. In many cases, the Empirics felt that, rather than a cause in the logical sense, these were premonitory symptoms of the disease. Their skepticism, which led them to doubt all opinions previously expressed, was at work in this field as well. Treatment was indicated by similarities among the various cases observed. If a new disease were to emerge, then it was proper to respond in the same manner, through comparisons and analogies. They emphasized the practical nature of medical practice: "It does not matter what produces the disease but what relieves it."[20] An empirical physician observed facts when the opportunity presented itself, repeated personal experience, and also took advantage of accumulated experience. At no time would he turn to experimentation proper. Experience alone lay at the foundation of medicine; it was conceded that this word could have many different meanings—three to be precise, the "tripod" of the sect, according to Glaucias of Tarentum. There is individual experience: direct observation, *autopsia*, which comes about either through the happenstance of life, or through intentional provocation, "in order to see," or else by recreating or imitating a situation. There is also a second form of experience, based on the "passage from the same to the same" or, to be more precise, from the nearly similar to the nearly similar. Thus, analogy allows a physician, in the absence of a certain plant, to use another similar plant in its place. The effect of a certain plant on a certain part of the body might lead the physician to try that same plant on another part of the body. Yet again, the resemblances between two diseases might authorize the physician to use the same treatment in both cases. The third meaning of empirical experience was collective experience, or "history"—one therefore knows what everyone knows, one gathers from what others say, and one relies on the repetition of observation, which can be done with greater or lesser passion and discernment.

The empirical sect, indeed, believed that medicine was a practice, above all a form of therapy, and that it was completely separate from speculation. Empirical medicine held up the useful in opposition to the superfluous; this medicine was not based on hidden things *(ab rebus latentibus)*, which engender doubt and are less than certain. Rather, it was based on those things which could truly be studied *(explorare)*.[21] The product of a mental state rather than of a positive doctrine, the empirical sect, on principle, possessed no holy text, and paid far less reverence to its master than did other sects.

The Penetration of Greek Medicine at Rome and the Doctrine of Asclepiades of Prusa

Following the establishment and development of military and political contacts between Rome and Greece, Greek medicine made its entry into Italy.[22] First appeared the god Aesculapius, who in 292 B.C. sent a serpent in his stead to the Tiber Island. Then came humans: in 219 B.C., the renowned Archagathos, initially praised to the heavens and later disgraced with the vengeful nickname of "carnifex." The medicine of the "paterfamilias," described for us by Cato, Varro, and Pliny the Elder, was scarcely altered. Far greater ramifications, however, ensued in the wake of the conquest of Corinth, in 146 B.C. Asclepiades left Prusa in Bithynia and took up residence in Rome. He formed part of the wave of physicians—some genuinely fond of Roman ways, others moved solely by self-interest—who were then abandoning Greece.[23]

The fundamental concept underlying Asclepiades' innovative system was that the human body (just as, in all probability, the world at large) is made up of *onchoi*, corpuscles visible only to the mind. Inside the body, these corpuscles move through equally theoretical *canaliculi*.[24] The great originality of this explanation lay less in its corpuscular nature and more in the divisibility of the exceedingly fragile corpuscles. When subjected to shock, they could easily break and continue breaking without limitation. To put it simply, the corpuscles are not atoms, an aspect that sharply differentiates this doctrine from those of Democritus and Epicurus.

Moreover, Asclepiades saw the human body as more or less "porous," varying from part to part; the corpuscles circulate in a network of "pores," or canals. These canals vary in number and are themselves hollow, permitting movement and, hence, change. If nothing blocks the regular flow, then a sort of equilibrium is established between the particles and the canals, and the body is in good health. If the corpuscular flow is interrupted, then blockage and engorgement ensues. Disease develops in a given part of the body. If the blockage is sufficiently great, then a counterflow from the diseased part of the body may ensue, in reaction, in the opposite direction. If the corpuscles break down too easily, then the infirmity can only be a disease of flux. The pores, too—which in their natural state are not the same size throughout the body—may contribute to the course of a disease, if they are too narrow or too wide.

While Asclepiades had a following of Asclepiadian physicians, few if any of them were renowned; the best known was Cassius the Iatrosophist (first century A.D.). The true heirs to the legacy of Asclepiades—ungrateful heirs, one might add—were the Methodics, hostile though they claimed to be to all speculation. There is a clear link between Asclepiades' concept of engorgement due to the blockage of the particles and the methodic notion of a state of tension in the body.

Methodic Medicine

A third medical sect developed, in Rome this time. Innovative and prolific, the most brilliant sect of the imperial period, this was the methodic sect.[25] Like the Empirics, the Methodics were well aware of their own originality, and they named themselves. If the Empirics had taken no interest in hidden things, neither did the Methodics. In the tradition of the Dogmatics, the Methodics had a system for the explanation of diseases; they followed a specific line of reasoning that led from observation to treatment. Deriving as they did from the two major sects that preceded them, but without forming part of those sects, the Methodics—despite their deserved reputation as outstanding clinicians—were badly misunderstood in their own time. They were subject to ferocious attacks, in particular from Galen, who heaped insults on them. It is difficult to set forth the basis of the methodic system, both for reasons inherent to that system, which introduced new ideas through the vehicle of old terminology, and for historical reasons, because none of the writings of the earliest Methodics survive. We should mention two names, around which swirl chronological controversies: Themison and Thessalus. Themison of Laodicaea, who was probably a direct pupil of Asclepiades, died sometime between 50 and 40 B.C.; Thessalus of Thralles reached the peak of his career during the reign of Nero, let us say about A.D. 55. Both of these physicians played a part in the development of new ideas but over a fairly long span of time and without any real continuity.

In the nonmethodic medical literature that mentions the Methodics, from Celsus to Galen, we encounter nothing but mistrust and even outright hostility. It may be that the mistrust was engendered by the Methodics' avowal that theirs was not an established science but rather an ongoing work of research, an inquiry, a body of knowledge still in formation. The methodic sect strongly opposed dogmatism, a well-established science of hidden things, offering a line of reasoning that led to a specific therapy; it equally opposed empiricism, which was not a science at all but merely an accumulation of fortuitously acquired knowledge.

The Methodics won a mass following by the apparent simplicity of their doctrine. Two major works of the group have been handed down: the *Gynaecia*, in Greek, by Soranus of Ephesus, and the *De morbis acutis et diuturnis* in Latin, by Caelius Aurelianus (an adaptation of a work, now lost, by Soranus of Ephesus). It is therefore much easier for us to examine the method of these later authors, whose work is directly accessible to us.

The teachings of the Methodics are marked by three fundamental ideas: "phenomenon," "community," and "indication."

The "phenomenon" is that which is apparent, though to whom and in what way we must infer. When we note the importance that Soranus of Ephesus attributes to the sensory education of the midwife, we can clearly understand that the phenomenon is provided not only by one's sight, but through other senses as well. A methodic physician can assist his own senses—broadening, in other words, the field of phenomena, by making use of instruments, such as the speculum, in the field of gynecology. And nothing prevents him from examining, should he have the opportunity to do so, the entrails of a wound victim, even though the methodic physician denies systematically practicing anatomy.

"Community" is a less accessible idea for us. It was a difficult idea even for the Methodics, who found in it an ideal ground for their *diaphonia*, or disputation. At least two methodic authors attempted to define "community" in their writings: Thessalus, in the early days of the sect, and Soranus at its acme. Despite the different points of view expressed and the development that the concept underwent, it is clear that the Methodics conceived of the existence of two principal communities: the state of relaxation and the state of tension. Quite soon a third state was added, that of mixed community, followed by yet others. Community is something quite concrete, which the physician perceives in the patient; it was also something abstract, which he conceives. Grasping the communities on the basis of the phenomena is a rapid, though not immediate, process. It depends on a mental operation, and it is here that methodism clearly appears as a form of dogmatism.

Given, however, that the ultimate objective of medicine is the restoration of health, what is the purpose of the observation of the phenomena and the recognition of the communities? They both lead to "the indication." In other words, the methodic phenomenon is a signal, operating at the level of the senses and then integrated into a broader set of references through the exercise of reasoning. A habit of observing these phenomena made it possible to classify them in this or that community—both the observation and the classification are indicators of the treatment to be selected.

Treatment aimed at suppressing the pathological state, by bringing tension to a relaxed body or relaxing a tense body. "Once it has been recognized, then, which it is of these, if the body is constricted, it has to be relaxed; if suffering from a flux, that has to be controlled," Celsus summed it up.[26] In reality, things were not so simple. First of all, treatment developed in accordance with the four periods that characterize all illness: the onset, the period of growth, the peak, and the decline. The period of illness was another indicator of what the physician should do. Treatment was often—though not always—broken up into periods of three days. For example, three days of fasting constituted the treatment to be adopted in case of indigestion, but the same three-day fast could serve as a preliminary—by ridding the body of harmful substances—to a treatment expected to be more complex. Following this fasting, or in its place, might be a cycle of recuperation, involving apotherapy, or gentle exercises through ointments and rubdowns, and so-called passive gymnastics, moderately or decidedly active exercises, such as vocal exercises or horseback riding; all this would be accompanied by a good diet. During this period, the patient would regain enough of his strength to be able to withstand the ordeal that awaited him, the so-called metasyncritic cycle. This cycle combined a strict diet with topical treatments that could be quite harsh: the ingestion of drastic substances, vomiting, bloodletting, cupping glasses, jolts, exposure to heat. These measures were meant to create profound modifications in the state of the body, thus causing the illness to disappear. Despite what the critics of the Methodics had to say, the application of this system was in no way automatic, and it was applied while taking into account a great many other factors: the acute or chronic nature of the disease, the psychology of the patient, and so on. Caelius Aurelianus, for instance, explained that only in cases in which neither diet nor persuasion succeeded in improving the state of an obese patient would one decide to apply the cycle in question.

Despite what the detractors of methodism would have us believe, there was a full-fledged methodic nosography, above and beyond the three pathological states—relaxed, tense, and mixed. What was disease in the eyes of a Methodic? Disease was generally defined under four main head-ings: name, generally with its etymology; description, which served as the true definition; the place or part of the body affected, or more precisely, the part of the body *particularly* affected, when the entire body is sick; and treatment. Let us focus on the place, a concept that provoked the majority of attacks on the Methodics. It is true that this sect's overriding principle was that in any disease, the entire body was sick: "communiter totum corpus patitur," as Caelius Aurelianus said concerning lethargy,[27] although cephalea took its name from the part of the body that was affected ("a parte corporis quae patitur nomen accepit").[28] When Soranos spoke of the set of digestive difficulties related to pregnancy—*kissa*—he clearly demon-strated that the overall conception of disease was in no way incompatible with the localizing conception of a given illness in particular. The unity of the method was a product of the adoption of a few simple principles, in particular, the doctrine of community. Nonetheless, the Methodics never had a unitary corpus of rigorous, demanding, and hierarchical rules. In a certain sense, one can say—to a greater degree than is true of other sects— that there were as many methodisms as there were great methodic physi-cians.

In the modern era, methodism enjoyed a new development in the eighteenth and the early nineteenth centuries. During periods when the rivalries among schools once again became fierce, a neomethodism devel-oped. Linked to it were such names as that of Prospero Alpino (1553–1617), author of a treatise entitled *De medicina methodica,* Philippe Hec-quet (1661–1737), Friedrich Hoffmann (1670–1742), and Giorgio Baglivi (1668–1707). All of them were in some sense forerunners of François Broussais (1772–1838).[29]

Pneumatic Medicine

The pneumatic sect is unique in that it took its name from neither a method nor a founder, but rather from the element that it considered an essential constituent part of both the human body and the world at large. This problem was already mentioned in the *Definitiones medicae:* "The first two sects of medicine are the empirical and the logical; the third is the methodic. It seems, however, that Agathinus of Sparta invented a fourth one, which some called 'episynthetic,' others 'eclectic,' and others still 'ectic.'"[30] We can see that there was some doubt as to the legitimacy of this sect, which might be nothing more than a variant of the logical sect, yet which stood apart because of the great quality of certain of its members. In effect, Anonymous of Bamberg maintained the older standpoint, according to which physicians who described themselves as pneumatic were also rationalists: "[after Hippocrates] as important rational physicians [*rationabiles*] there were Diocles, Praxagoras, Herophilus, Erasistratus, Asclepiades, Athenaeus, Agathinus, Ariston, Archigenes, Herodotus, Philumenus, and Antillus."[31]

As had been the case with methodic medicine, the physician who launched the innovative idea was not the founding father of the new sect. In this case, the great innovator was Athenaeus of Attalia, while the founding father was Agathinus of Sparta. The innovator, inspired by the Stoics, was of course particularly sensitive to the role of pneuma and can be dated with some degree of approximation. Athenaeus was surrounded by a "chorus" of disciples, among them Agathinus of Sparta and Magnus of Ephesus.[32]

Agathinus of Sparta, often quoted by Galen on the subject of the pulse, is known to us as a member of the circle of L. Anneus Cornutus, who was persecuted by Nero. Agathinus was the true founder of the new school, although he did continue—like the Empirics—to assign great importance to the role of experience in medicine. Magnus of Ephesus, too, who seemed to have the same relationship as Agathinus of Sparta with Athenaeus, "also claimed to be a member of the pneumatic sect."[33] All the same, unless Caelius Aurelianus committed an error in translating Soranos, Magnus was *ex nostris,* that is, a member of the methodic sect. Agathinus himself had a number of disciples: Herodotus, often quoted by Oribasius, and a remarkable clinician; Leonides of Alexandria, known chiefly for his work as a surgeon, who exercised considerable influence on the surgeon Heliodorus, a specialist in delicate operations and a prolific author. Foremost among the disciples was Archigenes of Apamea, the most illustrious representative of the school (sometimes considered the founder of the eclectic sect). An extremely refined theoretician of the pulse, Archigenes was greatly indebted to Herophilus, as Galen points out in certain of his books.

Archigenes in turn influenced Antyllus, who was a clinician, a pharmacologist, and doubtless one of the greatest surgeons of antiquity. Antyllus flourished around 150 B.C. Famous as he may have been, only a few scattered fragments of his work survive, chiefly concerning the extraction of cataracts, bronchotomy, the incision of hydrocele, and so on.

According to the Pneumatics, the pneuma, or *spiritus*, is the great principle of life and health, a concept that links this medical school to the philosophical school of Stoicism. The state of the pneuma, however, is not directly visible, and reasoning is required to judge it: in the human body, it can be detected through the pulse, which the pneumatic physicians described according to numerous and elaborate criteria, more detailed than their predecessors'. Referring to the definition of the pulse, Galen wrote, "The Herophileans began this refined research, and later it was carried forward by a number of Erasistrateans, followed by those who are known as Pneumatics and by certain Methodics."[34]

The various reconciliations that the Pneumatics themselves authorized with other sects or subsects and their desire to incorporate everything—or at least to reject nothing—resulted in their widely being considered eclectics. This hurt the sect over the long run, in spite of their success in the field of therapy and surgery. Furthermore, Pneumatics showed a lively interest in doxography, to the point that much of what we know about sects in general—whether through Galen or others—comes ultimately from sources deriving from this group.

As for the subject of their writings, much speculation has been indulged in. In particular, the *Definitiones medicae* has been attributed to them, certainly an error, even though that text contains much of what was being said at the time, which would be roughly when Galen was beginning his studies. The *Introductio sive medicus* was attributed to them; it is surely pseudo-Galenic, though that does not make it pneumatic. The same is true of *Ars medica*, which, despite what anyone may say, is clearly the work of Galen. What remains is Anonymus Parisinus (also known as Anonymous of Daremberg, or Anonymous of Fuchs). This text was once attributed to Herodotus; nowadays it is believed to come from a premethodic circle, prior to the conception of the communities.[35]

The Anonymous Sect

There also existed a later sect, nameless, that appeared in Alexandria at the beginning of the second century. Galen carefully eliminated it from history, astutely disguising its consistency to show only a collection of fragments with no apparent link. Until our recent investigations, the school in question had completely eluded the notice of medical historians.[36]

Medical research and teaching enjoyed a veritable renaissance in the second century A.D. Marinus, Quintus, and Numesianus were the force behind this renewal, which reached as far as Pergamum, Corinth, Rome, and even Macedonia, through four generations, from master to disciple. The members of this unquestionably dogmatic sect had five main fields of interest: anatomophysiology, Hippocratic exegesis, clinical medicine, pharmacology, and a conscientious and well-organized teaching activity. They wished to reconcile humoral pathology with a location-oriented conception of disease; they wanted to temper speculations of a physiological, pathological, and pharmacological sort with a systematic and in-depth observation of living structures, pathological symptoms, and the effects of medicines. The chief new aspect in their approach lay precisely in the integration of discoveries concerning the human body into a single system, along with classical Hippocratism (especially the theory set forth in the treatise *De natura hominis,* the practical applications set forth in the *Epidemiae,* and the clinical method found in treatises on nosology and prognosis).

An anecdote set at the beginning of Galen's Alexandrian studies gives an idea of the group's practices in the presence of a specific case—in this instance, a certain type of tremor. Galen wrote:

> I once knew a young man who was one of my fellow disciples in Alexandria, to whom this happened at the very moment when the boat had delivered us, at the beginning of the autumn. He had eaten for several days running large quantities of tender fresh dates, as he left his bath and before entering the bath. Moreover, many of these dates were not yet fully ripe. And here is what happened to him: after exercise and bath, he began to experience violent shivering, which made him think that he had a fever. He took to his bed and there stayed, in repose, well covered with bedclothes, but he passed the night without fever, and in the morning he arose to attend to his habitual occupations. Once again he was taken with trembling, and so he went to bed and remained at rest until it was time to go to the bath. No sooner had he reached his bath, than he was seized by a powerful trembling: in this case, he had the symptoms of *rigor,* though not yet very markedly. Therefore, thinking that in any case he would be taken with fever, he once again took himself to bed. During the whole day and during the following

night, he made observations, noting that he experienced trembling if he made moderate movements, but literally shivering with cold if he made more marked movements. He followed my advice concerning what he should do. I remembered a woman from our Asia, to whom something of the same sort had befallen, and I freed my comrade of fear, urging him to make free use of food, drink, and warming remedies, which could free him of the density of his humors. It was thus that he recovered.[37]

This story shows the convivial relations among the pupils, who undoubtedly belonged to a group inspired by the teachings of Numesianus. Above all, however, it shows their systematic training to make critical and controlled observations. Galen's fellow disciple thought that the violent shivering that seized him as he emerged from the bath was the result of an outbreak of fever. This prediction, Hippocratic in derivation, proved faulty; at that point, he proceeded to make observations and even performed tests to establish the link between the extent of movement and the force of the shivering or trembling. And it was through a heuristic process based on reason (warming remedies against a cold sickness) and on empiricism that an effective remedy was finally arrived at. Galen claimed the credit for himself, but we can clearly see that the success was the result of a way of thinking, a mind-set, which was common to the group. The group had a preexperimental approach, a trial-and-error method in which pure chance played a major part, yet which was guided by doctrinal reasoning.

We can try to form an idea of the chronology of this sect: Marinus, who restored anatomical studies in Alexandria, had Quintus as a pupil; Quintus was "the best physician of his time," although he was a much-discussed practitioner. Quintus in fact took up residence in Rome and was forced to leave the city as a result of the jealousy of his colleagues; Galen therefore never knew him personally. Quintus had as pupils Satyrus, who had been Galen's master in Pergamum, and Numesianus, who lived and taught principally in Alexandria. It is likely that Galen was unable to meet Numesianus in person, but he did listen to the teachings of his pupil Pelops (during his stay in Pergamum); he likewise heeded the teachings of Herecleianus, son of Numesianus, who also taught in Alexandria. The chief pupils of Herecleianus were Antigenus—whom Galen met in Rome—and Lycus of Macedonia, an ungrateful disciple, whom Galen knew only indirectly, through his writings. Thus, we have classified all the members of the sect in relation one to another, and in relation to Galen, without whom they would not have been well known and might not even have left a trace, despite their great importance. In effect, even though Galen did not consider this to have been a medical sect—and as a result, no one after him so considered it, for his view of things naturally tended to be adopted by all—the intellectual movement expressed in the teachings of the Alexandrian anatomist physicians of the first half of the second century A.D. was indeed, de facto, a sect. It exerted a decisive influence on Galen; it thus exerted a similar influence on the formation of the medical system that was later to be known as Galenism, a veritable philosophy of medicine; its choices and doctrinal options were entirely consistent. It was, however, in a stagnant, repetitive, and entirely sterile form that this philosophy was to dominate medicine in the West and Near East for more than a millennium, in the fields of both theory and practice. In scholastic Galenism, the history of the sects was to play a particularly important role.[38]

Physicians without a Sect

Certain physicians, and not the least estimable among the profession, were affiliated with no group at all, or at least did not proclaim any such affiliation. This certainly did not prevent historians from applying labels to them.

Aretaeus the Cappadocian is, even now, most often considered a Pneumatic.[39] He indeed may have taken both pneuma and *tonos* into consideration, in his treatise on acute and chronic diseases—divided into two books, one on clinical medicine *(De causis et signis acutorum et diuturnorum morborum),* and the other on therapy *(De curatione acutorum et diuturnorum morborum),*[40] but this is not enough to establish his adherence to that doctrine. It is equally inappropriate to date him as a late writer: Aretaeus the Cappadocian most likely lived in the first century A.D., and historians were deceived by the willfully archaic style of his language, a linguistic choice that seemed typical of a dying civilization. The Ionian style of his prose is the immediately visible sign of a return to Hippocratism (particularly the humoral doctrine). This intellectual approach, his nosological sense (which led some to link him with the Methodics), and his remarkable descriptions (if we wished to name the most remarkable, we would be torn among his descriptions of diabetes, migraine, melancholy, and phthisis) all captured the imaginations of many of the great neo-Hippocratic physicians of the nineteenth century. These physicians produced a flurry of editions and translations into all the European languages. Laennec himself undertook a translation: the original manuscript of his work, still unpublished, is in the collection of the Bibliothèque Universitaire of Nantes.[41]

Aretaeus the Cappadocian may have been a rough contemporary of Scribonius Largus, author of a collection of pharmaceutical prescriptions, or *Compositiones*, dedicated to an emancipated slave of the emperor Claudius. Marcellus Empiricus of Bordeaux drew copiously upon this work. From the standpoint of the present work, the most important aspect of this treatise is to be found in its preface. In effect, Scribonius Largus established an ethical code for a prescribing physician; he was clearly aware of the heritage of Hippocratic ethics. He established this code much as Celsus had done for the surgeon, and much as Soranos of Ephesus had done for the midwife.[42] Galen made reference to them in his *Quod optimus medicus sit quoque philosophus*. In a period when the populace—or at least the mighty of the world—lived in constant dread of poisoning, Scribonius Largus made a plea on behalf of drugs, urging that the art should not reject any assistance it might find. In effect, he was to write shortly thereafter, medicine is the art of curing and not harming ("scientia sanandi, non nocendi"); medicine must therefore come to the assistance of those who suffer, be useful to the sick, in short, offer its help to all those who ask, and never desire to harm anyone; and the physician is guided in his practice by the two human virtues of *humanitas* and *misericordia*.

Rufus of Ephesus lived during the reign of Trajan and was a prolific scientific writer; unfortunately, his work has been poorly preserved. Daremberg and Ruelle (1879) were therefore obliged to draw on the works of Oribasius, Aetius of Amida, Paul of Aegina, and Rhazes for their edition, because all that was then known to survive included *De renum et vesicae morbis* and *De corporis humani appellationibus*, in Greek, and *De podagra*, in Latin. More work by this author seems to have been found, if it is true that the remarkable accounts of clinical cases, preserved in Arabic, were indeed written by him.[43]

Medical Writers Who Were Not Physicians

We must accord a share of attention as well to those medical writers who were not themselves physicians; essentially, we refer to the Roman encyclopedists, Celsus and Pliny the Elder, who played a crucial role in the

medical education of the Latin-speaking peoples, in the wake of the introduction of Greek medicine.

Aulus Cornelius Celsus, who probably lived during the reign of
Tiberius, in the first century A.D., was in all likelihood not a member of
the medical profession; rather, he was an exceptionally well-educated ama-
teur. His treatise *De medicina* formed part of a vast anthology that included treatises on agriculture, the military art, law, rhetoric, and philosophy. In a history of medical ideas, it is interesting to note Celsus's efforts in
the area of linguistic creation. Scientific medicine, as it was practiced in
the Roman world, was Greek, both in foundation and form. Celsus had to
invent a language in which to explain medicine to those who did not speak
Greek; this was an absolutely unprecedented undertaking, further hindered by an adverse social context: Pliny the Elder noted that "medicine
alone of the Greek arts we serious Romans have not yet practised," adding,
"If medical treatises are written in a language other than Greek they have
no prestige even among unlearned men ignorant of Greek."[44] There was
nothing to help Celsus in the works of Cato or Varro; the only partial
effort in this direction was to be found in the writings of Cicero.

Celsus was truly the first medical popularizer in Western history. He
wrote for the interested general public; he indulged in the typically Roman
idea that one should in some sense be one's own physician. His effort to
develop a technical language in some ways fell short: quite often, for
example, Celsus gives the names of diseases in a transliterated version of
the Greek. This sort of transposition continued throughout Latin antiquity, but all of the required linguistic schemes had already been set in place
by Celsus. He showed a remarkable understanding of the Greek authors
who were available to him—directly or indirectly—and seems to have
produced virtually no glaring contradictions in his body of writing. It is
true that only the simpler aspects—if we may venture to so state it—of
medicine are treated in his work, namely, the field of therapy, quite
sufficient for those who wished to be their own physician.

Pliny the Elder, who cited Celsus among his sources, often wrote in a
reactionary spirit, was hostile to most Greek contributions, and particularly opposed "modern" medicine. He was all the same an eminent figure
and curious about everything; these two characteristics led to his death.
While commanding the fleet of Misenum (modern Miseno), he died
probably of heart failure, trapped on a beach where he had ventured in
compliance with duty and out of curiosity, during the eruption of Mt.
Vesuvius that destroyed Pompeii, Herculaneum, and Stabiae in A.D. 79.

Pliny the Elder's *Historia naturalis* is an enormous work, in thirty-seven volumes; many of those volumes are devoted to medicine, especially to remedies and the numerous natural sources of remedies. The work was a compilation of general knowledge; it added nothing new to that body of knowledge. All the same, it played a major role over the ensuing centuries as a source of widely read treatises concerning the therapeutic virtues of plants and animals, in particular, the *Medicina Plinii* and the *Physica Plinii*. The former, compiled in the fourth century, drew chiefly on books 20 to 32. The latter was a new version of the former; many subsequent versions still survive.

Galen of Pergamum

Galen's life is fairly well known:[45] he himself provided numerous scattered details in his massive written work, as well as dedicating two books to his own work, *De libris propriis,* and *De ordine librorum suorum*. There is no reason to cast doubt on his accounts, even though a few points remain doubtful and unclear.

Galen was born during the rule of Hadrian, in A.D. 129, in Pergamum, a lovely city in Asia Minor, renowned for its temple to Aesculapius and for its library. His father, Nicon, was wealthy and educated, a competent practicing architect and excellent teacher. Apparently the only son, Galen throughout his childhood and youth was supervised by his father. Endowed with a traditionalistic piety, Nicon urged Galen to take up medicine following a dream, and Galen always accepted the idea of a divine inspiration to the medical art. Charles Daremberg, who was exceedingly well versed in Galen's work, was full of bitter criticisms of this "man who was the very definition of inconstancy, philosophical and superstitious by turns."[46] Daremberg copied out, in a letter to his friend Ernest Renan,[47] a number of arguments taken from his book *La Médecine: Histoire et doctrines:* "In reading his works, one is soon aware that this man accepted mystical ideas in his writings, and even in his practice. Just the title of his little treatise, *De dignotione ex insomniis,* clearly reveals that irritating tendency, which one is sad to find in a man whose understanding in other matters was so notable."[48]

In any case, the father guided his son's studies with prudence and sound sense, never failing to provide Galen with money or his personal dedication and time. When Galen fell ill, his father hurried to his side. Galen's earliest studies were done in his beloved Asia; in A.D. 144–145, he studied philosophy under four masters belonging to as many different schools: a Platonist, a Peripatetic, a Stoic, and an Epicurean. His earliest medical studies, too, were marked by an open and antisectarian spirit. In Pergamum, while still quite young, he wrote his earliest works, a treatise titled *De uteri dissectione* and the three books of *De motu thoracis et pulmonis.*[49]

Following the death of his father in A.D. 149, Galen finished his studies at Smyrna, then at Corinth, and finally at Alexandria. He lived in Egypt for a considerable time and worked hard to distinguish himself. In A.D. 157 he returned to the city of his birth, where he had the good fortune to be chosen as physician to the gladiators. Given the serious wounds that were regularly inflicted on his patients, it was a daunting task, but, for the same reason, it was remarkably useful training. He was so successful at his work that his contract was renewed. After Marcus Aurelius took the throne in A.D. 161, and in the wake of local political problems, Galen went to Rome in 162 to try his luck. The trip offered him an opportunity to make observations and considerations of every sort. In Rome, he took center stage in refined public debates and through remarkable anatomical demonstrations. During this period, he wrote his first works of anatomophysiology and of the history of philosophy and of medicine. The notable success that he enjoyed with the powerful won him the solid and lasting envy of many of his colleagues, whom he repaid with the same coin. In A.D. 166, for a complex set of reasons, he hastily departed Rome just as an epidemic of the plague broke out. He reached Pergamum in short stages and lived there for some time. Then he was summoned back to the capital by Marcus Aurelius and his fellow emperor Lucius Verus, who were both campaigning against the Germans and who supposedly desired Galen's presence and assistance in their military operations. In A.D. 168 Galen was in Aquileia, where he stumbled into the plague that he had fled just a few years before. Marcus Aurelius at that point entrusted the health of his son Commodus to him, and in 169 Galen began his second stay in Rome, a much longer stay than his first had been. This situation offered him the opportunity to write his books on hygiene. His young patient became emperor in A.D. 180 and proved to be a detestable and brutal tyrant. Septimius Severus, founder of a new dynasty, succeeded him in 192, a horrible year for Galen, because of the fire that destroyed both the temple and the library of Peace, where Galen's books were stored. During all these years, save for occasional voyages in search of simples, Galen had never left Rome. It was there that he wrote his books on pathology. Contrary to the indications given in the "Suda," according to which Galen died sometime before A.D. 200, Arabic tradition[50] suggests that between A.D. 200 and 210 Galen decided to return to his birthplace, and that he died sometime between 210 and 216, either during the course of the voyage or following his arrival in Asia.

Galen was one of the last great creative physicians of antiquity, the second "founding father" of ancient medicine after Hippocrates. A prolific writer, he left an enormous body of medical and philosophical work that, despite some major losses, now consists of over twenty volumes in Greek, along with work that survived only in Arabic, Hebrew, Syriac, and Latin. With some approximation, since many subjects overlap, his work can be broken down into various groups: biography; the medical art in general; philosophy, logic, and history of the sects; anatomy; physiology; nosology; diagnosis and prognosis; therapeutics; hygiene and prophylaxis; and Hippocratic studies.

Health and Aesthetics: Galen's Natural Philosophy and Religion

We shall attempt to understand Galen's god through his medical aesthetics,[51] which would not be out of line with the sensibility of Galen himself, who was not much interested in taking positions on mere problems of metaphysics. He "never attempted to define the nature of the soul. Is it totally immaterial or material, is it eternal or corruptible?" And he "never met anyone who had given logical proof of same."[52] In Galen's view, having an opinion on the essence of God was unnecessary, since it was of no particular use in dealing with the practical problems that one must face in reality.[53] Experience, which Galen always worked hard to link to a dogmatic reasoning, can tell us nothing new concerning problems of this sort. He was uninterested in pure speculation, or at any rate was unwilling to engage in such. This relative skepticism prevented him from belonging to a philosophical sect, despite his admiration for Plato[54] and the strong ties of respect that bound him to Aristotle.[55] Similarly, he steadfastly refused to join a medical sect.

Galen saw health as being made up of successive equilibriums linked one with the other.

> Among healthy bodies, some are purely and simply healthy; others are healthy currently, which, to be precise, we call good health. Among the bodies that are purely and simply healthy, let us say that

there is a double distinction, since the ones are always that way, while the others are that way most of the time . . . As for that which depends on the being itself, in those with the better constitution, there is an equilibrium among the homeomerous parts with respect to heat, cold, dryness, and humidity; and there is also an equilibrium of the organic parts with respect to the number and the size of the elements that make them up, and also with respect to the shape and the position of the part of each organ and the organ as a whole. As for that which is necessarily the consequence of the homeomerous parts, in the area of the sense of touch, for instance, it is an equilibrium in terms of delicacy and hardness; in terms of sight, it is a good complexion and an equilibrium between smooth and hairy. As for the possibilities of action, their complete character is that which we call their perfection. With respect to that which is related to the organic parts, this perfection consists of the equilibrium and beauty of the body as a whole, but also in the perfection of the possibilities of action which they are given.[56]

In other words, one falls sick when one can no longer freely devote oneself to one's proper occupations.

Ideal health does not exist in this world. Rather, it is an idea to which one can refer in order to evaluate the state of health of an actual person. No one, for example, can possess all natural functions in an excellent state. Real health has a certain depth, "an appropriate breadth,"[57] and it is in this margin between absolute good health and full-fledged disease that one can place the aesthetic action of the physician. The *Definitiones medicae*, although pseudo-Galenic, offers a good illustration of Galen's way of thinking: "that which is in keeping with nature, is health, while that which is opposed to nature, is illness. But there exist natural things that are neither in keeping with nature nor opposed to nature, such as the fact that one is too thin, or too dry, or too thick, or too fat, or that one has a hooked nose, or grey or blue eyes, or a snub nose."[58]

A state of health can be specified by adding a personal determining factor, the health of X or Y, or by adding a categoric determining factor, such as the state of health of athletes. Paradoxically, at first glance, the latter is a precarious state of health, inasmuch as it is pushed to extremes: the athletic disposition does not exist in nature.[59] True health possesses attributes that make it immediately noticeable: beauty, good constitution, and integrity. The first of these three attributes itself has three attributes: good coloring, good proportions of the limbs, and harmony. In other words, health, beauty, and the faculty of action could not exist one without the other. The treatise *Thrasybulus sive utrum medicinae sit an gymnasticae hygiene* insists on this especially:

> If there is a faculty of action, then there will necessarily be health and beauty as well. In effect, this latter cannot exist without the cause that produces it, and without the beauty that necessarily ensues from it. And so, if one has health, then one will immediately also have the faculty of action and beauty. These two qualities in fact derive therefrom. In the same way, if one were to create beauty, it is absolutely certain that first one would create health; by doing this, one would likewise have created the faculty of action.[60]

Who, in reality, creates, who can create, to what extent can one create, and why should one create? Galen found that "none of those formed for the sake of life itself or for a better life could possibly have been constructed more excellently if they were different from what they actually are."[61] In the body, everything is wonderfully suited to its function, and each set or assembly contributes wonderfully to a broader purpose, that is, the propagation of the species (genital organs of both sexes), the maintenance of life (brain, heart, liver), and the quality of life (eyes, ears, nose, hands). No detail of the body fails to fulfill this teleology, since each and every one of them behaves according to anthropomorphic rules. Galen does not realize that he is in fact describing a free man (and beneath him, woman) of a city of the Greco-Roman world, living in a temperate climate. He fails to distinguish between social and natural. The example of the hairs of the face and head is particularly indicative.

> Well, then, the hair of the beard not only protects the cheeks but also serves to ornament them; for a man seems more stately, especially as he grows older, if he has everywhere a good covering of hair. This is also the reason why Nature has left the so-called cheekbones and the nose smooth and bare of hair; for so [if they were hairy] the whole countenance would become savage and bestial, by no means suitable for a civilized, social animal . . . On the other hand, for woman, the rest of whose body is always soft and hairless like a child's, the bareness of the face would not be inappropriate, and besides, this animal does not have an august character as the male has and so does not need an august form . . . And the female sex does not need any special covering as protection against the cold, since for the most part women stay within doors, yet they do need long hair on their heads for both protection and ornament,

and this need they share with men . . . As regards the eyelashes and eyebrows, however, if you either added or subtracted anything, you would destroy their usefulness. For the former are set like a palisade before the open eyes so that no small bodies may fall into them, and the latter must provide shelter like a wall and be the first to receive all that flows down from the head. If, then, you made them shorter or thinner than they should be, you would to that extent impair their usefulness; for whatever they formerly kept out would be allowed by the eyelashes to fall into the eyes and by the eyebrows to flow into them. But again, if you made them longer or thicker, they would no longer be a palisade and a wall for the eyes, but coverings very like a prison, hiding and darkening the pupils, which ought least of all instruments to be obscured. Has, then, our Creator commanded only these hairs to preserve always the same length, and do the hairs preserve it as they have been ordered either because they fear the injunction of their Lord, or reverence the God who commands it, or themselves believe it better to do so?[62]

And so, how does agreement take place between nature and the providential deity? Matter is not the creation of the deity, and the deity, far from being able to use matter as it pleases, encounters a number of quite specific limitations. Galen's god is good, wise, and provident, but neither omnipotent nor capricious. No divine caprice can modify the natural order, and thus all the more, no caprice of a physician should do so.

We, however, do not feel this to be true, saying rather that some things are naturally impossible and that God does not attempt these at all but chooses from among the possible what is best to be done. Accordingly, when it was better that the length and number of the hairs of the eyelids should be always the same, we do not say that he willed it and straightaway they were made so; for though he willed it times without number, they would never become such as they are if they grew out from soft skin.[63]

Galen did not speculate concerning the limitations of divine power; he noted them and took his inspiration from them, establishing his line of conduct in the matter of aesthetic medicine, when faced with minor deviations, unquestionable failures, or mishaps of life. He made corrections, recognizing what was legitimate, and where it was forbidden to intervene attempting to impose his opinions on a less learned public, a public therefore far more presumptuous. Precisely because there is a certain rationality to nature can the physician understand it and can medicine be a relatively certain science.

In this way, the quite remarkable problem of authentic beauty and the legitimate means with which to restore it should not be considered a secondary problem, because medical aesthetics belongs to a nearly exact science, the science of nature. And this science is the foundation of theology, an "exact theology," according to the felicitous expression of Paul Moraux. Beyond the problems of medical aesthetics, Galen's religious positions barely interfered with his practice and his research. In particular, they imposed absolutely no limitations on his anatomical research.

Anatomophysiology

Galen's anatomy was based on a body of accumulated knowledge, the subtle criticism of prior discoveries, and on dissection, which unfortunately was practiced on animals rather than human cadavers: usually on monkeys, specifically, the monkey that most closely resembles man, the *Macacus rhesus;* or else on pigs, small mammals (especially for the female genitalia), and, occasionally, other animals still, such as the renowned imperial elephant. His great discoveries concerned the bones (bones with or without medullary space, apophyses, epiphyses, diaphyses, brainpan), muscles and tendons (thoracic muscles, Achilles' tendon), nerves (seven pairs of cranial nerves, recurrent nerves, rachidian nerves, cervical nerves), and the nervous system in general (neural ganglions, the sympathetic nervous system).[64]

His physiology, too, was the product of a complex combination of tradition, observations, and discoveries.[65] Galen wished to preserve the old theory of humors handed down from Hippocratic medicine:[66] ideal health implies that the four humors, and thus the related organs, qualities, and elements, are in balance. On the one hand, however, depending on the age of the person and on the seasons, there is a predominance of this or that humor: blood in the spring and in childhood; yellow bile in summer and in youth; black bile in autumn and in adulthood; phlegm in winter and in old age. On the other hand, the relative predominance of a humor, short of reaching a state of pathological imbalance, explains the existence of four temperaments: sanguine, phlegmatic, choleric (or bilious), and melancholic.

Nor was Galen willing to renounce the Platonic heritage, according to which the *pneuma* was the regulating factor of life. More precisely, three types of pneuma interacted: psychic, which governs the brain and the nervous system; vital, or animal, which regulates the functioning of the heart and arteries; and natural, or vegetative, which controls the liver and the kidneys.

To all this, one should add special forces, or faculties *(dynameis)*, responsible for contributing to the major biological functions of digestion, nutrition, and growth, namely, the alterative, attractive, retentive, expulsive, secretive faculties, and others. These faculties are in some sense the concrete appearance assumed by the intervention of the divine in the human body; they are the instruments of divine design.

Experimentation

Despite these teleological ideas, which were to seduce future physicians to such sterile purposes, Galen in reality made observations and performed experiments.[67] His experimental methodology was marked by alternating reliance on experience and reason, which he described as the "two legs" of his method. He claimed the considerable merit of being aware that the subject of medical experimentation is of an incomparable fragility and social importance:

> No one fails to realize that testing is dangerous, because of the subject upon which one exercises the [medical] art. In effect, unlike the other arts, where one can experiment without risk, the materials of medicine are not hides, logs, or bricks; it experiments instead on the human body, upon which there is a certain risk involved in trying the untested; especially because the experiment may lead to the loss of an entire living being. This is why, where the tasks of the art are concerned, such as in the proper preparation of remedies and the judging of what has been written by our predecessors, we must require that things be put to the proof, and hold that this is useful. Indeed, medicine in a sense has two legs, experience [*empeiria*] and reasoning [*logos*].[68]

In *De locis affectis*, Galen recalls that he wrote a book entitled "On the Dissection of Living Animals," and points out that this is preferable to the dissection of humans.

Of particular importance are Galen's ideas concerning the movement of blood, respiration, and the functioning of the nervous system. He had practiced the experimental cutting of the spinal cord at various levels on monkeys and pigs; he repeated the experiment on the muscles, as well, thus observing the effects of a partial destruction of the organism. He also noted that the ligature of a nerve will paralyze a distant muscle; he knew this already from his clinical experience, when a patient of his, who had fallen on his back, suffered the paralysis of a number of fingers on his hand.

By combining clinical method with experimental method, Galen systematically explored the topography of innervation and the mechanisms of respiration and phonation. It is odd that his fundamental book on this research and on the results, the *Adminstrationes anatomicae*, should not have been preserved intact in Greek. Nowadays, we are forced to rely on the Arabic version. When that version was discovered around the middle of the nineteenth century by the Englishman William Alexander Greenhill, it astonished the entire scientific community.[69] Let us also recall that a few years earlier, in 1841, Greenhill's future friend Charles Daremberg had devoted his doctoral thesis in medicine at the University of Paris to an analysis of Galen's knowledge of the anatomy and physiology of the nervous system *(Exposition des connaissances de Galien sur l'anatomie et la physiologie du système nerveux)*, after spending years in a laboratory in the Muséum d'Histoire Naturelle, verifying Galen's declarations.

Likewise, Galen attempted to understand the true nature of the pressure pulse wave, by inserting a solid metal tube into an artery. The experiment, repeated after him, was not conclusive.[70] He further contributed to clearing up the controversial matter of the contents of the arteries (blood or pneuma).[71] According to Galen, there are two types of blood, venous and arterial. Venous blood is constantly being renewed by the contribution of food. From the liver it nourishes the whole of the body—including the lungs, which it reaches through the "arterial vein"—as well as the heart. Arterial blood distributes vital heat, from the heart, or to be more precise, from the left ventricle, where it mixes with the pneuma brought by the "venous artery." Once they reach the periphery, the two types of blood are consumed, hence the need for constant renewal. In other words, the two types of blood run parallel, by virtue of the repulsive faculty of the liver and the heart, and by virtue of the attractive force of the parts of the body that require them. These conclusions of Galen's were pondered carefully by William Harvey when the English scientist began the research that was to lead to the discovery of the circulation of blood.

We should also recall Galen's conclusions concerning the elimination of urine:[72] in his opinion, while solid excrements derive directly from gastrointestinal digestion, the kidneys, by virtue of their attractive faculty, attract the serous components of the blood meant to nourish the kidneys, as well as all the blood processed by the liver, thereupon transforming it into urine. If one measures the quantity of urine eliminated each day—here is an interesting example of quantitative reasoning—it is clear that this waste material derives from the total of all liquids taken in.

Lastly, in the field of therapeutics, Galen did not hesitate to perform experiments on himself: he tested a plant-based remedy for nerve damage;[73] he tested lemnian earth;[74] and he burned himself with thapsia in order to test various possible remedies. His account of this last experiment is worth reading:

> If one is burned by an application of thapsia, vinegar will soften the burning. Anybody that wishes to do so, may learn this from experimentation, as we have done upon ourself, to have a precise test of the potency of the drug. We spread [*thapsia*] on our thighs in different points, and after four or five hours, when they began to burn and to become inflamed, we bathed one point with vinegar, another with water, another still with oil; on a fourth, we spread rose-oil, and other specimens of this or that product that we believed was capable of ameliorating acute pain or to lower a temperature. Vinegar proved to be more active than all of these products.[75]

It is easy to see the difference between Galen's experimentation and spontaneous experience, as described by Pliny the Elder, likewise concerning vinegar:

> Its great efficacy as an antidote for asp bite was unknown to physicians, but recently a man who was bitten by an asp on which he trod while carrying a skin of vinegar felt the wound every time he put the skin down, but at other times it was as though he had never been bitten. He inferred that vinegar was an antidote and was relieved by taking a draught of it.[76]

Things become more complex when dealing with pharmaceutical compounds: reasoning plays an important role in this case, because even complete familiarity with the properties of each of the ingredients of a compound does not necessarily allow one to predict their combined virtues. In most cases, one can form a rough idea of the compound's efficacy, but certainly not of its strength.

Diagnostic Reasoning

It has often been said that the physicians of antiquity never engaged in diagnosis. This statement contains only an element of truth. In fact, what the physician performed at the patient's bedside was called the "prognosis," the observation of those symptoms that, on the one hand, provide information on the past and present course of the disease and, on the other, allow the physician to predict its future development. These signs were then evaluated in relation to their causes. Concerning this fundamental activity,[77] Galen wrote an original book, *De praenotione ad Posthumum*, and three books of commentary on Hippocrates, *In Hippocratis prognosticum commentarii I–III*. He also mentioned it in many works, such as *Ars medica*. One of his chief concerns was distinguishing this effect of the art from that of the diviner:

> Indeed, by high summer I had made many praiseworthy predictions and cures in cases involving leading Romans: my reputation stood high among all, as you know, and great was the name of Galen. But envy grew apace with fame, especially among those who thought they were somebody and were vanquished by me in every aspect of their art. They ran round the city spreading various rumours; one that I had cured this or that man by good luck . . . ; another that my predictions derived from divination, not medical theory.[78]

It is probable that chance or luck played a part in Galen's prognoses; in a certain number of extreme cases, working against the wiles of patients who had their own reasons for wishing to elude the attention of their physician, Galen used all his skill, his "common sense," his culture, his psychological intuition, employing them in a material examination that verged on detective work, while keeping both his patience and his temper. One of the most amusing cases is that of a *pharmacophilos*, a drug addict,

> a wealthy man who took remedies at very short intervals . . . When I realized that his pulse was rising, I ruled out all the other causes that he had hypothesized, and I considered only one last alternative: either that which was happening to him was caused by a warming remedy, or else it was the result of an outbreak of fever . . . I asked him to show me his tongue, I saw that it was colored by a remedy, and once again I tested his pulse still entirely unsuspecting. At that point, I remembered that the previous day I had forbidden

him to take the drug that he wished to drink. And I immediately told him that he had drunk the remedy in question. When, however, he realized that I had based my idea on the fact that his tongue was colored, he again prepared little round pills of that drug, and he swallowed them, making quite sure that his tongue was not thereby stained. But I found out this cunning trick of his . . . I guessed what had happened and I did not hesitate to tell him: "It seems to me that you have taken that drug." At this point, the patient defended himself purely to save face.[79]

Sensory perceptions, as we have seen, played a certain role in scientific discovery; the physician made note of them before taking the fundamental step in his art, which consisted of placing—or deciding not to place—a patient in the category of the sick, and then in time removing him from that category by treating him according to the rules of the art. The most important sense was that of sight, used to evaluate the general appearance of the patient, his behavior in bed (whether he slept or remained awake), the coloring of his face and of the rest of his body, the state of the eyes and nails, the movements of respiration, the appearance of the spit, vomit, and excrement (color, consistency, abundance), the state of the blood in bloodletting. The sense of taste played practically no role (Galen did not taste the urine), while hearing and touch had their importance. The sense of touch was used to evaluate the warmth of the patient—his external warmth, not his internal temperature. Warmth could be determined only by the hand of the physician, which was also used to take the pulse. Galen was exceedingly refined in the field of clinical sphygmology. The Galenic corpus, in fact, includes ten works devoted to this topic. Observation was made of the moisture of the skin and of the mucus; palpation of the hypochondrium was practiced, allowing the physician to form an idea of the state of the liver, as well as palpation of the bladder. Finally, the sense of hearing was used to evaluate the tone of voice, the silences, the moans, and the sounds of respiration, coughing, and winds. The sum of all these sensory data allowed the exercise of judgment and reasoning in attempting to identify the disease and implement treatment.

Spoken words completed the sensory information: the physician would pose questions of the patient and of the people close to him and listen to their responses as well as to the quality of the patient's voice. A veritable dialogue was required for the development of the prognosis, covering the case history and any other details. This approach required a certain intellectual, cultural, and relational level in the patient, and it is striking that Galen had almost no interest in pediatrics of the newborn. His favorite patients, for various reasons, were men of high society, well aware of the problems of health, who attended sessions of anatomical demonstration or philosophical discussion. With these patients he could be sure of an accurate prognosis. The treatment could be implemented at precisely the right moment, the *kairos,* and continue in perfect agreement with a completely prepared patient.[80]

The Heritage of Galen and the End of Antiquity

In his own lifetime, Galen enjoyed remarkable glory in every walk of life, among every class of society, as both a practicing physician and a theoretician, but also as a philosopher.[81] His work covered all the branches of medicine, much of philosophy (which he did not distinguish from religion), and philology, especially his efforts in literary history and textual criticism.

He reached the height of ancient knowledge, for Galen read everything, understood nearly all of what he read, selected from it, analyzed and criticized it, and reorganized it. As a result, he established his work as a source, and increasingly it was felt that this source could just about replace all previous medical literature, with the notable exception of Hippocrates. He set himself up as a model to be followed, right down to the details, revealing his passion for science and truth, his disinterested devotion, his diagnostic cleverness, his own health problems, and the lessons that he drew from them. All of this helped to still any spirit of critical examination in his readers and encouraged the reigning principle of authority and dogmatism. Moreover, since Galen's god was not considered to be incompatible with the Christian God (save perhaps during the third century), medical scholasticism managed to survive—in spite of the discoveries of the Renaissance—right up to the seventeenth century.

Galen's portrait—undoubtedly fanciful—was preserved through the centuries. A poem from the *Greek Anthology* attributed to Magnus served as a legend beneath that portrait: "There was a time, Galen, when, owing to thee, Earth received men mortal and reared them in immortality. The halls of tearful Acheron were bereaved by the force of thy healing hand."[82] He was depicted in medieval manuscripts as well (beginning with that of Anicia Juliana, dating from the early sixth century, preserved in Vienna) and was portrayed talking with Hippocrates, or in the midst of other Greek physicians, or even—with the passage of time—with Arab physicians or physicians of the Latin Middle Ages. His portrait appeared on the frontispiece of first editions in the Renaissance. It was even frescoed, in the company of saints, in churches; notably, in the chapel of the Cistercian monastery in Olimje, in Slovenia. And Galen still walks through the Limbo of Dante's *Divine Comedy:* "Ipocràte, Avicenna e Galïeno,/Averoìs che 'l gran comento feo" ("Hippocrates, Galen, Avicenna, Averroës who discussed/the Philosopher in his great commentary").[83]

After Galen, ancient medicine was no longer creative: it translated, compiled, summarized, and stored scientific and folk knowledge. It became the art of preservation. At some extremely uncertain date, between the second and fourth centuries, Quintus Serenus created an anthology in scholarly form and in verse of the false treasures of folk medicine, in his book *Liber medicinalis.* Oribasius, the physician of Julian the Apostate (fourth century), amassed a similar body in his *Collectiones medicae;* for ease of consultation, it immediately became necessary to break that work into two manuals, the *Synopsis* and the *Euporista,* which became well known chiefly in their Latin translation, in the late fifth or early sixth century (at this time knowledge of Greek was disappearing in the West). These manuals have become a priceless treasure for modern editors of authors whose work has been badly or only partly preserved.

For the same reasons of distribution, Vindicianus (fourth century), a great personage and the proconsul of Africa under Theodosius I, facilitated the spread of methodic ideas, writing a number of simple treatises on human reproduction: *De semine, Gynaecia,* and *De natura generis humani.* Cassius Felix took inspiration from dogmatism in his book *De medicina* (published in A.D. 447). Similarly, Caelius Aurelianus (fifth century) translated and adapted the work of the greatest of all Methodics, Soranos of Ephesus: the vast treatise *De morbis acutis et diuturnis,* of which the original Greek text is lost, and a simplified and practical version of *Gynaecia.* Following that came Mustio's own *Gynaecia,* simpler still. And in his enormous book *De medicamentis liber,* Marcellus Empiricus of Bordeaux (fifth century) amassed everything that he thought might be useful to the populace at large—too often forced to make do without physicians—that they might heal themselves. There were even translations into Latin of Hippocrates and Galen.

Sects after the Sects

After the death of Galen, the disputes among the sects slowly died out; more accurately, the disputes ceased to be a living polemic and became the object of study, based primarily on the reading of and commentary on the treatise *De sectis ad eos qui introducuntur.* In the opinion of Galen himself, this book was a fundamental prerequisite to any serious study of medicine. In effect, it was to remain, in the centuries that followed, a breviary for young students of medicine, in East and West; next in importance was the compendium *Ars medica.* Many commentaries on this work survive, in Greek and in Latin, not to mention the commentaries and translations in eastern languages.

The school of Alexandria, to limit ourselves to the origin and the heart of everything, produced a certain number of ancient commentaries. A major article by Owsei Temkin[84] attests to the existence of a manuscript fragment attributed to Palladius; this fragment has since been published in part, and probably dates from the sixth century. It is quite incomplete; it consists only of an introduction, examining a series of general questions concerning the nature and value of medicine, a list of the three sects, and a breakdown of the medical art into its various component parts; it ends abruptly at the beginning of the commentary proper. A papyrus in Berlin preserves a fragment of an introduction to the treatise *De sectis ad eos qui introducuntur;* it, too, would seem to have been written in the sixth century, by a neo-Platonist. One may well wonder whether it is not an incarnation of the text of John of Alexandria. Lastly, the *Codex Vindobonensis med. 35* contains a number of folios that make reference to the work of Galen; it cannot be dated conclusively, but it is certainly of either direct or indirect Alexandrian origin.

The yield in Latin is also quite rich: the Latin edition of Galen, by Rusticus Placentinus, appeared in Pavia in 1515 and contains a Latin translation of the treatise *De sectis ad eos qui introducuntur,* with an introduction and a detailed commentary, attributed to John of Alexandria, translated directly from the Greek, and conceivably of earlier origin than the supposed author. Dating from the ninth century, a codex in the Biblioteca Ambrosiana contains Latin commentaries on *De sectis ad eos qui introducuntur* and *Ars medica,* as well as on the treatises *De pulsibus ad tirones* and *Ad Glauconem de medendi methodo.* A careful examination shows that this codex is nothing more than a copy of an earlier text, written in Ravenna, probably in the sixth century; this original was a Greek text written in the Alexandrian style; attributed to Agnellus of Ravenna, it is quite close to the text in the Pavia edition.

As for the authentic *Commentaria in librum de sectis Galeni* by John of Alexandria, it is preserved entirely in nine manuscripts containing a Latin translation by Burgundio da Pisa, dating from 1184 or 1185.[85] Without an adequate examination of the problem of his exact identity, the editor placed John of Alexandria between 600 and 642, which is hardly a universally accepted fact. There are good reasons to link his work with the manuscript from Ravenna mentioned above. These abundant commentaries offer a great deal of useful information concerning the teaching of medicine, which was then divided into a highly philosophical, theoretical medicine, the domain of iatrosophists, and a practical medicine, which was to survive in Byzantine medicine.

~ 5 ~

Reception and Tradition: Medicine in the Byzantine and Arab World

GOTTHARD STROHMAIER

During the Third Crusade, the Arab knight Usama ibn Munqid re-counted in his *Memoirs*[1] that the lord of the Frankish fortress of al-Munaytira in northern Lebanon sent a messenger to the narrator's uncle, who lived in the nearby town of Sayzar; the messenger requested that a doctor be sent. That request was fulfilled. The local physician, a Christian Arab named Tabit, set out, returning ten days later. Tabit told a horrible tale. He had been entrusted with two patients: a knight suffering from an abscess on his foot, which Tabit had managed to open with a poultice; and a woman suffering from "desiccation," or drying out, a state that he attempted to balance with a "humid" regimen. Thereafter, a Frankish physician began to interfere, ordering the knight's foot amputated with an axe; the knight soon died. As for the woman, Tabit recounted, the diagnosis of his Frankish colleague was that a demon lived in her head and had fallen in love with her. For this reason, the Frankish physician had ordered her shaved bald. This treatment obtained no positive results; moreover—Tabit pointed out with strong disapproval—the woman had resumed her customary diet, rich in garlic and mustard. As a result, her "desiccation" worsened. In accordance with the diagnosis of the Frankish physician, a cross-shaped incision was made on the woman's head, and the bare cranium was rubbed with salt. In time, too, she died.

The far less aggressive treatment suggested by Tabit was in accordance with Galenic medicine, which held that the mixture of the four elementary qualities of the human body—hot, cold, dry, and moist—could become imbalanced. To restore the necessary equilibrium, it was necessary to introduce into the organism—either with an appropriate diet or with medicaments—the opposite qualities. In the case of the woman, mustard and garlic were absolutely contraindicated: according to Galenic pharmacology, both of these foods were hot and dry to the fourth degree, which is the maximum of the pharmacological scale.[2] One distinctive aspect of this story is that the Arab physician was a Christian but was nonetheless steeped in Islamic culture, and that he viewed the Franks as foreigners and barbarians. The knight Usama ibn Munqid was a learned man; this is shown by the way he—no expert in the medical art—recounts Tabit's diagnosis. He was also willing to note cases in which the Franks had successfully cured the patient, as well as methods of therapy practiced by the Franks that he found reasonable.[3] This well-read knight showed marked intellectual curiosity, the same curiosity—widespread during the golden age of the caliphate of the Abbassids, in the ninth century—that had led to the reception of Galenic medicine and all of the Greek sciences, cultivated in late antiquity. This curiosity was lost with time. Thus, the medicine of Renaissance Europe, with all the new discoveries in the fields of anatomy and physiology, left not a trace in the East, aside from the late reception of Paracelsus in the seventeenth century, through the good offices of Ibn Sallum of Aleppo.[4]

An Imitative Medical Thought

In 1798, after the defeat of Aboukir, the French expeditionary corps under Napoleon's command was entirely cut off from provisions and supplies; the military doctors were forced to seek out local physicians. They found none of any worth. The hospital of Qalawun, formerly renowned, lay in ruins. There remained only a local folk medicine, tinged with superstition. Later, the pioneers of a new nationalism, foremost among them Mohammed 'Ali (who ruled from 1806 to 1849), relied on European physicians to fill the most important positions in the organization of health care. They rejected the local hakim and summoned European experts, who, with their microscopes and their understanding of modern biology, made major discoveries.[5] Promising young Egyptians were sent to study medicine in Europe. Thus ended an era in the history of medicine that had begun more than a thousand years earlier in Egypt, in the famous school of Alexandria. According to the information that has survived, it would seem that here alone, at the end of antiquity, a medicine still based on scientific thinking was taught and practiced. The school of Alexandria had a major influence on medical thought in the surrounding Mediterranean regions. The two chief traditions of Alexandrian derivation were the Byzantine tradition and the Syrian-Arab tradition. The Armenian tradition[6] and the Latin tradition from the Byzantine territory of Ravenna in the sixth century[7] were much less important. But the latter—which blended with the elements of Greek medicine that had survived in Latin culture—provided the foundation of the new reception of Galenism in western Europe, especially after the eleventh century.

In comparison with the golden ages of Greece and Renaissance Europe, this period of the history of medicine does not precisely sparkle with originality. The receptivity that had been so vigorous at first—both in Byzantium and in the Muslim world—lost its sheen over the centuries. An investigation of the causes of this phenomenon, however, makes it every bit as interesting as any of the periods marked by rapid changes in explicatory models or rich in discoveries of lasting importance.

Medicine in Byzantium and that in the Muslim world had a common foundation, partly because they both derived from the school of Alexandria and partly because they developed in similar social settings. Let us begin by examining the shared characteristics and then go on to analyze a few specific aspects of the medical thinking of the Arabo-Islamic world, aspects that allowed this body of medicine to surpass the Byzantine medicine of the same period.

The Influence of Galen in the Late Period of the School of Alexandria

The astonishing posthumous success of Galen began in Alexandria. At Rome, where he had practiced as a physician, done his writing, actively taken part in debates concerning medicine, and attracted attention for his public dissections of animals, Galen had never managed to found a school. He left virtually no trace in Latin literature; by contrast, Hippocrates and the representatives of the schools Galen had sharply opposed were widely quoted and accepted in Latin medical manuals, while their names and opinions were mentioned even by authors with no particular medical expertise. Nevertheless, the physicians of Byzantium and the Islamic Middle Ages formed a single Galenic sect. There was no other medical system to compete with Galenism. Medical thinking of this period amounted to minor corrections and calibrations, simplified summaries, and periodic returns to the original writings of Galen.

One can only guess at the reasons for Galen's becoming the leading medical authority of the school of Alexandria. His writings—which were full of polemic and largely unsystematic—made him a less-than-ideal author for use in teaching. It is not hard to imagine another physician emerging from the empirical sect or the methodic sect and attaining the standing of supreme medical authority. Galen was quite proud of the efficacy of his medical practice, but it could not have been responsible alone for the success of the Galenic system. His diagnostic precision, his mastery of medicaments, and his relatively effective forms of therapy all could be found in the context of other medical schools. The masters of Alexandria, who called themselves iatrosophists, favored Galen because of the theoretical advantages of his doctrine. In effect, Galen simply took the best of each school.

Galen had roundly rejected atomism and had instead seized upon Aristotle's doctrine of the four elements. According to this doctrine, the four fundamental substances—earth, water, air, and fire—generate *homeomeres,* substances that are perfectly homogeneous in their qualitative multiplicity. This is true, for example, of bones, cartilage, muscle fiber, membranes, humors of the eye, and all substances not composed of distinct parts. Galen, who considered this subject of special importance, devoted a treatise to it; only the Arabic translation survives.[8]

A further tie to Aristotle—and hence to Christianity and Islam—was established by Galen's adhesion to teleology. This doctrine linked diversity of substance to diversity of specific functions, which Galen considered a particularly fruitful heuristic function. All this constituted a strong encouragement to pursue anatomic research—which Galen practiced, performing numerous dissections of animals—as well as the physiological speculation that derived from it, speculation that caused him to differ from Aristotle on various points. This was the case with the tripartite functions of the soul, for instance; Galen situated those functions—based on the results of his vivisections—in the brain, the heart, and the liver. (Aristotle believed the heart was the sole site of these functions.) Galen also had ties to the thought of Plato; indeed, he summarized Plato's dialogues in a work of which only fragments survive, in Arabic translation.[9] This eclectic link-age with Aristotle and Plato was surely one of the reasons for Galen's success with the later Alexandrian school—that school's neo-Platonic orientation in time developed into a balanced synthesis, based on the thought of the two principal ancient philosophers.

Galen's vast culture—and his philosophical and astronomical knowledge, evident from his medical writings—surely impressed the iatrosophists of the Alexandrian school. The iatrosophists were in effect far less interested in a mastery of medical practice than they were in the establishment of a theoretical foundation of their art, linking it to all the other sciences. In this context, Galen also played an important role by recommending thorough study of logic and geometry. Johannes Philoponus expressly praised Galen as a great physician who had achieved a complete mastery of natural philosophy.[10] Alongside his theoretical requirements, Galen showed a high consideration of empirical thought and common sense. The materialistic foundation of his doctrine of the soul—which clearly underscored his reliance on somatic conditions and his skepticism toward the problem of immortality—presented difficulties for neo-Platonists, Christians, and Muslims. The most significant aspect of Galen's work, however, was his lack of methodological precision, his attempts to reconcile the results of his anatomical research and clinical observations with his theoretical schemes; this offered a fertile stimulus to further thought and research. Sadly, Galen's doctrine was later to atrophy in the context of scholasticism.

The biographies of the sophists, written by Eunapios in the fourth century, offer a tableau vivant of the movements of pupils and scholars from one center of teaching to another, proving that Alexandria had become the privileged site of medical research.[11] The growing influence of Galen is shown clearly in the *Collectiones medicae* written by Oribasius. Oribasius was a pupil of the Alexandrian master Zeno, as well as the personal physician and interpreter of dreams to the emperor Julian the Apostate. Most of the excerpts found in the *Collectiones medicae* are taken from Galen. In addition, there are others from authors whose work—significantly—has been forgotten by later traditions and is known to us only from Oribasius's citations. Oribasius also wrote, for the rhetorician Eunapios, mentioned above, a short medical synopsis.[12] Aside from the tendency to summarize knowledge in the form of manuals, designed for immediate practical application—a tendency exemplified by *Collectiones medicae*—there was another approach current at Alexandria. This approach placed medical theory above all other considerations. It was said of the iatrosophist Magnus that he was more skillful in theoretical debates than in the actual practice of medicine and that he could prove a patient other physicians believed they had cured was still sick.[13]

To make Galen's writings compatible with the educational purposes of the school of Alexandria, it was necessary to organize and abridge them. This was done in a canon of sixteen texts, to be read in a given sequence. The composition of this canon dated from a late period in the school's history; the canon has survived only in its Arabic version.[14] It is no accident that the first text is the treatise *De sectis ad eos qui introducuntur,* in which Galen attempted to demonstrate the superiority of his eclectic approach over various medical sects. Certainly, it would have been more appropriate to select some other text as the first, had the purpose of this canon been to provide an introduction to medical practice.

Hunayn ibn Ishaq, the great ninth-century translator, was familiar with the Alexandrian method of teaching medicine. According to him, the students gathered every day to read, together, one of the principal works from the Galenic canon. Each student could read the other works by Galen as he pleased; this is probably the reason that only a few Greek manuscripts of those works have survived.[15] The Alexandrian Galenic canon was completed by four treatises from the Hippocratic corpus.[16] Clearly, Hippocrates was completely overshadowed by Galen. This is confirmed by the Byzantine textual tradition of transmitting the writings of Hippocrates only according to the readings that Galen[17] made of them, and by the early disappearance from the Arab tradition of the texts of the Hippocratic corpus translated by Hunayn and his school. The Hippocratic writings that we still possess in Arabic, while presented as autonomous texts, are actually extracts from Galenic commentaries.[18]

Stephen of Alexandria (or Athens) wrote commentaries on two treatises by Hippocrates, *Prognosticon* and *Aphorismi,*[19] which were part of the four texts included in the Alexandrian canon. Stephen lived in Alexandria and in Constantinople, and his writings—save for a treatise on urine[20]—have survived entirely in Greek. Yet there are authors, such as Johannes Philoponus, mentioned above, and Paul of Aegina (who, at the time of the Arab conquest, drew up another systematic manual), who belonged to both branches of medical tradition: Byzantine and Arab. One can say the same thing about the Galenic corpus itself: most of it was handed down through both branches, and only a few relatively short texts have survived only in Greek or only in Arabic.[21]

The Arab-Syrian Reception of Galenic Medicine

Before we examine the features of medical thought shared by Byzantium and the Islamic world, we should briefly consider the conditions under which Galenism was received in the Arab world, a reception that was equal to, if not greater than, the survival of this medical system in the Byzantine world. The Alexandrian school, which died out following the Arab conquest,[22] had adepts as far away as Syria, as is shown, for example, by the exceedingly fruitful activity of Sergius of Reshayna (who died in A.D. 536). He studied in Alexandria and translated into Syriac at least twenty-seven works by Galen; the bulk of them came from the Alexandrian canon.[23] As late as the ninth century, when Hunayn ibn Ishaq left Baghdad to travel to Alexandria, he went by way of Syria, Palestine, and Egypt; in the course of his travels, he gathered many Greek manuscripts of Galen.[24]

In the sixth century, Sergius of Reshayna was a living example of the synthesis of Galenism and Aristotelianism, a synthesis distinctly characteristic of the Alexandrian school. He wrote a work titled "About the Universe, according to Aristotle," and composed a complementary text to the third book of *De diebus decretoriis* by Galen. (In that text, Galen clearly showed a certain affinity for astrological doctrines; he stated that to deny a link between the phases of the moon and the cycles of fevers showed a sophistic subtlety.)[25] This conjunction of Galenic medicine and Aristotelian philosophy, combined with a certain penchant for astrology, was to exert a decisive influence over Arab medicine.

The Christian Syrian physicians who worked in the court of the Abbassids, established after A.D. 756 in Baghdad and Samarra, venerated Galen. With the wealth they had accumulated in the service of the caliph, they were willing to pay dearly for good translations of the Galenic corpus into Syriac. Hunayn ibn Ishaq was able to satisfy their needs. Of Christian Arab descent, he had spent many years of his life in Byzantine territory, in pursuit of his studies, most probably in Constantinople.[26] Hunayn's master, the Christian Syrian physician Yuhanna ibn Masawayh—for whom Hunayn did a number of translations—described Galen as a man "who was assisted by the hand of God, and was solidly versed in wisdom."[27]

The reception of Galen in the Arab world began in the ninth century, at a time when official medicine was still entirely dominated by Syrian physicians. This was probably the result of efforts by nonphysicians, principally high court officials who wished to enrich their libraries with works of Greek medicine, as well as the works of philosophers, astronomers, and mathematicians. The translations of Galen into Arabic, done by Hunayn himself and by his pupils, have largely survived; owing to the decline of Christian culture under Islam, not much survives of the Syriac versions.

The Arabic versions by Hunayn allow us to glimpse his methodological principles. The translation was faithful to the meaning of the original text, though he paraphrased slightly when necessary in order to completely render the meaning in the target language. Arabic translations officially replaced the original texts for the physicians of the centuries that followed. Although the Syriac language was heavily contaminated by its borrowings from Greek, Arab scholars cultivated the purity of their language. Hunayn complied with this tradition; he shunned transliterations and created a new terminology, in conformity with Arabic means of expression. Particularly useful in this connection was the possibility of transforming a verb into a substantive with the use of a *masdar*, the Arabic infinitive. It was thus possible to create abstract concepts: for example, from *rakkaba*, meaning "he composed," it was possible to obtain *tarkib*, or "composition."[28] This terminological groundwork was a major condition encouraging the development of scientific thought in Islamic Arab culture. The procedure followed by Hunayn fit in perfectly with the linguistic principles of Galen, who rejected sophistic subtlety and employed the common usage of Greek.[29] Hunayn transferred these principles to his mother tongue, Arabic.

The passage to Arabic was especially facilitated by the preference among many influential Muslims for an encyclopedic education, in which medicine enjoyed a select standing, along with philosophy, mathematics, and astronomy. "All those who felt strongly about culture" came to Baghdad to attend the courses taught by Hunayn's master of medicine.[30] Their interest was particularly excited by the presence of Christian theologians and philosophers who, with their ready rejoinders and their air of self-assurance, gave the Muslims the feeling that they still had a great deal to learn.[31] These Christian scholars hearkened back to the tradition of the school of Alexandria. Most of them were Peripatetics, more often than not clerics rather than physicians.[32] They had facilitated the Arabic reception of Galen, because his doctrine was close to that of Aristotle; Galenism in Alexandria had undergone a similar consecration.

By virtue of the skill of the translators, the Syriac and Arabic versions successfully replaced the Greek texts, which were inaccessible in their original language. This opened the way for a parallel development of medical thought in the Byzantine and the Islamic worlds. In regions where Islam dominated, intellectual life was quite homogeneous. It should come as no surprise then that Galenic medicine, received in the ninth century in Baghdad, spread in much the same fashion from Cordoba in Spain to Bokhara in central Asia.

Features of Medical Thought Common to Byzantium and Islam

A Broad Public

In both Byzantine and Arab culture, an educated public, much broader than that of antiquity, took interest in medicine. Even the monarchs collected remedies. When the Arab legate Umara ibn Hamza was received by the emperor Constantine V Copronymus (741–775), the emperor took him proudly on a tour of the medicaments in his storehouses.[33] In the Islamic East, the imperial treasury contained the famous *mumia,* a rare pitch that was believed to heal broken bones miraculously.[34] The codification of the *materia medica* in the work of Dioscorides also aroused great interest. The famous Viennese codex of Dioscorides, which dates from the turn of the sixth century, was dedicated to Anicia Juliana, wife of the anti-emperor Olybrius. When—during the reign of the caliph Abd ar-Rahman III (912–961)—it appeared that a political coalition might be feasible between the Byzantine throne and the Omayyads of Spain, in opposition to the Abbassid dynasty of Baghdad, diplomatic gifts were sent to Cordoba; among them were books, and alongside the *History of the Church* by Paulus Orosius was a codex of Dioscorides. To interpret this codex, a commission was formed; with the aid of a Greek monk, the commission revised the ancient Arabic version established in Baghdad with the assistance of Hunayn.[35] The surviving Arabic manuscripts of Dioscorides were illustrated with the same luxury as the codex of Anicia Juliana; this suggests that they were commissioned by personages of great rank. Anna Comnena, daughter and biographer of the Byzantine emperor Alexius (1081–1118), described her father's last illness and the discordant and confused behavior of the physicians. It is clear from this description that she was very familiar with Galen's humoral pathology.[36]

It is significant that the many-faceted scholars who took up medicine never seem to have done so in a superficial manner. This was the case with Avicenna (980–1037), on the one hand, and Michael Psellus (1018–1078), on the other.[37] Literature showed an increasingly evident interest in medical theory and practice. The *Timarion*,[38] an anonymous Byzantine dialogue that imitates the style of Lucian with humor and skill, recounts how the protagonist (Timarion) is conveyed to Hades. Because he has lost all of his yellow bile in the course of an illness, he no longer has the right to live, according to Galen's rules of humoral pathology. A rhetorician and friend of Timarion's demonstrates, before the court of the dead, that the liquid that had been excreted was not the bile necessary to life; Timarion is thus acquitted and allowed to return to the world of the living. It is not clear to what extent the author was actually questioning the validity of the things he ridiculed; in this aspect he was fully at the level of Lucian, his model. In *Arabian Nights,* the current Galenic theories and the anatomical description of the human body are set at a far more modest level.[39] A slave girl, not only beautiful but also extremely well educated and well spoken, is offered for sale to the caliph Harun ar-Rasid. To establish her price, experts in many different subjects query her; the young woman proves as competent in her knowledge of medicine as of all other fields. She answers many exceedingly detailed questions concerning the number and the structure of parts of the body, as well as on dietetics and therapy: pure Galenic doctrine appears, only slightly contaminated by folk beliefs.

Empirical Tendencies and Magical Tendencies

Although the chief concern of medical literature was the systematic organization of the teachings of Galen, there was also a current that could be described as "new empiricism." This tendency derived from medical practice. Galen had zealously supported bloodletting. According to his humoral doctrine, it was possible to restore the equilibrium of the body by evacuating it of the two biles or the phlegm or by taking blood. The movement of blood was considered not a closed circuit but a sort of flow without return; therefore the selection of the spot in which to practice the bleeding was an important one. It was necessary to select that spot in accordance with the supposed location of the disease, so as to take blood precisely from that part of the body, or else to cause more blood to flow there. The development of these ideas in the medical practice of the Byzantines found its expression in the use of new terms to designate the veins tapped in bloodletting: the *basilike* (located on the inside of the arm, between the joint of the elbow and the armpit) and the *kephalike* (along the outer edge of the biceps).[40] The reason that the former vein was called "kingly" is not clear. The second vein was called "cephalic" because the bleeding done in this location served to cure headaches and nosebleeds.[41] The practice of bloodletting spread into Syria as well, as is demonstrated by the adoption of the Greek terms *basilike* and *kephalike* even before the major medical treatises had been translated.[42] An anecdote from *The Laughable Stories* by the Syrian bishop Barhebraeus ridicules the predilection of physicians for bloodletting. A man runs stark naked out of a public bath house. He is chasing a thief, who has stolen his clothing, but a doctor bars his way, advising him to be bled, a sure remedy against excess excitement.[43]

Sphygmology (which, with its exceedingly subtle distinctions among different types of pulses, was a legacy from the pneumatic tradition) had a distinctly empirical nature in the Galenic system. It underwent a refinement in the specialized writings of Byzantine and Arab physicians and took pride of place in the manuals.[44]

Empiricism dominated in the field of uroscopy; in Byzantine and Arab medicine, the examination of urine became a fundamental method of diagnosis.[45] Galen had developed no system in this connection. Patients at this point in history, however, expected that a physician should be able to read everything in their urine. The "Book of Medical Competence," attributed to Ibn Ridwan, warned against "madmen" who tried to test the ability of a physician by presenting colored water or animal urine. In this same book, mention is made of certain physicians who had trusted associates sit in the waiting room and persuade patients to discuss their problems. This stratagem gave physicians enough information to convince patients that they could make practically divinatory readings of urine samples.[46] Yuhanna ibn Masawayh had previously warned against the abuses of uroscopy. He said that a physician should not be ashamed to interview the sick to learn of the problems that afflicted them.[47]

An odd branch of symptomatology was that of prognoses of death based on the observation of cutaneous eruptions. This field is discussed in the pseudo-Hippocratic treatise *Capsula eburnea*, a text common in Alexandria during the fourth or fifth century, according to Karl Sudhoff.[48] The apocryphal character of this work is made abundantly clear from the beginning by the legend of its discovery. When Hippocrates sensed that death was approaching, he supposedly ordered that this treatise be placed in an ivory case and buried along with his body. Caesar himself, or a Byzantine emperor who remains nameless, then supposedly had the ivory case dug up and ordered the publication of the text contained therein. An example of the supposed empirical method can be seen in the thirteenth of the twenty-five rules of *Capsula eburnea:* "If a patient suffering from dysentery presents a black pustule behind the left ear and experiences intense thirst, that patient will die on the twenty-first day." The other rules of prognosis also feature so unlikely a combination of symptoms that the author of this counterfeit could rest assured that there was no danger of their being tested in a real case. The fact that such a blatantly counterfeit text could have enjoyed such widespread popularity—not only in Greek and Arabic, but even in Hebrew and Latin[49]—leaves us mightily perplexed about the level of medieval medicine. Even Avicenna made use of this text in a piece of didactic poetry.[50]

The penetration of deeply magical elements of folk medicine into medical literature is likewise linked to the new empirical approach. The remedies in question may have had a certain effectiveness, if for no other reason than the placebo effect, much like those medications recommended in the context of humoral pathology for their imaginary properties (hot, cold, wet, or dry). Alexander of Thralles, a reasonable practitioner, accepted a number of magical remedies in his pharmacological compendium. Magical prescriptions were also common in Syrian medicine. Thus, 'Ali ibn Rabban Tabari in his "Paradise of Wisdom" advised placing a shard—upon which a magical square and two verses of a psalm had been inscribed—under the foot of a woman in labor to facilitate delivery.[51] This was written during the ninth century, when Galen's works were beginning to be disseminated. Although such methods were far less common in the medical literature of the later period, this change resulted less from a radical rejection than from the growing authority of Galenic medicine. These methods would reappear still later in a new form in Arab medical practice.[52] The theoretical justification was based on a specific technical term: *mugarrabat,* or "tested remedies." This term described remedies that worked, not by a logically determined property, such as cold, heat, moisture, or dryness, but rather "with all of their substance." This process could be seen only in practical application.[53] The concept of *mugarrabat* was linked to that of *hawass,* which designated the "special" sympathetic properties of certain substances, described in "lapidaries" and other magical texts.

Actual experience reinforced superstition; in particular, the mysterious attraction of iron by a magnet was often offered as an analogy. Galen himself used this example in an explanation of the effect that a certain purgative medication had on a humor in the human body.[54] The shocks imparted by an electric ray, and the state of dizziness they caused, were also the subject of great wonder. They were employed as cures for headaches; it was noted as a peculiar fact that the animals used had to be alive. Avicenna spoke of this practice, with reference to Galen.[55] All this led to speculations concerning the mysterious qualities of certain other substances. Not a matter of prescientific thought, these speculations were simply arbitrary extrapolations based on actual observations. It is worth noting that the great scholar al-Biruni, one of the most enlightened minds of the Islamic Middle Ages, firmly rejected the magical effect of stones, enchantments, and all such phenomena, and yet found it necessary to add this caveat:

> I know not what to say about this, because I place no reliance in these arts. All the same, a man once fell victim to poisoning, a man who did not even believe in uncontestable truths, much less the chatter of the public. Well, he told me that a group of Indians were sent to him, for they have a certain repute in this field. They pronounced a number of spells over him, and he had felt a sense of relief, to the point that he actually felt he was cured when they made a number of signs with their hands and with wands.[56]

Another component of this body of magical medicine was the "excremental pharmacopeia," which appears even in the works of physicians otherwise faithful to the doctrine of Galen. In the "Banquet of Physicians," by Ibn Butlan, the author wonders why the feces of the wolf and the excrement of the lizard are useful in treating sore throats and scars; the commentator on this treatise, Ibn Atarudi,[57] comes to the evident conclusion that there are "special" qualities of these remedies, qualities that are as elusive as the force of attraction of a magnet or of amber.[58] The placebo effect was reinforced in these cases by the understandable disgust of the patients. Perhaps we should attribute a similar effect to the use of certain innocuous magical remedies; here, religious scruples created a psychological obstacle the patient was forced to overcome. Alexander of Thralles hints, with prudent allusion, that he would gladly have incorporated still other magical procedures in his book, had the majority of his contemporaries—whom he deemed ignoramuses—not been opposed to the use of these "natural" medications.[59] The distinctions made by the exceedingly influential theologian al-Gazzali (1058–1111) in his "Restoration of the Religious Sciences" show the theoretical foundations of this attitude, at least for the Islamic world.[60] He divided remedies into three groups. The first group included the most obvious remedies, such as water to quench thirst and bread to satisfy hunger. The second group included cold remedies against hot illnesses, as well as all other medications and procedures with properties contrary to those of the illness. This provides yet another demonstration of the degree to which humoral pathology had impregnated the general mentality of Islamic culture. The pious man should eschew the third group of remedies, which included spells and magical cauterization, for the effects of these methods were not clear. Reliance on them was, in the final analysis, nothing more than a sort of idolatry. And yet this demonization might encourage certain desperate patients to make use of the procedures in question. The spread of cauterization in Arab folk medicine is clear evidence that al-Gazzali's urgings were without effect.[61]

The Attitude toward Religion

The attitude adopted by rational Galenic medicine toward the prevailing religion was virtually identical in Byzantium and in the Islamic countries. In both cases, there was a state of peaceful coexistence, all things considered. And the exception proves the rule. One exceedingly significant example is the fate of Gesius of Petra (ca. A.D. 500), the coauthor of the *Summaria Alexandrinorum,* known from a hagiographic account by Sophronius of Jerusalem (who died in 638).[62] Gesius had dared to mock the Christianized ceremony of incubation practiced in the temple of Menuthis (now Aboukir), which had been consecrated to Isis in ancient times. The saints worshiped in that temple had harshly punished Gesius when he himself—suffering from chronic back pain—sought a cure at the sanctuary in question. This account is surely not reliable in historic terms, and we are chiefly interested in it as an indication of the intentions of the writer. We should further note that Stephen of Alexandria, in his *Commentaria in Hippocratis aphorismos,* states that Gesius suffered from a deviation of the spinal column in his old age.[63] In any case, a certain hostility began to appear between religious medicine and rational medicine, a hostility that had been unknown in pagan times. The school of Alexandria seemed like a fortress under siege; it became impossible to defend it any further after it lost the protection of the Byzantine empire, following the Arab conquest in A.D. 642. And yet it did not suffer the fate of the Academy of Athens. It is certainly understandable that, under such conditions, no new and original ideas should develop, and that every effort should be made to preserve tradition.

In Islam, too, only rarely did hostility appear between physicians and the representatives of the dominant religion. In most cases, the individuals under fire were philosophers or astrologers, suspected of attempting to place limits on divine omnipotence. In his "Key of Medicine," Ibn Hindu complacently recounts the tragic case of the Mutazilite theologian al-Iskafi (ninth century); the theologian, suffering from a serious case of diarrhea, had asked his physician to prescribe a medication for the treatment of constipation. He had then taken it, to demonstrate the uselessness of Galenic medicine. The result had been fatal.[64] From time to time, there were indications of a certain resentment against scientific medicine; this resentment arose chiefly because scientific medicine was of foreign origin, and in some ways it is reminiscent of attitudes found in ancient Rome. Thus, Cato the Elder warned against Greek physicians, because they were foreigners, and advised relying on the tested remedies of Roman folk medicine. In the Islamic world, something comparable developed with the foundation of so-called prophetic medicine. Prophetic medicine attempted to assemble all the opinions of Muhammad—authentic or apocryphal—concerning health and sickness. This unsystematic corpus comprised a great deal of the ancient heritage of Arab folk medicine, as well as more than a little Galenic medicine.[65] Prophetic medicine in no way threatened the exercise of rational medicine.

In Islam, as in Christendom, some particularly devout people mistrusted the physician's help and relied wholly on God. This attitude existed among Christian and Muslim ascetics, heirs in this context to Eastern monasticism. A legend recounted by al-Gazzali offers a particularly characteristic portrayal of the state of mind of these devout men.

Moses asked the Lord: "From where do disease and healing come?" The Lord replied: "From Me." Moses asked again: "And the physicians, who creates the physicians?" The Lord replied: "They eat their daily bread and they impart courage to My servants, as they wait for death or healing to come from Me."[66]

Among both Christians and Muslims, only fringe groups looked upon medicine with mistrust, an attitude the fathers of the church and the great Islamic theologians disapproved of—or at any rate condoned only in exceptional cases. Animosity toward rational medicine was limited to a few sectarian communities—as is the case in the modern world—and could therefore pose no serious danger to the medical profession. In the worst case, this attitude might reduce the number of paying customers consulting physicians. The idea prevailed, in the heart of the two great religions, that medications taken from plants or animals, as well as the medical art itself, were gifts of God, and that the faithful should therefore not look upon them with mistrust.[67]

New Developments in Medical Thought in the Islamic World

Medical thought in the Byzantine world had no truly new features,[68] even though original ideas and actions did appear here and there in the countries under Islamic rule. Since Greek knowledge was of foreign origin, it prompted—at least among particularly alert spirits—the determination not to accept everything uncritically, and to subject this knowledge to a thorough critical analysis. The behavior of the caliph al-Ma'mun (813–833)—who was a great advocate of Greek sciences—exemplifies this attitude. He could not resign himself to the fact that the value indicated by Ptolemy for a degree of the earth's latitude—which implied the circumference of the whole planet—was not known for certain, since the conversion of the Greek "stadium" into Arabic units of measurement was not precise. He therefore organized an expedition that proceeded to make new measurements in the Syrian desert, in accordance with the method of Eratosthenes.[69] The debates concerning the theoretical foundations of medicine—which appear from time to time in Arabic literature—occupied a far higher level than those carried on by their Byzantine counterparts. One of these discussions, recounted by the great scholar al-Mas'udi, supposedly took place between the caliph al-Watiq and the physicians of his court, with the participation of the translator Hunayn ibn Ishaq and his master Yuhana ibn Masawayh.[70] With reference to the Galenic text on the medical sects, they spoke of the doctrines of the Empirics, the Methodics, and—finally—Hippocrates and Galen, who alone were considered acceptable. Al-Mas'udi said, in praise of this caliph, that he loved unfettered inquiry *(nazar)* and despised blind respect for authority *(taqlid)*.

Ibn Hindu, cited above as the author of the "Key of Medicine," mentioned in his book the four circumstances that he believed had led to the discovery of different therapeutic methods: fortuitous observation of specific medical properties; experimental trial and error; premonitory dreams; and imitation of animal behavior.[71] He offered as an example the story of an ibis that, with the aid of its long beak, gave itself a seawater enema.[72] His contemporaries thought that dreams were a legitimate source of knowledge. Caliphs often, in announcing decisions, justified them as oneiric revelations. The book of dreams by the Greek author Artemidorus in particular was highly esteemed. In the work of Galen, one could read how, in his youth, he dreamed of opening a vein between his thumb and his index finger in order to relieve his chronic abdominal pains.[73] Then it should hardly come as a surprise that Ibn Ridwan dreamed that Galen recommended he apply a cupping glass to the occiput as a treatment for migraines; Galen had simply forgotten to mention this remedy in his *Ad Glauconem de medendi methodo*.[74] In Ibn Butlan's "Banquet of Physicians," an arrogant banqueter declared that the selection of the spot from which to let blood, determined by analogy or by revelatory dreams, was within the ability of the very mice in the hospital.[75] And Ibn Hindu mocked an idea widely accepted among the common folk, namely, that all of medicine was based on divine revelation. He rightly attributed this belief to the Indians. In his opinion, the progress of medicine was the result of experience accumulated over several generations. As is stated in Hippocrates' first aphorism, the life of a single man is too short to accumulate the experience required for the establishment of the medical art; to found that art, a written tradition is required.[76]

With the passage of time, all the same, the idea prevailed that the Greeks had already discovered everything of importance. Even so critical an author as al-Biruni expressed his regret—in the introduction to his pharmacological work—that Dioscorides had never ventured into central Asia. If he had, all the plants of his country might then have become medicaments.[77] Al-Biruni presupposed that Dioscorides possessed a nearly superhuman perspicacity. According to Ibn Ridwan, medicine had at first been the exclusive possession of the family of Hippocrates; as it spread to the population at large, a deterioration ensued that was finally repaired by Galen, who purified medicine of all the harmful additions that had contaminated it.[78] This view is certainly related to the idea that medicine had roots in a sort of revelation. Arab physicians thus linked their art directly to the myth of Aesculapius, in this way responding to the very religious, who were hostile to medicine.[79] Medicine became a precious good that, much like the revelations of prophets, should be preserved intact in its pristine state.

This belief prompted an unprecedented interest in the history of medicine—to be more precise, an interest in the personalities of the possessors of that tradition and in their moral integrity, considered a sort of guarantee of the reliability of the knowledge handed down. In the context of the Islamic doctrine of tradition—which was a compendium of the deeds and words of the prophet Muhammad—the study of all the "classes" of scholars who, over the centuries and in various lands, had handed down this historical record became accepted as a complementary discipline.[80] The immense history of medicine by Ibn Abi Usaybi'a, which is rightly praised for the wealth and accuracy of the extracts quoted in it, had a particularly significant title: "Sources of Information concerning the Categories of Physicians." Ibn Gulgul gave his text a similar title: "Categories of Physicians and Scholars." In the introduction to a similar work, al-Qifti explicitly states his belief that all science—including medicine—can be traced back to the prophet Idris (corresponding to the biblical figure Enoch).[81]

It is in this context that we should understand the extraordinary interest in the biographies of Hippocrates and Galen, taken as models for the moral behavior of physicians. The apocryphal letters of Hippocrates and the little autobiographical elements that Galen liked to introduce into his writings were major sources. In addition to the other ethical writings of the Hippocratic corpus, the oath was particularly esteemed. A commentary by Galen on the Hippocratic oath, the Greek version of which is lost without a trace, has survived in Arabic.[82] For the first time in history, a state authority used the Hippocratic oath as the basis for swearing future physicians to a code of ethics. The manuals for the *muhtasib*—"guardian of the market"—offer a record of that obligation.[83]

The Hippocratism of Rhazes

The foundation of Islamic medicine in tradition is evident even in the author who can fairly be considered the most independent thinker of the Islamic Middle Ages. Muhammad ibn Zakariya' ar-Razi (865–925),[84] known to the Latin world as Rhazes, felt that all prophets were so many impostors who, with their teachings, had brought only discord to humanity. All the same, this lack of piety did not keep him from becoming the head of the hospitals of Baghdad and Rayy, the town in which he was born (in that time, a major Persian city, just south of modern-day Teheran); nor did his impiety keep him from assembling a sizable group of disciples. It comes as little or no surprise that even within the field of medicine, Rhazes was far less obsequious toward authority than were his contemporaries, not to mention his successors. One of his writings has a title that might as well be considered a program: "Doubts about Galen." Rhazes had a clear understanding of the concept of progress. Convinced that medical research should never rest, he felt obliged to criticize Galen just as Galen had criticized his own masters. The "Book That Contains All," translated under the Latin name of *Continens*, is an immense posthumous compilation of Rhazes' scattered notes; it was the work of Rhazes' pupils. It contains a vast number of clinical observations, partly made by Rhazes himself and partly culled from his encyclopedic knowledge of medical literature.[85] It shows his concern with assembling all possible empirical material and examining it, leaving aside any theoretical speculation. Rhazes, thus, is quite close to the spirit of the Hippocratic corpus, which was incorporated into the Arab tradition only as an appendage to Galenic medicine. In a shorter text, in which Rhazes lists thirty-three clinical cases he observed directly, it is possible to recognize the model of Hippocrates' *Epidemiae* even in the structure and the literary form of the narration.[86] The description of the rheum provoked by roses—an allergy from which his friend, the philosopher and geographer al-Bahli, suffered—reveals the interest that Rhazes devoted to the observation of clinical facts that were hitherto unknown. In this case, after indicating the cause of the sickness and its treatment—based on humoral pathology—Rhazes advised against sniffing roses.[87] His little work "Book of Smallpox and Measles," printed in London in 1766 in the original Arabic version, and later translated and published in a number of European languages, became famous. Rhazes distinguished perfectly between these two diseases; he provided a clear clinical description; he failed however to consider the possibility of contagion. He remained wholly within the context of humoral pathology. The appearance of the disease in young people was attributed to an excess of blood, which supposedly deteriorated, provoking a violent process of putrefaction. The recommended treatment made use of cold substances of all sorts.[88]

The Further Developments of Humoral Pathology

During the years that followed, the principles of humoral pathology—generally accepted and consolidated—were used to explain certain phenomena, such as the euphoric effects of hashish. Physicians focused on the hot and dry properties of the plant; they deduced that it was less danger- ous to consume hashish in areas with a cold and wet climate.[89] Even questionable observations—such as that diamonds were poisonous—were supported by humoralist considerations and by the belief that this stone was cold and dry to the utmost degree. Avicenna stated this in his "Canon of Medicine,"[90] while al-Biruni told of having seen a dog fed a diamond, without noticing the slightest effect.[91]

The debate over the classification of foods—a debate that seems quite pointless to us nowadays—could be quite heated. For example, con- sider the literary debate, studded with personal insults, between Ibn But- lan and Ibn Ridwan, over this question: do chicks have a warmer nature than other young birds?[92] Similarly, 'Abd al-Latif al-Bagdadi (1162– 1231), initially a follower of Avicenna, became his adversary in time: Avicenna advised diabetics against eating quinces—classified as cold and dry—while 'Abd al-Latif recommended them.[93]

The eclectic ninth-century philosopher al-Kindi had the idea of cre- ating a pharmacological scale for compound medications, thus perfecting the Galenic doctrine of the four degrees. This task required exceedingly complex calculations. Galen had renounced the project, declaring it served no useful purpose in terms of medical practice. And, in fact, the Muslim physicians were unable to derive any practical results from it. All the same, the quest for mathematical precision made a considerable impression in certain circles, and even reverberated in the Latin world.[94]

An Arab physician could learn about the influence of environment on the health and on diseases by reading Hippocrates' *De aere, aquis, locis*. He was more likely to read Galen's commentary (the original Greek version of which has been lost) in which the apodictic statements by Hippocrates are reinforced by a narrow application of humoral pathology.[95] Hippocrates derived from the seasons and the type of climate not only the appearance and nature of different diseases, but also the physical constitution of entire populations and even certain traits in their collective characters. These ideas later found fertile ground in a number of Islamic thinkers, who combined them with the doctrine of climatic zones, a doctrine they had also taken from classical antiquity. In their view, civilized life was only possible where the climate is temperate and only attained a complete state in the median zone, the fourth between the pole and the equator. As if by happenstance, this zone corresponded to the territories of Islamic expan- sion westward from the East. Some went so far as to say that the appearance of the various prophets had in some sense been influenced by this favorable median location.[96] The philosopher al-Farabi did not accord human dignity either to the inhabitants of the far north or those of the deep south. The best that he felt could be expected of them was to serve as slaves.[97] Al-Biruni held similar opinions, although he disputed an Indian doctrine which stated that not all humans shared common origins, given the differences in language, customs, and skin color. In clear reference to the title of the Hippocratic treatise *(De aere, aquis, locis)*, al-Biruni argued that it was possible to explain the differences by the diversity of the soil, water, air, and regions. Thus, he was able to remain faithful to the biblical and Koranic doctrine that all humanity descended from a single pair of ancestors.[98]

A special connection was established between the concept of endemic disease—as it is set forth in *De aere, aquis, locis*—and the opinion, attributed to Muhammad, that there was no such thing as contagion. The concept of contagion was well known and had developed from experience in breeding camels, but the prophet had ruled it out, rejecting it as mere superstition. This rejection was deeply rooted in religious tradition.[99] Still, it was important to know whether or not to conquer a town in which a pestilence raged,[100] or whether one should simply consider a pestilence to be a divine scourge from which there was no escape, as had early Christian theologians. Al-Gazzali recalled the demands of charity: fearing infection, people hesitated to help their neighbors. He tried to allay this fear by referring to respected physicians who said that pestilences were caused by miasmas that did not take effect until they had been inhaled for quite some time.[101] When the plague began to spread through the lands bordering the Mediterranean, in 1348, opinions changed. The vizier Ibn al-Hatib, author of a history of Grenada, was no physician, but he had come to the conclusion that contagion was empirically demonstrated, and that Muhammad's statement to the contrary should be considered in allegorical terms.[102] In the earliest period of Arabic reception of Galenic medicine, we find in the work of the translator Qusta ibn Luqa a defense of the theory of contagion. This translator was a Christian and felt no particular allegiance to the statements of Muhammad.[103] Qusta ibn Luqa explained the unseen action of contagion by comparing it to the transmission of certain psychic manifestations, such as yawning, laughing, or the need to urinate. He supposed the existence of a material substrate, similar to a spark, that traveled from one body to another. This substance, called *buhar* ("vapor"), was exhaled by a patient's entire body. A sort of miasma, this substance failed to explain infectious ophthalmia, for example, in which only the eyes were sick. Qusta ibn Luqa was forced to fall back on the idea of a ray emitted by the eye, which—in this case—transmitted the disease through the gaze, a sort of "evil eye." The fact that many people had suffered damage to their vision while watching a solar eclipse seemed to confirm this theory. It was thought that the diminished and almost diseased light of the sun must be the cause.[104] Clearly, theoretical aberrations could result from the integration of empirically obtained information. On the whole, the attitude that was adopted by Arab physicians concerning epidemics differed sharply with the resigned attitude of Byzantine physicians.[105]

The brutal outbreak of epidemics that clashed with the traditional endemic concept of disease was also explained by astrology. The reasoning of the Arab physicians of the Middle Ages went well beyond the thinking of the physicians of antiquity. During a stay in Constantinople in 1054, Ibn Butlan witnessed an epidemic and linked it to the appearance of a supernova in the constellation of Gemini, while Saturn was entering the house of Cancer. He described this phenomenon with the term *al-kawkab al-atari*, an expression we may translate as "meteorological star."[106] Since the celestial spheres were considered to be immutable in Aristotelian cosmology, all phenomena that appeared to contradict this principle were placed in the sublunary sphere of fire. In this connection, we may mention the title of a treatise by al-Biruni, though the treatise, sadly, has been lost: "Refutation of the Opinions Developed by Certain Physicians concerning the Stars That Form in the Air."[107]

Galen had encouraged the penetration of astrological ideas in the field of medicine. While he had rejected the practice of horoscopes ("judiciary astrology"),[108] he had drawn a connection between cycles of fever and lunar phases, stating that an attempt to deny such a connection was sophism, pure and simple.[109]

Islamic physicians believed that the moon, with its rapid course through the sky, governed acute diseases, while the sun, slower to shift its course, governed chronic diseases.[110] It was a commonplace to quote from *De aere, aquis, locis*, to the effect that astronomy had contributed greatly to medicine.[111] This was actually a misreading of the Hippocratic text: it states, in fact, that the heliacal cycles of the fixed stars (last setting before and after the first rising after invisibility due to conjunction with the sun) indicated changes in season, and thus changes in corresponding diseases. Nothing explicit was said about any causal links between the constellations and the human body. Galen and, after him, al-Biruni, both attributed to Hippocrates the belief that the zodiacal position of the sun, marked by heliacal risings and settings, brought about only the change of seasons.[112] A small group of scholars, on the fringes of legitimate medicine, sustained the predominance of astrology over medicine, along with the notion that all medical prescriptions should take the horoscope into account.[113] Not even Ibn Ridwan subscribed to that belief, though he simultaneously practiced—separately—the professions of medicine and astrology. The doctrine whereby different parts of the body were linked to the signs of the zodiac—there was an exceedingly schematic association of the head with Aries, the Ram, and the feet with Pisces, the Fish, at the two extremities of the body—did not develop independently from medical thinking. Rather, it was an offshoot of astrology alone.[114] Later, however, this Arabic conception was to play a major role in Western medicine.

In Arabic medicine, the entire array of environmental factors took first place in the list of what were known as the "necessary" or "non-natural causes." These factors were described in Latin terminology as the *sex res non naturales*. The originator of this doctrine was Galen, even though he never formally propounded it.[115] In this series of causes, first place was occupied by the air that surrounds us; next came food and drink; third came sleeping and waking; fourth was motion and rest; fifth, filling and voiding; and sixth, psychic phenomena. The natural causes, by contrast, were the processes that take place in the interior of the body; these are regulated by nature itself, and it is impossible for man to modify them in any manner. The *sex res non naturales* are necessary for survival, and yet they are not natural, to the extent that they can be in some sense manipulated by humans in order to prevent or treat sickness.

The sixth category is quite interesting, as it is evocative of a psychosomatic approach that is peculiar to Arabic medicine. Galenic medical thought gave virtually no role whatever to the human soul. Galen had in fact openly disputed the view of the Platonists of his time, and had posited that one's state of mind depended on the mixture of the humors of the body. The title of one of his books, *Quod animi mores corporis temperamenta sequantur* (literally, "that the state of the soul reflects the condition of the body"),[116] clearly reflects this opinion. It was echoed in the tenth century by Ishaq ibn 'Imran, physician at the court of an Aghlabite sovereign at Kairouan, in North Africa. In a treatise on melancholy (which survives in Greek as well, thanks to Constantine of Africa),[117] Ishaq ibn 'Imran recognized that an excess of black bile would produce a psychic disposition that led to melancholy. He also admitted the possibility that purely psychic forces might be at play as well, and he further stated that melancholy and intellectual activity tended to stimulate one another. This belief, associated with the astrological concept of the saturnine temperament, was to play a major role during the European Renaissance. Avicenna, however, felt there was nothing good about sadness, save for the fact that it helped one lose weight.[118] Yuhanna ibn Masawayh intentionally reversed the title of the text by Galen and declared that the constitution of the body tended to follow the psychic disposition. It followed that he urged the physician to encourage his patients, even in situations that were serious or uncertain.[119] Physicians were so highly respected in Muslim society that a doctor could confidently offer an optimistic prognosis, without fearing for his reputation should the patient's condition worsen rather than improve.

Psychosomatic treatment featured prominently in anecdotes about renowned physicians.[120] A female slave whose modesty had been severely offended—the doctor had lifted her skirt—regained the use of her paralyzed arm through this psychic shock. In another instance, a patient was suffering from hallucinations and became convinced that he was a cow. He demanded to be slaughtered but was persuaded by the physician (traditionally said to have been Avicenna) that he could not be slaughtered until he had been properly fattened. A proper diet and an improvement in his physical state caused the man to recover from his state of folly. Avicenna is also mentioned in connection with the anecdote about the physician who took the pulse of a lovesick prince and properly diagnosed his condition. This anecdote, which in antiquity had featured Erasistratus, was widely known. According to what Avicenna states in his own book, he may indeed have used this procedure.[121] Galen also made successful use of this procedure in his time.[122] The unanimous opinion of Muslim physicians was that unrequited love constituted a serious sickness.[123]

Manuals, and the Return to the Sources in the East and the West

The modest innovations of medieval Arabic thought had only the slightest influence on Western medicine. The reception of Arabic medicine, which began at the end of the eleventh century with the Latin translations by Constantine of Africa, marked a revival of intellectual activity in western Europe, a revival that corresponded to growing economic development and increasing military might. On the one hand, the Crusades—despite their ultimate failure—were a remarkable military and logistical performance. On the other, the episode recounted by Usama ibn Munqid, cited at the beginning of this chapter, illustrates the level of barbarism found in European culture, and in particular in the medicine of that period. Thus, the medical school of Salerno—renowned throughout Europe; Constantine of Africa worked here—sought access to only the most common medical literature, that familiar to ordinary practitioners in Arab lands. The spread of Arabic medicine was facilitated by the fact that the literature that existed in translation was essentially restricted to the work of Galen. It was therefore compatible, on the one hand, with the remains of the medical culture of antiquity that survived in Latin, and, on the other hand, with the new translation of the work of Nemesius of Emesa, done by Alphanus, one of the patrons of Constantine of Africa.

The most important translation done by Constantine of Africa, published under his own name, with the pseudo-Greek title *Pantegni,* was the "Complete Exposition of the Medical Art," by 'Ali ibn al-'Abbas al-Magusi, the personal physician of the Buwayhid emir 'Adud ad-Dawla (949–983). In his introduction the author lists all of the attempts, prior to his undertaking, at composing an exhaustive account of medicine. He criticizes the shortcomings of these previous attempts, thus highlighting the merits of his own work.[124] Success proved him right. The Jewish physician Ibn Gumay' (who died in 1198) wrote a work entitled *Treatise to Salah ad-Din on the Revival of the Art of Medicine.* In it, he mentions the great popularity of the manual by 'Ali ibn al-'Abbas as a demonstration of the decline of medicine and exhorts his readers to study the original works of Galen.[125] For European physicians, however, so systematic a body of work offered considerable advantages, both as a reference work and as a scholastic manual. Much the same thing happened with Avicenna's celebrated "Canon"; translated a century later in Toledo by Gerard of Cremona, it supplanted the manual of 'Ali ibn al-'Abbas. These two manuals had an influence on Western medicine that would be impossible to overstate. Like nearly all medical literature translated from Arabic into Latin, the two great manuals were inspired by the philosophy of Aristotle—especially the doctrine of the four elements; but they also insisted on the importance of an exact knowledge of the interior of the human body. These scientific requirements allowed the integration of medicine into the nascent university structure, in contrast with what happened to many other arts, such as architecture, alchemy, and agriculture. Galen had hearkened back to the ancient school of Alexandria, and had opposed the empirical and methodic sects, by maintaining that anatomical investigation should be one of the foundations of medicine, even though he himself had been forced to limit his work to comparative animal anatomy. In Islamic culture, the idea of dissection was not acceptable. It is noteworthy, all the same, that only half of Galen's manual of dissection should have survived in Greek, while the version in Arabic has survived virtually intact.[126] The teacher of Hunayn, Yuhanna ibn Masawayh, known as an eccentric, had once dissected an ape and had declared that he would have done the same to his son—a weak-spirited boy—if he had not been afraid of being punished by the caliph.[127] Chance assisted 'Abd al-Latif al-Bagdadi; in 1200–1201, near Cairo, he happened upon an enormous pile of human skeletons and established that the mandible and the sacrum were not made up of two and six bones, as Galen had claimed. 'Abd al-Latif al-Bagdadi felt that he did not dare put his objections to Galen in writing before examining more than two thousand skeletons and having his friends confirm his findings with their own independent observations.

As a general rule, anatomical knowledge remained at a fairly bookish level. But the manuals that spoke about anatomy in some detail kept interest in the subject alive. Julius Hirschberg and Julius Lippert have shown—concerning the anatomy of the eye in the work of Avicenna[128]—to what degree his information was taken from Galen, right down to the tiniest details. 'Abd al-Latif thus underscored his own daring: "Everyone agrees that the maxilla is formed of two bones, solidly joined. When I say, 'everyone,' I mean by that Galen himself, for he personally performed the dissection." It is particularly noteworthy that 'Abd al-Latif set forth his criticisms of Galen not in a medical treatise but rather in a description of Egypt;[129] his fellow physicians paid no attention whatsoever to his discoveries.

The case of Ibn an-Nafis (who died in 1288) is controversial. He may have been the first to postulate the passage of blood through the lungs. Galen had already taken this possibility under consideration. When he observed, however, that the vena cava and the pulmonary artery had a different diameter, he came to the conclusion that at least part of the blood passed from the right ventricle to the left ventricle through invisible pores in the interventricular septum. Galen himself stated explicitly that the interventricular septum is compact and impermeable in appearance. Ibn an-Nafis required no anatomical investigations of human or animal cadavers, even though it is logical to think that he could easily have examined the heart of an animal at the slaughterhouse. In the introduction to the section concerning this topic, in his commentary on Avicenna's "Canon,"

Ibn an-Nafis is careful to state that religious law and his innate love of his neighbor prevented him from performing dissections himself.[130] P. Catahier believes, nonetheless, that the author was simply covering his back with precautionary rhetoric, because many of the details in Ibn an-Nafis's anatomical descriptions go well beyond Galen's text. Ibn an-Nafis thus supposedly performed his own anatomical research.[131] The matter has not yet been settled. It is worth pointing out that Ibn an-Nafis was not only a physician, but also a pious theologian, who must certainly have felt strongly bound by religious precepts. He demonstrates that clearly in a short literary work, whose publisher titled it, quite aptly, "The Self-Taught Theologian."[132] The book tells the story of a man who grew up all alone on an island; through pure thought, he developed a respectable body of rational knowledge and familiarity with the Islamic religion. The author clearly shows a bent for speculation in this work. It is likely that Michael Servetus, renowned for his mention of pulmonary circulation (published in a philosophical work), was at least indirectly familiar with the opinion of Ibn an-Nafis.

Orthodox Peripatetics were the source of most of the criticism of Galen; they felt obliged to combat Galen's corrections of Aristotelian biology and psychology. A period that was so deferent toward authority simply could not accept disagreements between these two revered masters. It occurred to no one that both might be wrong. Yuhanna ibn Masawayh stated naively in his "Medical Aphorisms": "When Galen and Aristotle agree upon something, it is true; when they are in disagreement, it is exceedingly difficult for the mind to determine the truth of the matter."[133] There was a danger that this synthesis of medicine with philosophy (and hence with logic and the natural sciences, inasmuch as they were part of philosophy)—a programmatic synthesis, developed by Galen—might once again collapse. This synthesis had secured the inclusion of Galenic medicine into the course of study of the school of Alexandria, and— later—its integration in European universities. In the Arab tradition, the synthesis was at risk. It was not until Avicenna that a final judgment was reached.

The Compromise of al-Farabi and the Synthesis of Avicenna

Avicenna's doctrine is so closely tied on numerous points to that of the philosopher al-Farabi (who died in 950) that, at the time, it was common to refer jokingly to the "two al-Farabis." Al-Farabi attempted to resolve the contradictions between medicine and philosophy with a generalized attack on the philosophical ambitions of doctors, an attack aimed at Galen in particular. We should note that Galen's numerous philosophical writings have been better preserved in Arabic than in Greek. In his criticism of Galen's thinking, al-Farabi refers to an ancient author who, in the Arabic tradition and in Galen's own writings, had the name of Alexander of Damascus. It is now thought—though there is still some doubt—that this was the renowned Alexander of Aphrodisias.

One highly controversial point had to do with the role of the brain. Aristotle considered the brain an organ that served in the cooling of the blood; he believed the seat of consciousness lay in the left ventricle of the heart. Galen observed the phenomena of paralysis that ensued from his experiments in vivisection; he recognized the real functions of the brain and the nerves that originate in the brain. Thus, he returned to the opinion of Plato, who felt that the rational soul was located in the brain, the irascible soul in the heart, and the concupiscent soul in the liver.[134] In the Alexandrian school, as is evident from Stephen of Alexandria's commentary on the *Prognosticon*, there was no clear determination as to which of the two was right on this point.[135] Al-Farabi attempted to show that Aristotle was right on all points by undercutting—with subtle and logical reasoning—the conclusions that Galen had reached empirically through his observations in the dissection of nerves.[136]

Al-Farabi opposed the theoretical ambitions of medicine; instead he placed it with farming, joinery, and cooking, as a practical art. According to him, all these arts concerned changes in the physical world, while the true vocation of man and his real happiness derived from pure rational knowledge. Not even al-Farabi could deny that the practice of medicine requires knowledge of the organs of the human body, and that the determination of sickness and of health shared certain points of interest with the natural sciences. He solved the problem by dividing medicine into seven parts. The first part, common to medicine and the natural sciences, was the knowledge of the organs of the body. The second and third parts concerned the state of health and the different diseases of each organ, or of the body as a whole. These parts were also common to medicine and to the natural sciences, though each pursued through them different goals. By contrast, the last four parts—symptomatology, the knowledge of foods and medicaments, hygiene and dietetics, and therapeutics—pertained solely to medicine.[137] Al-Farabi wished to demonstrate that physicians, who must concentrate on their practical tasks, are not competent to formulate judgments of a purely theoretical nature, concerning the functions of the body's organs, for instance. This scholar attempted to create a general system of the sciences, whereby each discipline was organized in the context of a hierarchical structure. The fact that his writings were even translated into Latin, with the titles *De scientiis* and *De ortu scientiarum,* demonstrates that his efforts were to some degree crowned with success. Remaining consistent with his beliefs, he left medicine out of his catalog of the sciences.[138] He also reproached Galen for having neglected the use of hypothetical syllogisms in his logic; these logical tools would have been particularly appropriate in clinical practice, where certain details always escape the physician. Galen, al-Farabi continued, had tried to construct a body of medicine based on a mathematical ideal, and therefore in accordance with a rigorous logic, in the certainty that what was still unknown would sooner or later be discovered.

The rivalry between medicine and philosophy is particularly clear in a dispute that took place around 1037–38 in Bassora. An unidentified philosopher set forth the thesis that the passion of love was not a sickness, and that emotions were not within the field of expertise of a physician. The physician Abu Sa'id ibn Bahtisu' (who died in 1058) replied with a polemic, in the text of which he stated that a sickness can begin in the soul or in the body, and can then spread from one to the other. Physicians, inasmuch as they are "true philosophers," could intervene effectively in either case. All the same, this stance did not constitute, as the modern editor of this text seems to believe, a declaration of war on the part of medicine against the domination of philosophy, since there is no questioning of the natural foundations of humoral pathology. The author simply expressed his opposition to an extreme neo-Platonic position that rejected any and all ties between the soul and the body.[139]

There did exist an eminently practical body of medicine, distant from all philosophical theorizing; it was chiefly to be found in numerous books of medical prescriptions. These works, often described as *aqrabadin,* listed the medicaments recommended for each part of the body, from head to foot, and described how to prepare them. According to what al-Farabi said, this body of medicine never managed to go beyond the culinary arts. Ibn Ridwan condemned this primitive form of medicine and compared it—in disregard of the facts—to the teachings of the Methodics, previously refuted by Galen.[140] All the same, it was Avicenna who made the decisive step. Much like al-Farabi, he considered himself a philosopher; it was his habit to speak with mistrust of physicians and their master, Galen.

He made no exceptions, not even for the renowned Rhazes. In connection with Rhazes' creation theory, heavily influenced by mythology and highly unusual, Avicenna pointed out that Rhazes would have done better to stick to observing bottles of urine and excising wounds.[141] The precocious *enfant prodige* of Bokhara studied medicine, as well. According to his autobiography, Avicenna did not consider medicine a difficult science.[142] After being banished from his own hometown, he found refuge in the courts of numerous Persian princes, both as a physician and as a minister. He had assembled a number of pupils around him, and they assured that his ideas and his vast body of writings were widely known for many years. His medical writings had the same importance as his philosophical writings, especially his "Canon of Medicine." In the East this work was held in unrivaled esteem till modern times. For a number of decades (at the end of the fifteenth century and the turn of the sixteenth) the Latin translation was the most widely printed book after the Bible.

When it came to reconciling the works of Galen and Aristotle, Avicenna decided in favor of the latter, whenever possible. He did not hesitate, for example, to state that the heart had three ventricles, an opinion that had been roundly refuted in Galen's anatomical observations.[143] Avicenna was reluctant to depose the heart from its position of supremacy, though he did make an effort to take into account Galen's work by stating that the heart delegates certain functions to other organs, especially the brain. A physician might well believe that impulses causing movement and sensory perceptions originated in the brain.[144] A treatise on "cardiac remedies" examined a range of medicaments, among them several we would classify today as neuroleptics.[145] Avicenna felt he could ignore the medical authorities in his anatomical description of the human body; instead he relied on methods that deserve the name of speculative anatomy. Although he never performed dissections, he went so far as to describe different anatomical structures based on their supposed functions. In this manner, he determined that there were three differentiated conduits in the penis: one for the sperm, one for the urine, and one for the secretion of lubricants.[146] Galen, in open disagreement with Aristotle, had postulated the existence of a female seed, endowed with formative properties. Avicenna instead reduced the female contribution to generation; all the same, he maintained certain new ideas of Galen's.[147] His theory of embryonic development was speculative in nature.

Galen was at first uncertain about the order in which the three principal organs were formed; in the end he concluded that the liver is formed first, followed by the heart and then the brain. He thus hearkened back to the threefold hierarchic partition of the heart that had first been formulated by Plato.[148] Avicenna abandoned his Peripatetic convictions and accepted the prior formation of the heart. Although he took a number of anatomical details from Galen, he denounced Galen as an "inopportune gossip" *(fuuli)*.[149] Avicenna's theory of the three embryonic bladders[150] became a commonly accepted dogma. So widely accepted was it that Ibn Tufayl, a friend and teacher of Averroës, wrote a philosophical novel, *Hayy ibn Yaqzan,* in which the hero of that name—born not of mother and father, but of fermenting mud—was formed in accordance with the canonical sequence of embryonic bladders.[151]

In his fusion of philosophy and medicine, Avicenna prevented either of the two disciplines from pursuing its search for truth independently of the other. In Muslim Spain, Averroës returned quite resolutely to the standpoint of al-Farabi and rejected yet more sharply the new ideas of Galen.[152]

Scholastic philosophy considered Avicenna to be the true interpreter of Aristotle, despite certain neo-Platonic tendencies that had been noted. In the matter of individual immortality, Avicenna's philosophy had none of the heretical connotations found in the work of Averroës. Avicenna's "Canon" was accepted enthusiastically, and even such nonphysicians as Albertus Magnus took to quoting him in connection with matters of natural philosophy. Over time, however, the excessively systematic and polished presentation of Avicenna's work led scholars back to the source, which is to say, to the original text of Galen. An independent thinker like Arnald of Villanova (who died in 1311), knowing both Greek and Arabic as he did, was capable of grasping the breadth of Avicenna's and Averroës's debt to Galen. Arnald came down clearly in favor of Greek medicine.[153] The return to the original Galenic text, even with its verbosity and its sometimes pathetic efforts to reconcile the assumptions of theory with clinical and anatomical knowledge, was a fecund move. The Galenic text was more stimulating than Avicenna's firm and complacent presentation. This return to Galen led to a renewal of the appeal that Ibn Ridwan and Ibn Gumay' had launched among their Arab colleagues and resulted in the salvaging of a fundamental portion of medical thought. In Europe, attention focused on the original Greek texts of Galen's work preserved in Byzantine libraries. There was no fundamental difference between Galen's work and the medical literature translated out of the Arabic. The chief claim to credit of Byzantine science—which had developed even fewer new ideas than Arabic science—was that it had preserved the original Galenic texts.

～ 6 ～

Charity and Aid in Medieval Christian Civilization

JOLE AGRIMI AND CHIARA CRISCIANI

Caritas and *infirmitas* are two concepts and values central to Christian spirituality. The relationship that evolved between them at various levels (doctrinal, religious, social) gave origin, during the course of the Middle Ages, to specific forms of behavior, both in the individual Christian and in the charitable institutions fundamental to the structure of society as a whole. The new value and concept of charity, in its varied and manifold accepted meanings, as expressed in the Gospels and as it was developed in patrology, marked the most evident watershed between the belief system of the *philanthropia* of late antiquity and the charitable precepts of Judaism, on the one hand, and the new Christian tradition, on the other.

The Meaning and Value of Christian *Caritas*

Numerous terms—*dilectio, misericordia, pietas*—while not truly synonymous with *caritas*, overlap with the semantic content of the word, clarifying various of the word's characteristics on diverse levels. We should also note the broad polysemy, or diversity of meanings, of the word *caritas* itself. *Caritas* can be used to mean—to cite only two extreme cases—the nature of the living God (*Deus caritas est:* 1 John) or a place of charitable intent *(domus caritatis);* or, less loftily, it can simply mean "charity," as a synonym for almsgiving. In this fluidity of terminology, however, *caritas* essentially signifies the bond[1] of love that—simultaneously and reciprocally—establishes a paternal link between God and humans, and hence a bond of brotherhood among all mankind. The novelty of these concepts introduced by Christ, when compared to the precepts of Mosaic law (as John and Paul emphasized particularly), lies in the reciprocity of the relationship (our love for God and God's love for mankind); it further lies in the familiarity and intimacy of the affection evoked—at once paternal, filial, fraternal—which implies closer and more reliable relationships than those that prevail between a creature and its Creator and Lord. Another innovation is the universal and, at the same time, personal nature of the bond. God's love makes us all his children and makes all humans our brothers. Yet each individual is a child and brother in his own individual personhood. Finally, the last innovation involves the reciprocal conditions that attach to the bonds established by charity: only by loving others do we love God; if we love God, we cannot fail to love our brothers.

Charity is unanimously considered to be the "queen" of virtues. In particular, it rules the theological virtues (faith and hope are the others). Charity is the unifying foundation, roof, and bond of those virtues. Above all, charity gives them life and directs them toward their true purpose. Without charity, they are worthless (Paul). Charity represents the proper path toward perfection for all Christians. There are degrees of charity, and it must attain realization in works and behavior ("Inasmuch as ye have done it unto one of the least of these my brethren, ye have done it unto me": Matthew 25:40). Lastly, charity extinguishes sin, the sin that marks the earthly voyage of man, the *viator* (wayfarer).

It is in the collective dimension, in the community sphere, in the acts of giving and in good works—that charity and justice come together; in this sphere there is more properly an exercise of mercy than of charity, and it is here that questions arise about which works can best achieve the imperatives of charity. The issue of identifying the proper recipients of charitable works also arises. And one wonders whether there are certain agents better suited than others for overseeing the distribution of "gifts."[2] All these questions are linked to the "works of mercy." The Gospels had already given some specific indications.[3] The first of the two mnemotechnical verses—"Visito, poto, cibo, redimo, tego, colligo, condo,/Consule, carpe, doce, solare, remitte, fer, ora"—offers a summary of merciful works that involve physical actions of assistance toward the body, following the indications of Matthew 25: visit the sick, give drink to the thirsty, feed the hungry, take care of the imprisoned, clothe the naked, take in strangers and pilgrims, and bury the dead. The second verse lists the acts of succor toward the soul, accomplished through spiritual actions, primarily through communication (counsel, teach, console, and pray).

The particular attention paid to matters of classification by scholasticism resulted in the seven works of mercy being listed with other groups of seven (the seven virtues, the seven deadly sins, the gifts of the Holy Ghost, the petitions of the Lord's Prayer, and so on). On the one hand, this understanding of mercy helped keep open the life-giving relationship between spiritual development and the doctrinal speculation of masters of theology, between the pastoral directives proposed in the synodal texts to the parish priests and the exhortations of those parish priests to the simple faithful. On the other hand, the systematic organization of the acts of mercy was one of the forms into which the spirituality and the religious generosity of laymen was channeled between the twelfth and thirteenth centuries. Married couples who worked in the temporal sphere found in this system rules to be followed, suited to their married status, indicating the path toward salvation. This path might be more sharply marked by the values of the here-and-now, with "works" viewed in their concrete form of charity, but the various steps could also be linked to the values of the afterlife, in accordance with an ascending path of the soul and the acquisition of beatitudes. Sermons delivered on these subjects in the thirteenth century by the Dominican Humbert de Romans and the Franciscan Gilbert de Tournai—especially those preached to the sick, lepers, and assistant nurses—clearly expressed this twofold form of spiritual perfection that the seven merciful works offered to the layman.

In the correlation between *caritas* and merciful works, between charity and aid,[4] we are able to glimpse with particular clarity the "paradoxes of charity."[5] First of all, it is clear that an imperative of charity, affecting the personal salvation of individual Christians, is integrated into the collective institutional structures of the church. The church, a practically inevitable link between the benefactor and the great number of the needy, acts as a mediator in the evaluation and distribution of the impulses toward charity and aid. Furthermore, whoever helps the needy must do so in a disinterested manner. Only—and precisely—because an act is disinterested will it be "recompensed," will it be "weighed in the scales" on Judgment Day. If there is any "interest" prompting a benefactor, that must be a spiritual interest.

The *Infirmus* in Christian Society

What role is played by the *infirmus* in terms of salvation—his own and that of others? How can we characterize, in ideological and social terms, the specific suffering of the sick? Between charity and aid, between suffering of the body and health of the soul, what space is recognized for the particular relief that medicine and its operators can offer, and on what conditions?

In relation to these questions, we find a "long-term" approach over the course of the high Middle Ages. The terrain covered by the term *infirmitas* appears to be quite broad and has no sharp boundaries. The very concept appears to be undifferentiated. By this we mean that, according to a great number of texts, there was no sharp distinction among the poor, the sick, and the pilgrim, and that there was no specific attention to individual diseases or specific pathological entities. In social terms, *infirmitas* had a negative connotation, as weakness, inability to work, lack of status and dignity, and state of dependency. Fluid though the boundaries may be between the condition of the healthy and that of the *infirmi*, the *egroti*, and the *languentes*, those boundaries are also suddenly and incomprehensibly easy to cross. (All that is necessary, in fact, is a famine, a flood, or an epidemic to make the boundaries uncertain in so precarious a society and ecosystem.) The presence of the sick in the social spaces of the community—squares and markets, churches and ceremonies, roads and pilgrimages—appears common, everyday, and obsessive. In these spaces the *pauperes infirmi* mingle with the healthy, in no way isolated from the rest or subjected to specific therapy. There are, in other words, no places specifically set aside for the ill as such, in which they can be properly treated with purely medical techniques. In this context, *infirmitas*—in which the most evident factor is the overlapping identity between sickness and poverty—and more specifically disease and physical weakness are perceived and presented in material reality and in the collective imagination not as an occasional and momentary imbalance with respect to the natural state of health, but rather as the normal state of affairs, that is, as the natural condition of man after the Fall. Disease, in fact, is one of the *tria mala* that entered nature and history with Adam and through his sin.

In its manifestations and in its various aspects, disease was made the subject of a radical religious set of values that remains, nonetheless, profoundly ambivalent. The *pauper egrotus* is not the incarnation of a body of symptoms, arrayed by a neutral and scientific observer, but, first and foremost, the incarnation of religious admonitions. He, the invalid, becomes, therefore, the subject of a pedagogy of suffering and charity, which is as much—or even more—about the healthy people who surround him as it is about him. The sick person thus becomes at once an outcast and a chosen individual. He is the image of the sin that caused his disease, but he is also the remedy and the physician, and therefore admirable in that he is a living example of direct, blinding divine justice, which strikes in him flaws of which not even he is aware.[6]

The invalid is odious, in that he incarnates and displays sin, at the same time provoking salutary reflection and repugnance; but he is also the object of our love, for he reproduces and multiplies endlessly the image of Christ's suffering, a wandering and needy pilgrim. It is therefore necessary to turn toward him with pity and charity. The invalid reveals to us, in the suffering of his flesh, his resemblance to Christ, who donned on our behalf the "abominable clothing of the body." This same invalid manifests the stern justice of God the Father, who, though stern, is nonetheless merciful, for He corrects even more harshly with the "flagella" of disease the one He loves most. As if He were squaring a block of rough stone, He hacks away at the body of the invalid in order to strengthen his soul against temptation and sin. This message, particularly insistent in the *admonitiones ad egros* of Pope Gregory I, the Great, can be found also in numerous patristic and monastic texts concerning *patientia*,[7] the virtue par excellence of the poor and especially of the sick. And the invalid can only harvest the spiritual fruit of his physical suffering by supporting them in silence—*tacitus*, just as Christ was, and Job before Him—while remaining aware of the great privilege bestowed upon him by God in the form of spiritual correction or therapy.

From these brief indications, it becomes clear that the perception of disease was ambivalent. Its position between body and soul was also ambiguous, divided between the sign and the meaning: disease manifested at the level of the body the defects of the soul. The assignment of religious value to *infirmitas* gave a certain ambivalence to terms that have for us only a single meaning, such as disease, therapy, and healing. Given the absolute priority of the *salus animae*, a Christian had to beg God to correct or cure him with disease and regret not being afflicted with sickness more often. He had to recognize the degree to which the "salus cordis sit molestia corporalis" (Gregory the Great). The transformation of the *infirmitas* (of the body) into *salus* (of the soul) and of *sanitas* into mere opportunities to sin were frequently mentioned, especially up to the twelfth century. Nevertheless, disease was also a spiritual medication for those in good health, who comforted the suffering invalid with acts of mercy and material assistance, acts destined not only to promote the recovery and health of the invalid but also to further the spiritual well-being of the healthy person who performed them. The *pauper egrotus,* then, need not be socially isolated, for he was, in both the spiritual community and in the economy of salvation, the chief instrument of the restoration of sinners in good health. The role of the invalid was one of assisting in redemption. The invalid at the same time was himself a penitent and offered an opportunity to perform penitence, to accomplish acts of charity that heal others. From this point of view, the true "physicians" were the sick, the deformed, the diseased beggars who cried for alms.

Since *infirmitas* remained undifferentiated, and as long as the first purpose of assistance was not the bodily health of the person being assisted but the salvation of the soul of the person providing the assistance, throughout the Middle Ages there developed a charity that was as completely devoid of discrimination as the *infirmitas* was undifferentiated. There were consequently no specific forms or sites of assistance, according to whether it was a poor person, an old person, an orphan, or an invalid being helped; a pilgrim who fell sick and an invalid making a pilgrimage from sanctuary to sanctuary were treated in the same manner. There was no specific aid to be given for certain diseases or infirmities, nor were there precise distinctions as to who might have a greater "right" to help than others. There were likewise no distinctions among those who were to offer that help. All Christians, even the most miserable, had a duty—short of being able to heal—to imitate Christ in His acts of mercy, which the Gospels portray as being entirely unencumbered, dictated wholly by compassionate charity.

In more general terms, Christ was the tip of the pyramid used to portray the religious conception of *infirmitas* and *caritas.* He was the symbolic unity in which the ambivalence and conflict that characterize the perception of disease, therapy, and recovery found coherence. Christ, in fact, was the "physician" in the most complete sense of the term, not only because of His miracle cures, but also because He brought true salvation to humanity, made infirm by sin. Christ, moreover, was a medicament ("ipse et medicum et medicamentum"),[8] because He was used to heal the wounds of people's sins. Through his incarnation, Christ took onto himself the *infirmitas corporis.* Christ teaches humanity, then, that the body can be used to attain salvation; He also shows the invalid the value of suffering and silent patience as medicines for the soul; and He teaches us patience and charity, entrusting us all with the means for the redemption of the flesh as well.

Of course, one can detect a number of significant variations in this amalgam of different symbols. Thus, during the high Middle Ages, Christ was first and foremost the model for the acceptance of suffering; after the twelfth century, there was a greater emphasis on the human aspect of Christ, suffering the torments of the flesh, and particularly on His compassion and loving care for the poor and the sick.

The Ambiguous Status of Profane Medicine

This aspiration to the *salus animae* clearly left little room for the appreciation of research into the *sanitas corporis*, the health offered by medicine through human and profane means. These means were clearly perceived—and rightly so—as uncertain, haphazard efforts when compared with the rapidity and certainty of the miraculous curative intervention of God. Moreover, these were means that often—in their impartial appeal to laws of nature—put the soul at some risk. During the course of the twelfth century, many religious authors, writing from monasteries in particular, pointed out that remedies and delicate foods *perhaps* helped the body of a sick person but certainly could do no good for the soul. This indifference, and sometimes hostility, toward profane medicine translated into a topical question: why rely on a physician when Christ, the true physician, has supplanted the Aesculapius of the pagans?[9] This same tension characterized the equally frequent opposition between the *schola Salvatoris*, whose goal was salvation, and the *schola Hippocratis*, which strove to attain physical health.

These repeated reservations and worried admonitions were joined by critical narratives that—especially in hagiographic texts and chronicles—pointed out complacently the inevitable failure of medical therapy before the inscrutable will of God, which governs disease and healing. These accounts, along with the strict, rigid, and restrictive version of the prerogatives of the physician, as drawn up by the bishop Raterius,[10] suggest the continuation, however scattered and weakened, of a profane tradition of medical doctrine and the presence, limited though it may have been, of both secular schools and operators. Even the monastic currents, overwhelmingly concerned with the *salus animae*, were themselves quite solicitous of the physical health of the members of the monastic community, as we can see from Raterius's rules. In other areas, monks were engaged in the preservation and transmission of texts of classical medicine and pharmacological knowledge. Consider, for instance, Cassiodorus's exaltation of the nearly sacerdotal role of the physician, whose oath he compared to the vows of the priest, and his instructions to his monks to preserve and transcribe classical medical texts.[11]

In the East as well as in the West, alongside the criticism of profane medicine (mostly in the ninth to eleventh centuries, and even then only in certain currents of monastic thought), we see evidence—admittedly in the larger framework of an emphasis on spiritual values—of a parallel structure of functions, indeed an implementation of overlapping roles between those who care for the body and those who care for the soul. It is no accident that a priest's tasks included the *visitare languentes,* and that among the responsibilities of the church we find the management of places—sanctuaries, collegiate hospices, monastic infirmaries—where care is offered also to the body. And it is no surprise that a religion based on the pursuit of salvation from degradation and sin should find in medicine a reservoir of terms, concepts, metaphors, and allegories. Theologians and preachers drew freely from medical texts. This practice continued without interruption from Augustine to Pope Gregory I, from Alain de Lille to Humbert de Romans, leading to the development of a "spiritual medicine." Even at the end of the Middle Ages, someone like Jean Gerson could point out just how fertile the hermeneutics of that spiritual medicine was, and how useful for those who had the care of human souls.[12] As both Humbert de Romans and Jean Gerson, among others, noted, in the Middle Ages at least three forms of spiritual medicine were established and consolidated. One placed value on disease and suffering, considering them to be remedies for the soul (typical of the high Middle Ages). A second used the categories of medicine better to interpret the structure of the soul and the spiritual "treatments" that it requires. And a third form held that pastoral activity itself—in particular confession and preaching—should be seen as a spiritual therapy.

The Reevaluation of Medical Knowledge

The renewal of both society and culture that made the twelfth century such a crucial time in the development of the medieval world had its effects on the landscape we have just described. In the vast undifferentiated area of *infirmitas,* we begin to see distinctions made between various components and conditions. It begins to become clear that *paupertas,* although often found alongside *infirmitas,* is not entirely the same thing. *Infirmitas* itself no longer designates a generic feebleness, or only the depressing but "normal" and constant situation of humanity. Rather, it has come to indicate more specific, identifiable, and temporary failures of the body, failures that are clearly detectable. In part, these failures or short-comings are susceptible to remedy (not only through charity, but also, for example, through suitable techniques or "mechanical arts"). Indeed, the values and conditions that form part of *infirmitas* begin to break free of their intertwining bonds. At the same time, charity begins to acquire a more complex articulation. Whereas charity once appeared as a virtue and a gift, it has grown into an attitude that is almost naturally proper to humanity, which is *mansuetus* and *pronus ad misericordiam*.[13] Thus, it is no longer *infirmitas*, but now mercy that appears "natural." In the new society of the twelfth century, this disposition was to be analyzed and articulated, as other natural characteristics of mankind had been. Once indiscriminate, charity had become orderly. This meant that the destitute should be helped not all in the same way but *secundum ordinem caritatis*.[14] A hierar-chy thus developed, ranking duties of assistance, with privileged status for the circle of one's blood relatives. A distinction was made between the truly poor and the false poor, the truly sick and the false sick, or between the sick who were ethically acceptable and those who were not. For exam-ple, hospitals were not to accept those persons who, though truly sick, were infamous or dishonest. There was a body of case histories of vices, defects, and even faults of the poor, who might themselves be the negligent cause of their own condition. A minute analysis of orderly charity took these factors into account, along with the quality of those who received assis-tance and the way in which the giving was done. As Humbert de Romans pointed out, few merciful works were as meritorious as that of aiding the sick in hospital. This was both because they were in greater need of charity than others (they were in fact both sick *and* poor), and because all of the senses of those who cared for them were mortified.

Likewise, in the stratification and overlapping of tasks and functions linked to acts of assistance and care (wholly concentrated in the operative hegemony of men of the church), a process of distinction was underway. The ecclesiastical hierarchy itself, in the face of the new and increasingly demanding pastoral tasks arising from the growing diversification of soci-ety, felt the need to distinguish among the different areas of intervention. The church assigned priests specialized fields of jurisdiction, making them veritable "professionals" of the care of the soul. The deliberations of vari-ous councils[15] were moving in this direction, as they forbade men of the church to engage in the practice of medicine or other profane disciplines. This policy was not prompted by a scorn for medicine itself; rather, the idea was to encourage the clergy to pursue deeper theological studies, improving its preparation and preventing overlapping roles. Moreover, the intense commitment and involvement in the world that so marked the activity of the new mendicant orders, while they did require these specific fields of expertise, also increased awareness of the need for and value of physical health and energy, indispensable requirements for the new concrete commitment to society. Saint Francis's praise of "brother body," Humbert de Romans's recommendations to the monks against physical mortification and "hygienic" neglect, considered both debilitating and a sign of arrogance—these were all indications of how the body had acquired value, something to be used for spiritual purposes, but not through suffering and patience only.

The physician attained in this period a broader and more complex definition of his scientific and professional prerogatives. His education now took place—first in schools, later in universities—according to preestablished, homogeneous institutional paths, which sanctioned with public examination the acquisition of a specialized doctrine and expertise. The physician's knowledge had been enriched through translations that restored the ancient acquisitions of Greeks and Arabs. It had become difficult, therefore, to write off this impressive and institutionalized body of knowledge as a pack of vain or uncertain notions or as merely ineffectual practices. Philosophical and theological thinking was increasingly introducing into the relationships between nature, God, and mankind forms of mediation that portrayed natural phenomena as less immediately dependent on a circumscribed act of divine will. This idea of mediation allowed—indeed, obliged—humans to make use of the rationality that God had infused in them, as well as in nature, to study and understand the regularity of natural phenomena. All this meant—in that area of thought revolving around *infirmitas*—that health, healing, and disease were no longer viewed solely as direct results of divine intervention, or only as the direct expression of the vicissitudes of the soul, but were seen as phenomena that depended on natural and regular events, which the physician might and must investigate.

Medicine, in this new outlook, was itself seen as a gift of God. God had endowed mankind with the capacity of understanding the organism, and He had endowed herbs with curative properties the physician must study. Nothing gives a clearer indication of this shift in perspective than the frequent quotation—by physicians and nonphysicians—of the understated exhortation of Ecclesiastes 38:1: "Honor physicians for their serv-

ices, for the Lord created them," which progressively supplanted the impe-
rious admonition of Exodus 15:26: "For I am the Lord that healeth thee."
Confident of the value now recognized in the science of the body, a
physician—in making use of his command of doctrine—could reconcile
his Christian obligation to perform charity with his special social standing,
both as a scholar and as a professional. He could therefore receive payment
for the therapeutic acts he performed. So reasoned even preachers and
moralists, who were attentive to what was licit and proper and what
constituted illicit behavior for the various categories and professions.
Medicine and health were fundamentally considered to be gifts of God;
thus it was not right to sell them, although the physician, beneficiary of
the gift of "talents" (intelligence, the capacity for study), had the moral
obligation to render these talents fruitful through rigorous and profound
studies. If he demanded payment, it was not for the result obtained
(knowledge or healing, for which he is nothing more than an intermediary
of God), but rather for the preparation and work that cost the physician
much zeal and effort. Charity demanded that he ask his rich patients to
pay more so that he could care for the poor free of charge. Henri de
Mondeville commented that surgeons exercise an *ars beatissima,* in that
they can give *floridae* and *maiores* alms, closely bound up with health, and
not limited to such extraneous considerations as food or clothing, of relatively little use if the body is sick. If a surgeon demands his due from a
wealthy patient *(salva conscientia)* and operates on the poor out of charity,
then he need not perform pilgrimages: "quoniam ex scientia vestra potestis
salvare animas vestras."[16]

On the one hand, medicine was organized on a solid foundation
inasmuch as it was a discipline and a legitimate profession; on the other
hand, the material and symbolic stratifications of the high Middle Ages
had begun to dissolve. And it was at this precise juncture that two experts,
the priest and the physician, could begin to exchange and cooperate,
abandoning their traditional conflicts and territorial squabbles. Both of
them—in the words of Archimatthaeus of Salerno in his instructions to
physicians visiting patients—have a right to an honored presence in the
house of the patient they are summoned to visit.[17]

For his part, the physician agreed to respect the *mandata* and the
praecepta Ecclesiae, which affected his soul, as a professional, and the soul of
his patient. He would treat the poor free of charge; he would offer all his
knowledge, neglecting nothing; he would not deceive his patients concerning their infirmities in the pursuit of lucrative treatment; nor would he

organize frauds with the complicity of apothecaries; nor would he practice abortions or provide any poisons. These last two precepts had long formed part of the professional ethics of the physician, already cited by Cassiodorus. The physician would be ready to summon a confessor (conciliar deliberations required this) before commencing therapy, especially in serious cases. Lastly, he would take into account the considerations and advice of the moralists concerning communication with the invalid, determining the difference between culpable silence, fraudulent lies, benevolent half-truths, and exhortations intended to influence the patient in a favorable manner.

Men of the church, in turn, were able to appreciate and recognize the doctrinal and professional competence of the physician, and to some extent attempted to imitate it. They also ensured the monopoly of the Christian physician in cases where ecclesiastical deliberations forbade recourse to Jewish doctors, or in cases where the church condemned the *illicite practicantes,* those who practiced medicine without the right to do so and without supervision. Priests and physicians, intellectuals educated in the shared values of scholasticism, exchanged valuable reciprocal assistance in warding off the pretenses and practices of charlatans, Empirics, and fortune tellers—all those who lacked the sort of institutionally sanctioned doctrinal education that ensured authentic and legitimate competence. The priest, then, saw specifically the *scientia* of the physician as the stoutest bulwark against magic and superstition. It should therefore come hardly as a surprise that when a priest was called upon to evaluate the sins a physician might commit, he would rank in the first place, ahead even of fraud, the lack of skill, the failure to study, inadequate or haphazard preparation, the lack of knowledge, and the failure to keep up with the latest scientific developments. A physician might be guilty of murder through lack of knowledge. The *recta scientia,* therefore, was an indispensable prerequisite for a *recta conscientia.*

The physician, too, considered the acquisition of knowledge the highest value toward which he could strive and toward which, as a Christian *medicus-philosophus,* it was his duty to strive.[18] *Scientia* was the path by which he could become one with God. More than any other, the physician was aware that, in the exercise of his difficult, daring, and sometimes uncertain profession, he had need of the grace of God. Medical science thus "saved souls," for the physician's knowledge allowed him to do good, to practice charity, and to attain truth, all at the same time, in a sort of *consortium divinum.*

The Medieval Hospital

"Philanthropy is a fine thing, the zeal of helping the poor and bringing succor to human frailty. Leave the city; immediately outside the gates you can admire a new city; I am referring to that stone dispensary, that commonly held treasure, always rich and available to all . . . in which disease is accepted with the serenity that comes from wisdom; in which misfortune is considered a blessing and mercy is striven after and put to the test." This is the earliest known description of a Christian hospital; the author is Gregory of Nazianzus,[19] the city is Caesarea in Cappadocia, and the new citadel of charity that has sprung up at the city's gates is the hospital, adjacent to the monastery. It was built (around A.D. 370) at the order of the bishop, Saint Basil, to succor the poor and the aged, to give haven to lepers, to treat the infirm.

Between the late Middle Ages and the early Renaissance other hospital citadels, designed to respond to the growing need for specialization, developed in Pistoia and in other cities in Tuscany and Italy. Founded in the thirteenth century by the association of Santa Maria del Ceppo of the Poor—taking its name (*ceppo* means tree trunk) from the trunk in which alms were gathered for the needy—the hospital of Pistoia had won particular distinction in housing and caring for those infected with the plague, during the terrible early rise and spread of the disease. In the frieze by Giovanni Della Robbia that decorates the Renaissance loggia, the seven works of mercy are emblazoned, reiterating and emphasizing, through the simple and direct language of images, the Christian ideal of charity and the all-encompassing character of aid, which provides the context in which the organization was caring for the poverty-stricken sick.

The medieval hospital was first and foremost a space established to fulfill, concretely, publicly, and free of charge, the obligation of charity. We can see this clearly from the two examples mentioned here, widely separated by geographical distance and historical time, set one at the beginning and the other at the end of an era, thus documenting a certain continuity. The hospital originated as and remained a fundamentally religious structure. This was so even when it was no longer run in accordance with the pastoral and social obligations of the ecclesiastical hierarchy, but instead maintained by the religious impulse of solidarity of laymen. In any case, it remained a "pious" place, even though as early as 1439 the Ceppo was described as *locus profanus*[20] and an increasingly secular administration responded to the more greatly differentiated requirements of the material and spiritual needs of the poor.

The Western medieval hospital was neither originally nor chiefly a specifically therapeutic social space—unlike the Byzantine, and especially the Muslim hospital, in the same period of time in the East. The Western hospital was not, therefore, a place in which it was possible to activate and organize "that array of acts by which disease, in a society, is encircled, attacked medically, isolated, distributed into privileged and closed areas, or assigned to places of healing arranged in such a way as to encourage that healing."[21]

Universal and undifferentiated—like the religious sites it long adjoined (sanctuary, bishop's home, cathedral, monastery)—ideally destined to house and care for every man (who was by nature *viator* and *infirmus*), the medieval hospital soon became a space set aside for those on the social edge. Social differentiation appeared among the sick as well. Initially a place in which private and public charity was offered, especially for the poor and the weak, the hospital took on as one of its goals that of helping the infirm: not simply the sick and infirm per se, but the sick poor, and the poor elderly infirm. The hospital thus brought about an important first distinction in the social space of disease: a "familiar and domestic" space for the well-to-do. This made it possible to define the sick person as a patient, and to organize, in a private space, a therapeutic process overseen by the knowledge of the physician. But there remained a "public" space, where the sick person received material help and, above all, spiritual comfort, more than any specific therapy. The space of illness was considered a medically oriented space only in unusual circumstances, or very late in history.

At the end of the Middle Ages, at any rate—though with considerable difficulty, gradually, and with delays in certain areas—a new image of the hospital began to spread. The hospital became a place of treatment, if not healing; it was no longer limited to offering consolation and preparation for a good death. This new orientation better fit the secular aims of medicine, which was increasingly involved in the operation of the hospital. Two events triggered decisive new orientations in the process of institutionalization of aid. The first was the urban, religious, and cultural rebirth of the twelfth century; the second was the eruption of the plague into Western history. While the first event revolves around a phase (from the twelfth to the middle of the fourteenth century) that André Vauchez and Michel Mollat describe as the period of "revolution" or "urgency" of charity, the second event marked the emergence of a need for more effective public control of the economic and social effects of the epidemic, thus accelerating the process of secularization of charitable institutions.

Xenodochea, Infirmaries, and Hospices-Hospitals

In the East, where the ecclesiastical hierarchy was involved in the foundation of hospitals as early as the fourth century, forms of diversification and specialization of aid—which would not be attempted in the West until much later—were being tested during the fifth and sixth centuries. If the idea of man as a stranger and a pilgrim on earth remained at the center of the practice of Christian charity, the church devoted growing attention to specific aspects of social reality—the poor, the old, orphans, and foundlings, as well as the sick. Public charity was organized in an anthropological and religious context that emphasized the links—not the opposition— between body and soul, between spiritual medicine and profane medicine. It should come as no surprise, then, that the most common term for the Byzantine hospital should have been *xenodocheum* (*xenos* meaning, in fact, "stranger"). Nonetheless, we cannot ignore the variety of names used, from the sixth century onward, to describe the functional diversification of the hospital: hospices for the poor *(ptocheion, ptochotropheion),* for pilgrims *(pandocheion),* for the elderly *(gerontokomeion);* the orphanage for foundlings *(brephotropheion);* and the hospital for the sick *(nosokomeion).*

In Rome, the forms of social assistance tied to diaconal organizations consisted largely in charity, in particular the giving of alms. The growing numbers of the needy, the feeble, and the sick in time forced the bishops of Western Christendom—who played a central role in the political and social life of the cities of the period—to adopt more efficacious forms of charity and more stable institutional solutions. Still, for all the expressions of admiration of how things were done in the East, the West took no steps to emulate those forms. The term *xenodocheum* is virtually the sole inheritance taken from the Byzantine tradition. A succession of councils throughout the sixth century urged bishops to fulfill their duty to provide hospitality and social aid, especially for the poor; the *Liber diurnus* (of the seventh and eighth centuries) urged the same thing. In particular, they advised that suitable rooms be established, *intra muros* and adjacent either to the bishopric or the cathedral, furnished with beds, where the sick and the needy could be housed and provided with care and assistance. The progressive decline in urban population clearly shows how inadequate this form of social assistance really was. Between the seventh and eighth centuries, these older hospital structures underwent a general decline. The idea of ritual charity and the obligation of undifferentiated hospitalization prevailed during this period. The term "hospital" appeared alongside the term *xenodocheum*, becoming common from the ninth century onward.

In this largely undifferentiated area of disease, sin, and poverty, patients were essentially expected to play the role of repentant pilgrims. The sanctuary was a place where the power and mercy of God were revealed. In such a setting, the "scientific" distinctions between a curable and an incurable disease, between states of chronic or acute illness, between sickness and deformity, really had no meaning at all. Likewise, it made no sense to think of a time for illness and a time for the accompanying therapy and convalescence. The instantaneous nature of divine intervention was substituted for the timing of the physician.[22]

Hence there were religious reasons for making the sanctuary the most important center of healing. At the same time, there were ideological reasons, as well as social and economic ones, for making the *hospitalia* the only structures for assistance in the Middle Ages. They were built chiefly at the behest of the bishops, *promotores charitatis*,[23] and at first they were located primarily within the urban boundaries of a bishop's see. Later, as the cities began to decline, and growing numbers of the sick were to be found in the countryside, the *hospitalia* were located in country parish churches, along various roads (especially pilgrim routes), in monasteries, or, in some cases, such as that of Saint Martin de Tours, near major sanctuaries. The assistance involved little more than providing all comers with a place to rest and a meal. Treatments were generally limited to a series of generic, undifferentiated services, intended to reduce pain and suffering.

Secular charity had not yet come into existence, except for the specific case—likewise undifferentiated—of the royal duty of hospitality (particularly the case in Merovingian France and Longobard Italy). A modest attempt to reorganize the way in which social assistance was provided was made during the Carolingian period, with ecclesiastical and royal power poised side by side. Charlemagne ordered "that there should be set up in various places hospices for travelers, places of accommodation in the monasteries for the poor and in the communities of clerics, since the Lord will say on Judgment Day: 'I was your guest, and you took me in.'"[24]

The religious ideal of hospitality and the liturgy of charity particularly influenced monastery hospices. The *Regula monachorum*, the monastic rule composed by Saint Benedict (480–547), devoted two chapters to these subjects (36 and 53). The text advises: "First of all, and above all else, it is necessary to provide for the care of the infirm, so that one serves them precisely like Christ in person, since He has said: 'I was sick, and you cared for me.'"[25]

At first, Benedictine spirituality made no distinction between rich and poor, between guest, pilgrim, and patient. An incipient differentiation, along social and economic lines, however, began to cause a division of the space in which monastic charity was undertaken, beginning as early as the Carolingian era. That space had come into being as a single, unitary entity, represented by "the Door" at which, previously, guests, the poor, and the sick had all been welcomed without distinction.

The monastic context allowed a distinction to be made between those who were sick and those who were healthy. The prosperity of the community and a strict adherence to the monastic rule thus led to the abolition of the rigorously identical treatment that had long been accorded the poor and the sick in the hospice. The monastic infirmary, with its *domus* and *claustrum infirmorum*, was created to accommodate those members of the community who were obliged by weakness or disease to cease observance of the rule. They were designated the infirm, requiring the same cares that were accorded a rich patient in his own home. These conditions permitted the development of a therapeutic activity that was for many years, at least until the eleventh century, to constitute the only organized collective form of medicine practiced.[26]

The architectural plan of the abbey of Saint Gallen (820–830) offers a typical example of the "hierarchic" development of Benedictine hospitality, as well as an instance of the development of medically oriented assistance.[27] Adjacent to the infirmary, which had a dormitory and a refectory for the sick monks, stood the *domus medicorum*. That space contained a room for the very sickest patients. The room of the physician stood next door; there was also a small pharmacy, equipped for giving therapeutic baths and for bloodletting, and a garden in which medicinal plants were grown. The earliest medieval manuals of medical botany, pathology, and pharmacology were written in this setting, in virtue of the close ties between the library, the *scriptorium*, and the infirmary. Suffice it to mention *Hortulus* by Walafrido Strabo, the abbot of Reichenau; *De innumeris morbis* and *De innumeris remediorum utilitatibus*, attributed to Bertharius, the abbot of Monte Cassino; the translations and compilations done in the same abbey by Constantine of Africa; and *Causae et curae*, by Hildegard von Bingen, abbess of Rupertsberg. Likewise, with a view to practical applications, generation after generation of *infirmarii* and physicians-monks gathered, compiled, and corrected prescriptions for the treatment of all sorts of diseases. By the end of the eleventh century, in a number of abbeys, distinctions were already beginning to be made among various professional roles concerning the care of the sick. In surviving documents we find increasingly frequent mention of *phlebotomi, minutores,* and *ventosarii* (responsible for letting blood), as well as the *infirmarii, medici,* and *physici.*

Of course, as Grmek points out,[28] the specific therapeutic connotations found in the infirmaries of the monasteries influenced no more than a marginal aspect of the countless hospices or hospitals that they administered. Between the twelfth and thirteenth centuries, prohibitions enacted by the councils and a rebirth of secular medicine together worked to discourage the spread of these forms of medicalization to the hospital structures. And yet, as Mollat has observed,[29] the influence that the monastic experience had on the newly founded hospitals that sprang up from the middle of the twelfth century on is undeniable. Movements for canonic and Benedictine reform marked the appearance of new denominations and new orders. The latter tended especially to encourage participation in works of corporal mercy, practiced by monks and nuns in the hospices adjacent to the convents, under the supervision of a *frater hospitalis.* Let us only mention the community founded by Robert d'Arbrissel to succor sinful women and lepers, or the order of Prémontré, whose program of charity included "pauperum curam et hospitalitatem." In more general terms, a new spirituality as well as a different attitude toward the body encouraged both lay and religious—without neglecting the care of the soul—to work to allay both poverty and physical suffering, wherever they might appear, outside the monasteries and in the cities. The exercise of this new spirituality also led both lay and religious to assemble in congregations for the foundation and operation of hospitals. New religious orders were formed for the sole purpose of providing assistance to the needy. A fourth vow was added to the traditional monastic vows: that of offering hospitality to pilgrims and to succor the infirm. Thus two new figures arose in the field of charity, beside the figures of bishop and monk: the *laicus religiosus*[30] and the Hospitaler friar.

The Hospital as a Place of Treatment and Assistance

In response to urgent new needs and according to conciliar instructions, the church undertook—as it had previously done in the sixth century, though with different forms and structures—to exhort the clergy to fulfill its duties toward the disinherited and the sick. At the same time, faced with ineffective management, inadequate forms of social assistance, and the decline of moral and religious values, all produced by this burgeoning germination of new hospitals, the church strove primarily to control and reform the internal functioning of hospital institutes both old and new. According to the councils of Paris (1212), Rouen (1214), and Lateran IV (1215), it was now the duty of the religious congregations and lay brotherhoods that ran hospitals and leper colonies to observe a common rule. An effort was made to standardize the ways in which charity was practiced, in order to make them more effective, while preserving the independence and individual features of these institutions. The rule that was adopted had been written by Saint Augustine, in actuality a simple pastoral letter with advice on community living; the same rule was adopted by reform canons and was to inspire the new Hospitaler orders.

The foundation of the Hospitaler orders was, moreover, a symptom of a larger push toward charity. The order of Saint John of Jerusalem (or the order of the Hospitalers) received its first statutes from Raymond du Puy between 1125 and 1153. One specific chapter describes "how their *highnesses* the sick should be received and served." This formulation can be found thereafter in the statutes of many Hospitaler orders. The specific attention of the order toward the needs of the sick, designated as a special category of guests, may have been inspired by the example set by the Byzantines. In precisely the same period, an exceedingly well organized hospital complex was founded (1136) near the imperial monastery of the Pantokrator in Constantinople.[31] The attitude evinced by the order of Saint John toward the hospitalized sick was laid out quite explicitly in the statutes drawn up in French and promulgated in 1181 by Roger de Molins. These statutes expressly recommend that "for the invalids in the Hospital of Jerusalem there should be made available four learned physicians, who are able to distinguish the quality of urines and the differences among the sick, so that they can properly administer medicinal remedies."[32]

At the end of the century, the influence of yet another Hospitaler order, that of Saint-Esprit (founded by a modest burgher, Guy de Montpellier), extended from the south of France down into Italy. The most important hospitals of this order were located in Marseilles and in Rome. The hospitals accepted and cared for pilgrims, the poor, the sick, pregnant women, and children. According to the *Liber regulae Sancti Spiritus*, "every day of the week a search is made in the streets and squares for the indigent and sick. They are then led to the Maison du Saint-Esprit, where they are cared for with the most attentive solicitude." All the same, no mention is made of physicians. The order of Saint John was soon to abandon the Hospitaler role it had originally evinced. This did little, however, to undercut the extent of the influence that both orders exerted on the reformation of assistance and especially on the reorganization of hospitals run by congregations and confraternities. From this time forward, the statutes of these sorts of organization featured specific regulations concerning the accommodation and treatment accorded to the needy and sick. Every aspect was codified: the kindness and courtesy of the nuns at the moment of hospitalization; the vigilant watchfulness over the sick, day and night; how frequently patients should be visited; how spiritual succor should be provided; hygienic and dietetic prescriptions; furnishing the beds with warm furs and bright lamps at night; the celebration of mass. The most vivid and involved description of this general reform can be found in the well-known pages of the *Historia occidentalis* (chapter 29), written by Jacques de Vitry a few years after Lateran IV. This author sang the praises of those congregations of "men and women who . . . have devoted their lives with humility and devotion to serving the poor and the infirm." Among the best-known hospitals, he praises those of Santo Spirito ("hospitale Sancti Spiritus in Saxia") in Rome, of the Venerable Anthony in Vienna, and of Sainte-Marie in Roncevaux, as well as the hospitals in Paris, Noyon, Provins, Tournai, Liège, and Brussels, "where one can see honesty and piety, workshops of holiness, centers of dignity and worship, havens for the poor, help for the miserable, consolation for the afflicted, nourishment for the hungry, and tender care for the infirm."[33]

In the context of economic expansion and population growth, during the thirteenth and fourteenth centuries, urban hospitals grew and flourished as they never had before. Their social role became increasingly important. The need for a more solid and permanent structure came to replace the older, "precarious" image of a *hospitale* as a center of temporary accommodation, "along the side of the road." Of course, hospitals remained primarily shelters and sources of generic assistance. They continued to have a powerful religious connotation even if they had been founded by secular organizations and even if they were run by municipal governments. The church itself was to reaffirm in the councils of Ravenna (1311) and Vienna (1312) its prerogatives concerning the assistance and the religious nature of hospitals.

Xenodochea, hospitals, and hospices all began to assume specific roles. Accepting only the sick, for instance, might become a prerogative of the major hospitals in the cities. Still, the boundaries between assistance and treatment remained vague and unclear. Most often, the hospitals accepted the sick without any distinctions whatsoever. A number of statutes expressly excluded not only those sick people who were considered dangerous or contagious (lepers, for instance), but also persons afflicted with ergotism (subject to horrible spontaneous amputations), as well as cripples, the maimed, criminals who had had limbs lopped off or branded, and the blind.[34] The reason for this was more ideological and social than it was medical. However vague, an idea of differentiation by the status of the patient, based on the nature of the disease, is expressed in the recommendation that "the cripples should not be taken in unless they are afflicted with serious illness, since disease in the limbs is not the same as disease that renders one incapable of work; therefore, as soon as they are better, they should be sent away."

The statutes of the Hôtel-Dieu of Montdidier (1208) allowed the sick to remain in the hospital for a week after their recovery, to prevent relapses; this provision seems to indicate a notion of a time of sickness and a time of convalescence. This rule was eventually incorporated into many different statutes, such as those of the Hôtels-Dieu of Tonnerre and Paris. During this period, the distinction between curable and incurable was reinforced, forcing a differentiation between hospices and hospitals. The Hôtel-Dieu of Valenciennes refused to accept paralytics and the deformed because "they occupy spaces that are needed for the curable ill, who require care and beds." Simultaneously, hospices were built to accommodate those excluded—the sick and the invalids who had no chance of becoming well—so that their needs could be provided for, without isolating them wholly from society.[35]

In Italy, during the second half of the thirteenth century, the processes of secularization and restructuring of assistance effected so major a change that it prompted the interest of chroniclers, becoming the material of a new civil and professional rhetoric. The hospital system was considered one of the factors in a city's prestige, a legitimate cause for *laudatio urbis*. To mention one example, we can quote Opicino de' Canistris concerning the city of Pavia,[36] and Bonvesin de la Riva on Milan. The latter wrote that in the Brolo, "all of the poor who are sick, with the exception of lepers, who have a separate hospital, are taken in and cared for. Here they find a bed and food, given with benevolence and generosity. All of the poor who require surgical care are scrupulously assisted by three surgeons who devote themselves to this activity, and who are given a salary by the municipality."[37]

There was only a minimal relationship between hospitals as institutions and the simultaneous development of scholastic medicine and the medical profession; indeed, the ties were negligible in almost every case. There were, however, nuances that should be pointed out. If Peter of Abano advised future physicians to visit hospitals often, because they could see every sort of disease there, even the strangest, he did so primarily to attain a rhetorical effect and for the pleasure of citing an authority. The recommendation in question, taken from the *Pantegni,* by 'Ali ibn al-'Abbas, was not based on Peter of Abano's personal experience.[38] It formed part of the professional rhetoric of the *doctus et expertus* physician who, to acquire practical experience at the bedside of various patients, was expected to visit convents, prisons, and hospices.[39] Physicians and surgeons, in some cases at the behest of municipal authorities, began to explore these places, though only on various occasions; finally they made them one of the customary settings for their profession—this was certainly the case with Guglielmo de Saliceto. Of course, the hospitals were fields of observation more than places of therapy for these physicians. Guglielmo, for example, tells in his *Cirurgia* of having seen and attended a hydrocephalic child in a hospice in Cremona, without attempting any of the surgical operations suggested by the authors he consulted, feeling that those operations were excessively risky.[40]

The hospice, then, remained a generic site of conservative therapy, and it was also seen as an exemplary place in which *natura medicatrix* held sway. In this ideal observatory, a physician could acquire valuable indications concerning the best *modum curationis,* which he could then apply to the cases of his own patients. Clearly this was rhetorical, but it is a valuable indicator. Another important development was the appearance, in Italy and in the cities of France and the Netherlands (unlike in other countries), of documents which demonstrate that there were increasingly common professional relationships between health technicians and administrators of structures of assistance. Thus, in 1297, Jan Yperman was engaged by the city of Ypres to provide the services of a surgeon in the hospital of Belle.

Just before the fourteenth century in Italy, and just after in France and Spain, many city hospitals opened their doors to health professionals and technicians of healing. A number of statutes—for instance, those of the hospital of Siena (Spedale di Santa Maria della Scala)—that date from the turn of the fourteenth century call for the regular employment of surgeons, physicians, and pharmacists. The same is true of the Hôpital du Saint-Esprit of Marseilles, whose statutes specify, among other things, that the physician should visit his patients twice daily (1338).[41] In 1328, an ordinance of Charles IV required the sworn royal physicians of the

Châtelet in Paris to provide care to the poor patients hospitalized in the town hospitals. The contracts of the salaried physicians *(medici condotti)* in Italy,[42] and the professionals paid by cities in France, Germany, and Flanders, began to include clauses requiring that they visit patients in the hospitals. In 1365, a surgeon was hired to work in all the hospitals of Avignon.[43]

The importance accorded to charity has led some not only to reject, rightly, the idea of the medicalization of medieval hospitals in general (at least until the fifteenth century), but also—less correctly—to proclaim the complete absence of any therapeutic aims. And yet, the idea of acting "for the health of the body," as the statutes of the hospital of Siena put it, gradually made its way into the awareness of the directors of these institutions. It was necessary, according to the statutes just mentioned, "that every infirm person should be cared for in their infirmity, in accordance with the decisions of the physicians and the guardians of the hospices; thus, those who are infirm should have syrups, soups, poultry, and all that which they may require, in accordance with the nature of their infirmity, so that none should perish for lack of some thing."

For the most part, this activity was limited to a series of hygienic prescriptions and a richer diet. The call for a special diet for the "poor who are sick" represents in our opinion a fundamental prerequisite to the medicalization of hospitals. It was through the existence of an alimentary regimen—nonpersonalized though it may have been—that the social setting of the poor opened up to the rules of medicine, with its partial assimilation, at least in theory, to the private space of the wealthy patient. In effect, the poor would not be able to follow the same diet outside of the hospital; poverty condemned them to inadequate dietary regimens. And if surgery entered relatively rapidly into the practices followed in hospitals, it was a simple, routine form of surgery; moreover, it was more commonly practiced upon members of the congregation and the staff of the hospital than upon the poor guests of the hospital. According to sources, the *potio*, which is to say the administration of syrups, ointments, and other medications, also formed part of the routine in hospitals,[44] though it was not as varied and refined as was the case with wealthy patients.

Leprosy and the Plague

Two diseases, with tragic consequences both for individuals and for the collective, should be considered separately: leprosy and the plague. They are important not only in terms of pathology and epidemiology, but also in terms of their social connotations and the ideological values they engendered.

Leper Hospitals

Leprosy is notable for its early and evident effects on "secularization" and "specialization," more markedly in the social procedures of isolation, exclusion, and control of the sick than in the implementation of any medical treatments. Leper hospitals and leper colonies represented, if you will, the archaeology of procedures of strong control of diseases, which were thought of in the same terms as deviance; beginning in the late fourteenth century and especially in the fifteenth century, those procedures resulted in the creation, by secular authorities, of lazarettos and hospices for the mentally ill. These were places of isolation and seclusion, not of healing.[45]

In the West, lepers became increasingly numerous from the end of the eleventh century on. This growth in their numbers, parallel with the development of cities, posed a new danger to public health. Leprosy was more than this, however. Certainly, the disease brought about the space that was created to contain it, but both the disease and its space of confinement came to acquire certain religious and moral connotations. Until the disappearance of leprosy as an endemic disease—whereupon its negative values were transferred to syphilis or transposed and sublimated to folly and madness—it maintained in the West the symbolic and exemplary content of a disease of the soul. The corruption of the body, therefore, was nothing more than an exterior manifestation of that internal corruption. The prescription of Leviticus (13:46) remained scorchingly up-to-date: "All the days wherein the plague shall be in him he shall be defiled; he is unclean: he shall dwell alone; without the camp shall his habitation be." Just like a heretic, for whom the leper became a metaphor,[46] a leper was shut out of the community and kept at arm's length from society. The leper became the symbol, par excellence, of sin, the exemplary mark of divine justice. The leper, however, was also (and here once again we see the fundamental ambiguity of Christianity), especially in the spirituality of the twelfth and thirteenth centuries, the image of Christ, who accepted the burden of all the filth of the body, becoming abject among the abject in order to save humanity. The kiss given to a leper by Saint Francis or Saint Louis marked this symbolic identification. Lepers—according to the statutes of the leper hospital of Lille—were those whom the Lord wished to visit more intimately than others. If, in the monastic infirmary, the rule isolated both the sick and the sickness, in leper hospitals the disease itself created the rule. This rule was conceived for communities of the sick and the healthy, in which the healthy were devoted to the service of the sick and organized—from the thirteenth century on—according to a strict discipline that often mirrored monastic discipline. The social practices implemented to isolate those suffering from this disease (following banishment, the earlier, primitive form of exclusion,[47] and following the segregation in free and spontaneous groups, typical of the eleventh and twelfth centuries) were now organized and administered by the municipal authorities.[48] They constituted a new direction in sanitary policy, and they were clearly developed with a view to protecting citizens from contagion rather than to treating those already sick. Physicians did not enter a leper hospital; they only began to go there after the number of lepers had declined drastically, from the fourteenth century on, and after the leper hospitals and colonies had been opened to other invalids, with more or less contagious diseases. There was a widespread belief that leprosy was a punishment for sexual transgression, and that the disease could be transmitted sexually. As a result, measures were adopted to restrict or repress sexuality, often sublimating it through a sort of vow of chastity.[49]

The Effects of the Plague

The outbreak of the plague epidemic in 1347–48, an epidemic that lasted for several centuries, engendered many new differences in the responses to the need for sanitary assistance but also served to unify the collective attitudes in this field. Ravaging populations without distinction, the plague united different countries and social classes in an imminent mortality experienced in apocalyptic tones. According to the French chronicler Jean Froissart, "a third of the world died." The Sienese writer Agnolo di Tura described an entire city awaiting, dry-eyed, death and the approach of the end of the world. The plague manifested itself everywhere as a sudden, unpredictable, and astounding laceration of the social fabric and of Christian brotherhood. "Charity was dead," declared the surgeon Guy de Chauliac.[50] "The son abandoned his father; the husband, his wife; the wife, her husband; one brother would flee from another; one sister, from another"—lamented, in virtually the same words, Marchionne de Coppo Stefani,[51] Agnolo di Tura, and Boccaccio. Relations between the community of the living and the world of the dead were turned upside down.

Traditional funeral processions and ceremonies had to be prohibited in many cities. The dead were stacked up before the doorways of houses; in some cases, they were simply abandoned inside the houses themselves. Burial, when it was possible, was done hastily and unceremoniously. To prevent the spread of fear, which was considered to be one of the causes that helped to facilitate the spread of contagion, in Orvieto and Tournai it was forbidden to dress in mourning.[52]

In the face of death, people fled their own homes in terror.[53] A common reaction among city dwellers, following the initial paralysis of terror, was flight. Since there was no cure, the only possibility of survival lay in prevention. It therefore became necessary to shun social contact and even the slightest possibility of contagion: "One should scrupulously avoid public debates and meetings, when possible, lest one's breath mingle with that of others, such that one person may infect many. One should remain alone then and avoid those who come from places where the air is infected."[54]

This advice was given by a respected professor and practitioner: Pietro da Tossignano. In the face of the epidemic, physicians no longer spoke of divine vengeance to explain this new scourge. The immense body of written literature concerning the plague ranges from the learned official reports of the university departments of medicine of Paris and Montpellier to the simple and anonymous prescriptions by unassuming health care professionals. This body of writing emphasizes the gap between an exceedingly elaborate etiology, which did not account for the actual manner of contagion, and an absolutely inadequate form of therapy.[55] It hardly seems surprising that the more developed portion of the treatises on the plague had to do with the regimen required *de preservatione a morbo*. A great emphasis was put on the measures that could be taken to prevent contagion, so as to control and limit the spread of the disease.

And if doctors were unable to treat or combat the plague effectively, priests were also unable to oppose this new scourge with any consistent form of behavior. They were torn between two approaches. The first was a religious response that tended to favor, especially at first, great processions of penitents, public masses,[56] and prayer vigils; the civil authorities soon opposed these gatherings, recognizing in them new opportunities for contagion.[57] The second attitude adopted by priests was to leave the sick and their families to engage in a private, individual practice of religion, since it had become clear that the traditional tools of religious therapy—administering the sacrament, sermons, funeral rites, and so on—had become dangerous or difficult to put into practice. "And it was so contagious . . . that people died without servants and were buried without priests," wrote Guy de Chauliac. In Rouen, for instance, it was forbidden to engage in behavior that might prove offensive to God, such as swearing, betting, or drinking. The bishops of Bath granted the laity the right to hear confession of one another, in the manner of the Apostles. Moreover, "if it was not possible to find a priest who could administer extreme unction, then faith had to suffer."[58] The plague brutally introduced a new type of death, sudden and "savage."[59] The disease was identified with death itself. Death was no longer considered a departure or a passage, but was seen rather as an end, as decomposition. There was no time to ready oneself for a good death; there was no one to look to, no one with the science, the art, or the divine power to domesticate death.

The bafflement of the two great specialists—in health and in salvation—was immediately noted and recorded, and not merely in "technical" terms, but also and primarily in terms of ethical repercussions. Chroniclers observed that physicians and priests were among the first to flee the plague-ridden masses, failing the precepts of both ethical duty and charity.

Clearly, the failure of scholastic medicine in the face of the plague triggered a major crisis in the fields of medical doctrine and the medical profession. Rivalry sharpened between physicians, surgeons, and barbers. Each of these categories, which some time previous seemed to have found a mutually satisfactory equilibrium in terms of roles, claimed to be the only one to know how to face death and to obey the requirements of ethical duty, while accusing the others of incompetence and cowardice. Guy de Chauliac admitted that he would have liked to flee the plague, as physicians did, but he wrote that he did not do so out of fear of discredit attaching to his name. In Avignon, at the insistence of Pope Clement VI, the practice of autopsies was encouraged, in the hopes of improving medical knowledge. Stricter requirements were imposed on the study of medicine and the exercise of the medical profession. During the first half of the fifteenth century, despite the adoption of these measures, which perhaps constituted the tangible sign of this growing awareness, numerous physicians, among them Michele Savonarola, Antonio Guaineri, and Jacques Despars, criticized the shortcomings of medical theory and the inadequacy of therapy.

~ 7 ~

Medical Scholasticism

DANIELLE JACQUART

"Set, or rather, crushed between Antiquity and the Classical Age, medieval thought is most often thought of as a vast list, or better yet, as a storehouse, as the Storehouse, of the questions that are no longer asked."[1] This observation, although expressed by a historian of philosophy, typifies a more widely held view of medieval medicine. In the entire history of universal culture, is there any other field that has more aptly served as a symbol of sterility of thought than that of scholastic medicine? During ensuing centuries, scholars have been unable—and unwilling—to free themselves of the image handed down by the Renaissance, by those wishing to enhance their own reputation for originality. Nonetheless, to judge by the evidence, and despite their own claims, the scholars of the Renaissance owed more to the Middle Ages than they did to antiquity. True, it is difficult to place the contribution of medieval medicine in a broad historical landscape or in a simplified reconstruction with any great precision. We can cite the establishment of an educational system, the official sanctioning of the practice of dissection, the originality of one author or another, or the development of some given problem. Its most distinctive characteristic, nevertheless, remains its unfailing persistence to examine its own progress: aside from any intrinsic historical interest, this can serve as fertile ground for an examination of scholastic medicine.

The medicine described as "scholastic"—from a term that originally meant only "scholar," or "pupil," and referred to the teaching done in cathedral schools—did not disappear with the end of the Middle Ages. In the sixteenth and seventeenth centuries, for instance, physicians continued to read Avicenna's "Canon of Medicine" and to employ the same methods of reasoning used in the thirteenth and fourteenth centuries. All the same, the continuation of this tradition can hardly be isolated from the new currents of thought that sprang up in the same period: the various components of a certain period's body of thought must all be taken together, lest we misread the meaning of one or the other of them. For this same reason, we will not consider the period after the middle of the fifteenth century; we shall draw a line at the years of the invention of printing and the earliest humanist translations.

The Establishment of Medicine as a Scientific Discipline: From Alexandria to Salerno

One of the accomplishments of the Western Middle Ages was to force society at large, and the world of scholarship in particular, to accept once and for all the intellectual standing of medicine. Of course, this standing had been advocated from earliest antiquity, through the work of major thinkers and celebrated schools, but alongside these thinkers and outside these settings free rein had been given to a practice based on no theoretical principles whatever, theoretical principles that would have had to be based on an interpretation of physical and biological phenomena. The decisive transition—which would lead to the establishment of scientific medicine and would thrust out into the no-man's land of charlatanism all practice that failed to conform to commonly accepted doctrine—occurred during the eleventh and twelfth centuries. At this time, one of the several currents handed down from antiquity to the Middle Ages prevailed: Western medicine chose in favor of Galenism.

In a well known article entitled "Von Alexandrien nach Bagdad" [From Alexandria to Baghdad], the Orientalist Max Meyerhof[2] demonstrated the importance of Alexandrian teachings during the fifth and sixth centuries A.D. in the development of Arab medicine. The Latin West drew upon the same heritage, at first directly, during the high Middle Ages and, later, through the vehicle of Arabic texts, during the eleventh century. Constantine of Africa undertook a number of translations, thus situating himself on the cusp of the two traditions and triggering a process that progressively came to affect all Western medical scholarship, dyeing it all in the same doctrinal hue. The concepts that his work triggered among the masters of the school of Salerno were the first manifestation of this process.

The High Middle Ages

We begin with Isidore of Seville (A.D. 570–636).

> Some ask why the art of medicine is not included among the other liberal disciplines. It is because whereas they embrace individual subjects, medicine embraces them all. The physician ought to know literature, "grammatica," to be able to understand or to explain what he reads. Likewise also rhetoric, that he may delineate in true arguments the things which he discusses; dialectic also so that he may study the causes and cures of infirmities in the light of reason. Similarly also arithmetic, in view of the temporal relationships involved in the paroxysms of diseases and in diurnal cycles. It is no different with respect to geometry because of the properties of regions and the locations of places. He should teach what must be observed in them by everyone. Moreover, music ought not to be unknown by him, for many things are said to have been accomplished for ill men through the use of this art, as is said of David who cleansed Saul of an unclean spirit through the art of melody. The physician Asclepiades also restored a certain insane man to his pristine health through music. Finally also, he ought to know astronomy, by which he should study the motions of the stars and the changes of the seasons, for as a certain physician said,[3] our bodies are also changed with their courses. Hence it is that medicine is called a second philosophy, for each discipline claims the whole of man for itself. Just as by philosophy the soul, so also by medicine the body is cured.[4]

When he was writing this passage of his masterwork, *Etymologiae,* European medicine, even in the few places where it was taught, was far from attaining this ideal of becoming a "second philosophy." The texts that survive from the period between the fifth and tenth centuries, so often described as the "dark ages," point to an exceedingly heterogeneous situation.[5] The manuscripts, largely transcribed in monasteries, abound in prescriptions and collections of pharmacopeia and feature works of a practical bent, offering summary descriptions of diseases and lists of treatments unsupported by any clear justification of their soundness. Nonetheless, bits of Greek medicine survived, fragmentary and heteroclite though they may have been. Translations were made of numerous Hippocratic texts (the treatises *Aphorismi, De aere, aquis, locis, De mulierum affectibus, De hebdomadibus, De natura hominis,* and *De diaeta* [*Regimen*]). The Galenic corpus was far more meager: it was limited to the treatise *De sectis ad eos qui introducuntur* and probably *Ars medica;* fragments of *Ad Glauconem de medendi methodo* and other works circulated, in the context of collections that were largely apocryphal. Soranus was more adequately represented, through adaptations by Caelius Aurelianus and a certain Mustio. Sections of the Byzantine encyclopedias by Oribasius, Alexander of Thralles, and, later, Paul of Aegina assembled some few elements of a body of knowledge that lay in shambles. It is difficult to make out in the whole of medical literature of the high Middle Ages—whether we are talking about translations, adaptations, or original works—the expression of any theoretical positions or of any clearly defined medical thought.

Without being able to determine the actual influence that medical thought exerted over the course of the centuries—a time that remains dim and unclear to historians—we can still make out a consistent tradition. If we are able to make out this tradition at all, however, it is by virtue of the continuity that was, in a certain sense, provided by the earliest translations from the Arabic. This tradition, which borrows its principal features from the late Alexandrian teachings, counted among its representatives a number of masters who taught at Ravenna, the capital of the Byzantine hexarchy from A.D. 568 to 752.[6] A certain Agnellus of Ravenna thus linked his name to a body of commentary on the works of Galen, which was used to introduce Alexandrian students to the study of medicine (*De sectis, Ars medica,* and *De pulsibus ad Theutras*).[7] A commentary on the *Ad Glauconem de medendi methodo* belongs, in all likelihood, to the same intellectual circle.[8] Of different geographical provenance (possibly from southern Italy, for example), a commentary on the *Aphorismi* of Hippocrates—which sometimes appears with attribution to Oribasius—as well as a number of pamphlets wrongly attributed to Soranus, served as introductions to the basics of Galenism and to the methods of philosophical and medical teaching practiced in Alexandria during the fifth and sixth centuries.[9]

These various works all reiterate the same concepts. In one commentary after another we find a general introduction to medicine. The preliminary method of exposition generally follows a well-established outline that dates back to the fifth-century philosopher Ammonius. One encounters again the idea first presented in the *Etymologiae* by Isidore of Seville:

"Medicine is the philosophy of the body, philosophy is the medicine of the soul." This statement is generally attributed to Aristotle. Despite the fairly arbitrary nature of this attribution, the fact remains that Alexandrian teaching did insist on the link—which typified medieval medicine— between the principles of Galen and the philosophy of Aristotle. If we take as an example the commentary on the treatise *De sectis,* attributed to Agnellus of Ravenna, we find the Aristotelian system of the four causes: the efficient cause is the medical act or the physician himself; the material cause is the human body; the instrumental cause is the lancet, the scalpel, or any other therapeutic instrument; and the final cause is the restoration of health. Applied fairly crudely here, this outline of the four causes was taken up again in more subtle ways throughout the course of the Arab and Latin Middle Ages. Among the reproofs that Agnellus addressed to the Methodics, we find that of failing to take into account another hierarchy that distinguishes among the immediate, the antecedent, and the conjunct causes. This hierarchy formed part of Western medical progress for a considerable period.

Alexandrian teaching also bestowed upon the Latin West a rigid division of the goals of medicine. First, we have the distinction—like that in philosophy—between a theoretical sector and a practical sector.[10] This division was not merely a matter of establishing the difference between thought and action; rather it meant singling out a purely speculative objective of the discipline of medicine. Theory strove to attain, for its own sake, knowledge of the function and malfunction of the human body. Practice, by contrast, partook equally of the realm of thought, but this thought was meant to lead to therapeutic action; such action was further broken down into the maintenance of health and the treatment of disease. Treatment included surgery, drugs, and diet.

The isolation of a sector that strove toward the attainment of disinterested knowledge gave medicine the standing of an intellectual discipline, among the very noblest. Theory included, in the most widespread classifications, three parts: "physiology," "etiology," and "semiology." Physiology concerned that area which the Latins called—beginning with the earliest translations from the Arabic—the *res naturales:* the four fundamental elements that make up the universe, the complexions, the humors, the solid parts of the body, the faculties or virtues, and the operations. The number and the role of the faculties or virtues that administer the chief functions of the human body were established by the Alexandrian physicians, who strayed from authentic Galenism on quite a few points.[11] We thus find definitions of an "animal" virtue (that is, of the *animus*, or "soul"), housed in the brain; a "vital" virtue, housed in the heart; and a "natural" virtue, housed in the liver. These three faculties corresponded to the tripartite nature of the soul, postulated by Plato and Aristotle. The study of the animal faculty offered medieval physicians an opportunity to venture into psychology and to skirt dangerously near the territory of theology. This faculty was broken down into rational, sensory, and motor functions. The rational sector was made up of imagination (which perceived and fixed the images provided by the senses), judgment, and memory. Each of these faculties was housed in one of the three zones into which the brain was divided, from front to back. Thus, beginning with the earliest Latin versions of the commentaries of Alexandrian origin, dating from the sixth and seventh centuries A.D., the idea of cerebral localization was introduced into Western thought. This idea was to have a long career ahead of it. Through a reading of these texts, we can see that the general principles on which scholastic medicine was based were already well known in Latin in the high Middle Ages. But it was not until the earliest translations from the Arabic that these principles were truly understood and used.

The Translations by Constantine of Africa

The figure of Constantine of Africa continues to fascinate historians.[12] Medieval biographers attributed to him linguistic knowledge and travels that largely belong to the realm of legend. From their accounts, however, it seems reasonable to believe that Constantine was born in North Africa, possibly in Carthage. It is not certain that he was of Muslim descent; it seems more likely that he formed part of one of the Christian communities surviving in the Maghreb. He reached southern Italy during the second half of the eleventh century, for reasons we have yet to determine. He took up residence in the monastery of Monte Cassino, where he became a monk. While living there, he translated a great many medical texts from the Arabic. He died prior to 1098.

Although southern Italy had undergone extensive Arab incursions—Sicily was under Arab occupation at this time—the strongest influence during the lifetime of Constantine of Africa was that of Byzantine culture. Despite the troubled relations with the Holy Roman emperor, at Monte Cassino, under the guide of the abbot Desiderius, Greek letters and arts flourished. The translator therefore undertook the introduction of Arab medicine in a powerfully Hellenistic setting. Long considered a shameless plagiarist, Constantine of Africa was blamed for putting his own name to the works he translated and for distorting the original text frequently and egregiously. Nowadays, however, he appears to have been like an author of remarkable skill. The Greek guise that he applied to Arabic texts, and the adaptations he made to fit the intellectual concerns of Western scholars, allowed them to be assimilated without great resistance.

Constantine of Africa translated the literature that had developed in North Africa during the tenth century, especially at Kairouan: treatises on dietetics, fevers, and urine, by the physician and philosopher Ishaq al-Isra'ili; a pamphlet on melancholy by Ishaq ibn 'Imran, which owed much to Rufus of Ephesus; a fundamental work on pathology by Ibn al-Gazzar, entitled *Breviarium dictum viaticum*. In this book, various diseases were presented according to their causes, their symptoms, and their treatments. He translated a treatise on the degrees of medicaments, that is, the four levels of intensity that each of the first qualities (heat, cold, dryness, and moisture) typifying them could attain. These works clarified and augmented Western learning considerably, in terms of diagnostics, description of diseases, and pharmacology.

If the texts written in Kairouan helped to enrich the stock of knowledge of Western physicians, two works from the Muslim east in the ninth and tenth centuries had a more profound influence, for they provided a theoretical framework. The framework was that of the late Alexandrian teachings, a faint echo of which had filtered through to readers of the high Middle Ages, in Greek and Latin versions. There can be no doubt that Constantine of Africa was well aware that he was contributing his translations from the Arabic to this context of continuity. In particular, he was familiar with the commentary, of Alexandrian inspiration, on the *Aphorismi* of Hippocrates; a tenth-century manuscript of this commentary still exists in the library of Monte Cassino.[13]

The earliest translation that we can attribute to Constantine of Africa is that of the *Ysagoge*, a text read by medical students until the end of the Middle Ages.[14] An abridged version of the *Quaestiones medicinae* by Hunayn ibn Ishaq, or Johannitius (a prolific translator from Greek to Arabic, working in the ninth century), this manuscript appears to be a plagiarism of the introductions to Galenism written by the Alexandrian masters of the fifth and sixth centuries. A comparison, for instance, with the commentary written by Agnellus of Ravenna on the treatise *De sectis ad eos qui introducuntur* reveals a number of features in common: postulation of the separation of medicine into theoretical and practical branches, the same further subdivisions of these two branches, an exposition of Aristotelian causality, and so on. We find differences as well, chiefly, the addition of a seventh *res naturalis*, or natural thing: the spirits, or *pneumata*, puffs of air that convey the faculties or virtues. Like the latter, they are three in number: the animal or psychic spirit, the vital spirit, and the natural spirit.[15] Although it had its obscure points—understandable given its concision—Hunayn ibn Ishaq's *Ysagoge* presented Alexandrian Galenism, as revised by the Arabs, more clearly than did its Greco-Latin counterparts of the high Middle Ages. The vocabulary was radically different as well, most of the Grecisms having been replaced by Latin words, understood by one and all.

Constantine also produced a free adaptation of the *Liber regius*, which had been written at the end of the tenth century by the physician of Persian descent 'Ali ibn al-'Abbas al-Magusi (known in the Latin West as Haly Abas). Entitled the *Pantegni* ("all the art"), it was to become one of the chief reference works, overshadowed only by Avicenna's "Canon of Medicine."[16] While taking into account the accomplishments of Arab medicine, especially the work of Rhazes, al-'Abbas also hearkened back to two traditions of the late Greek world. He borrowed from the Alexandrian commentators the subdivision into theory and practice. This subdivision served as the basis for breaking his great work into two parts; he adopted the Alexandrian method of exposition in eight principal points, the *accessus ad auctores* used by Latin authors in the Middle Ages.[17] Moreover, he emulated the ambition of the Byzantine encyclopedists of collecting in a single book all of the knowledge necessary to a physician. Constantine of Africa accentuated the Greek nature of this work by eliminating all the references made by al-'Abbas to his Arab predecessors. In the same spirit, he prefaced the *Pantegni* with a list of the sixteen books or groups of books that made up the Alexandrian Galenic canon.[18] Thus, a doctrinal direction had clearly been announced, and the West was now constantly questing after the ideas of Galen.

Aside from the theoretical framework that it provided, the *Pantegni* served as a manual, a source of fundamental knowledge in all fields. In particular, it offered information on the subject of anatomy, a science that had been poorly represented in the high Middle Ages; nothing more than a summary enumeration of the principal organs in a few works could be found, most notably in a number of pamphlets by the fourth-century author Vindicianus.[19] Should we view this erosion of anatomy in the high Middle Ages as a result of widespread adherence to the methodic doctrine, broadly diffused through the numerous adaptations of the work of Soranus? Or was it a result, more simply, of the difficulties encountered by translators faced with a technical vocabulary that they could not grasp? The works of classical Latin, and the language itself, were, in fact, particularly inadequate in this field. The *Pantegni* bridged a gap by offering an exposition of Galenic anatomy, no longer limited to just the principal organs. Still, this exposition was a summary and confused one, and the Latin translation in some places simply left out words that were essential to the meaning. Constantine of Africa never managed to provide a literal translation. In other fields, ellipsis and concision might have the fortunate result of lightening the style of the original, without any loss in meaning. In the field of anatomy, the resulting lack of precision could be quite unfortunate.

Let us take the example of the esophagus, which al-'Abbas described as follows: "The esophagus is an elongated structure, hollow and rounded in shape. It begins with the mouth of the stomach and terminates at the upper extremity of the larynx. There where it begins, at the mouth of the stomach, it is narrow, and then it widens constantly until it reaches the larynx, to that its widest section is located there."[20] Constantine of Africa twice neglected to translate the Arabic word *fam*, which means "mouth" or "orifice." The description was thus considerably altered: "*Meri* [from the Arabic word meaning esophagus] is a long, round, hollow corpuscle, that begins in the stomach, and runs to the upper part of the throat; at its origin, it is narrow, then it widens gradually until it reaches the extremity of the throat."[21] The earliest readers of the *Pantegni* therefore believed that the author made no distinction between the esophagus and the opening of the esophagus into the stomach (the cardia).[22] Despite these inaccuracies, a place was once again established for anatomy in the heart of Western medical knowledge. The description of the *membra*, or solid parts of the body,[23] became part of the study of the seven "natural things" that formed the foundation of theoretical medicine.

The Contribution of the Masters of the School of Salerno

Already renowned in the tenth century for the skill of its physicians, the school of Salerno[24] paved the way for the entry of medicine into the universities. It is likely that other circles contributed equally to this process—in northern France or at Montpellier, for instance—but they certainly left fewer surviving traces.[25] Salernitan works with a wide range of purposes survive from the eleventh and twelfth centuries:[26] brief anatomical treatises based on the dissection of pigs, books of antidotes and collections of pharmacopeia, *Regimens,* and *Practicae* that describe various diseases and illustrate their treatment. There was also a series of commentaries, particularly worthy of attention in this context. Dating from the second half of the twelfth century, these commentaries most likely reflect the content of the course lessons. They refer to a set of texts—a sort of medical canon—which the Salernitan masters had painstakingly assembled and which remained in use until the Renaissance, when it was published in numerous editions under the name "Articella" (or "Little Art").[27] The core of this work consisted of translations dating from the eleventh century, from the Greek or Arabic: the *Ysagoge,* by Hunayn ibn Ishaq; the *Aphorismi, Prognosticon,* and *De diaeta acutorum,* by Hippocrates; *Ars medica* by Galen; *De urinis* by the sixth- or seventh-century Byzantine writer Theophilus; and a treatise entitled *De pulsibus,* ostensibly by a certain Philaretes but largely derived from a pseudo-Galenic pamphlet. These texts were commented on at Salerno in the light of yet other translations, like Constantine of Africa's *Pantegni,* and the treatise *De natura hominis* by Nemesius, third-century bishop of Emesa,[28] turned into Latin from the Greek by Alphanus, the archbishop of Salerno from 1058 to 1085.

The commentaries on *Ysagoge* offered the Salernitan masters an opportunity to describe their vision of the medical art and to set forth the fundamental principles of their doctrine. They felt strongly, first of all, about establishing a place in the entire body of human learning for their discipline. Excluded from the seven liberal arts—subdivided into the *trivium* (grammar, rhetoric, and dialectics) and the *quadrivium* (arithmetic, geometry, astronomy, and music)—medicine was most frequently considered a mechanical art. This meant that it was ranked as a human activity directed toward useful and practical purposes, without a speculative vocation.[29] The classification of the sciences by the theologian Hugh of Saint-Victor, composed sometime in the 1120s, still treated medicine this way, among the disciplines that were not based on a study of causes. At the time that Hugh of Saint-Victor was writing his *Didascalion,* this classification was no longer tenable: the introduction of Galenism, through the translations of the eleventh century, had made the search for causes one of the fundamental features of medical procedure. The theologian himself cited the *Ysagoge.* But he did so in an abbreviated manner, which allowed him to preserve the consistency of his own system. One can see in the work of Hugh of Saint-Victor clear indications of a reluctance to accept the development of scientific medicine.

It is true that the qualification of medicine as a "second philosophy" or a "philosophy of the body" in the work of Isidore of Seville and in the Alexandrian commentaries was quite vague, since it was still necessary to extract medicine from its standing among the mechanical arts. With clear reference to a tradition of Stoic origin,[30] Constantine of Africa, in his prologue to the *Pantegni,* declared that human knowledge ("the generality of all science") was divided into three disciplines, physics (which incorporated metaphysics), ethics, and logic. He concluded that medicine did not belong exclusively to any of these three branches, since it was founded on logical arguments and since it treated phenomena that were both natural and moral. Medicine thus wavered, from one author to another, and at times even in the context of the same work,[31] from the rather ignoble standing of a mechanical art to the more eminent but still vague level of a discipline that included all the others.

The Salernitan masters of the second half of the twelfth century finally adopted a satisfactory solution. Following the various systems of classification used in the high Middle Ages, they subdivided philosophy (the whole of human knowledge based on reason) into three branches: ethics, logic, and "theoric," which gathered together metaphysics, mathematics, and physics (or the science of nature).[32] Medicine belonged to the branch of physics; its sister disciplines were the science of meteors (meteorology) and physics in the narrow sense. In turn, medicine was broken down into theory and practice, each of which was considered a science in its own right, that is, a discipline based on reflection and reasoning. According to Bartholomaeus of Salerno, theory was the science of causes, and practice the science of signs; it was not possible for practice to exist without the previous existence of theory. A formula that appeared in the work of one of the earliest commentators, Archimatthaeus of Salerno, was cited again by Maurus of Salerno: those who had no theory, such as certain apothecaries, could not be deemed *practicos;* they were simple operators *(simplices operatores).* At Salerno, therefore, the model was established of the learned practitioner, for whom therapeutic action was based on a search for causes, according to the principles of Galenic medicine.

The identification of medicine as part of physics was also the stance taken, in the same period but independently and slightly differently, by Dominicus Gundisalvi, a Toledan translator and philosopher. In his *De divisione philosophiae,* he relied on Avicenna's *Logica* to establish medicine as a science subordinate to physics or natural science.[33] Medicine was subordinate, and not an integral part, for it did not study the human body as such (which was one of the purposes of natural science), but rather sought to determine whether the body was healthy or sick. In the twelfth century, what was generally meant by "physics" corresponded to the definition given by Boethius: the study of the nonabstract things of matter subject to movement.[34] It included the science of the stars and that of the sublunary world, subject to generation and corruption. Since the Salernitans were not familiar with the zoological writings of Aristotle, which had not yet been translated into Latin, they essentially developed a medical physics, based on *Physica* and on the treatise *De generatione et corruptione*,[35] as well as on the neo-Platonic concepts found in Chalcidius's commentary on *Timaeus*.

The culmination of this thinking can be found in the work of Ursus of Salerno, the last great Salernitan master of the twelfth century. In the prologue to one of his theoretical works, *De commixtionibus elementorum libellus* [On the mixture of elements], he noted that the Latins were chiefly interested in writing books about practice, "which list the different methods of treatment, in accordance with the variety of diseases and the causes, deduced from the symptoms." Ursus of Salerno himself devoted many treatises to this practical branch: one on the effects of medications, the others on critical days, the pulse, and urine. These latter works did not limit themselves to listing the rules to be followed in establishing diagnosis and prognosis; according to the definition that the author himself provided, they tended to "teach, by the light of evident reasoning, how the pulse and the urine are altered by the different qualities that act, accidentally or naturally." The interaction of the first qualities lies at the center of Ursus of Salerno's philosophy. His adoption of the Galenic notion of complexion (the outcome of the mixture of first qualities in a natural body) was the most important consequence of the translations of Constantine of Africa. At Salerno, this notion was intimately tied to the physics of the elements, since humors were the "daughters" of the elements, as the formula went in the *Pantegni*. In *De commixtionibus* Ursus of Salerno took the logic of the underlying system used by natural philosophers and physicians of the twelfth century to an extreme.[36] Beginning with the first matter, the Creator formed the four elements, which themselves—by virtue of their substantial qualities (heat, cold, moisture, and dryness) and their accidental qualities (lightness, heaviness, mobility, fineness, and so on)—then blended to create the so-called elementals, which are the natural bodies. Although they never exist in a pure state in the tangible world, the elements—through their transformation or destruction, prompted by the interaction of qualities—guide all natural phenomena, including the functions of the human body. For instance, the faculty of digestion is implemented through the heat of fire and the moisture of the air, which work together to dissolve foods.

To explain the range of states and actions, Ursus of Salerno relied on a subdivision of each element into three "species" (superior, middle, and inferior), which correspond to the degrees of intensity of the qualities. The interplay of the species and their qualities was formulated in terms of mathematical combinations and served to explain the chief characteristics of the tangible world: color, odor, and weight, as well as stability and movement. In another work, a commentary on his own "Aphorisms,"[37] Ursus of Salerno placed the spirits, or *pneumata,* at the center of his account. Instruments of the soul of the world or, in humans, of the rational soul, the *pneumata* are largely formed of air and fire. They permit the accomplishment of desired actions, by establishing a link between soul and body. Thus, at the cost of altering the theory of the elements, Ursus of Salerno succeeded in providing a single explanation of the diversity of the real world, extending from matter to psychological states. His medicine can, without exaggeration, be described as iatrophysics.

Aside from this advance in theory, the Salernitan masters proposed methods of teaching that were forerunners of university scholasticism. Taking inspiration, on the one hand, from the medical tradition, especially the late Alexandrian tradition, and, on the other hand, from the new directions of Western philosophy, they developed the genre of the commentary, itself a reflection of the *lectio,* a study and interpretation of the authoritative texts. When the universities of the thirteenth century, at Montpellier or Bologna, commented in their turn on the *Ysagoge* of Hunayn ibn Ishaq or the *Aphorismi* of Hippocrates, they were doing nothing more than continuing the exegesis of the Salernitan masters, with whose work they were familiar. Another teaching method that was inaugurated at Salerno was the *quaestio.* Much like the theologians or jurists of the twelfth century, physicians began to make use of the procedure of the *quaestio* to present and resolve contradictory arguments, when the reading of a text presented a problem of interpretation.[38] Likewise, the Salernitan teaching methods continued the tradition of Aristotle's *Problemata* by formulating different questions, concerning medicine or natural philoso-phy, not strictly linked to a text.[39] The *Quaestiones salernitanae* continued to feed endless university debates.

The Debates of University Medicine

The admission of a discipline into the university framework implied the adoption of the methods of teaching that were accepted there. Medicine was no exception to this rule. Like their colleagues who studied and taught the arts, theology, and the law, masters of medicine based their teachings on the reading of authoritative texts and the division of those texts into *puncta*, or points—phrases that could be subjected to exegesis and discus-sion.[40] Despite their determination to preserve and reinforce the intellec-tual standing of medicine, they could not get around the difficulties in-volved in fitting into this framework the operative aspect of medicine, with its inescapable components of improvisation or skill. Is medicine a science or an art? This classic and eternal question returns like a leitmotiv over the course of the centuries, with different answers, depending on the age, the setting, and the individuals in question. At the heart of the debate lay the respective roles played by reason and experience, a fundamental problem that did not escape the notice of scholastics.

The Institutional and Intellectual Context

Until the middle of the fourteenth century, three main universities enjoyed a virtual monopoly on the teaching of medicine: Bologna, Montpellier, and Paris. In the thirteenth century, sporadic teaching was also done at Siena and Piacenza. The university of Naples, founded in 1224 by the Holy Roman emperor Frederick II, underwent an endless series of vicissi-tudes. Despite its renown in the fields of theology and philosophy, Oxford never attained a high level in medicine during the Middle Ages; neither did Cambridge. Inaugurated in 1222, medical teaching at Padua did not develop in full until 1350. At the end of the Middle Ages, centers of education developed throughout Europe: in Spain, in the Holy Roman Empire, and in other French and Italian cities.[41]

In Montpellier, there is documentary evidence of a school as early as the first half of the twelfth century, but the term "university" does not appear until 1220, on the occasion of the issuance of the university stat-utes. In Paris, physicians appeared in the context of the university in 1213.

The organization of their teaching was laid down in the statutes drawn up between 1270 and 1274. In Bologna, although an embryonic medical teaching staff seems to have existed earlier, the college of physicians did not establish its effective and organized presence until the 1260s, coalescing around the master Taddeo Alderotti. Despite minor differences between one university and another, these three centers developed a body of medical thought that drew on the same sources and reflected the same concerns. The exchange of ideas and methods occurred through the circulation of manuscripts and of people.

Historians sometimes contrast the rather professional orientation of Montpellier and Bologna—both subject to the influence of leading departments of jurisprudence—with the more intellectual orientation of Paris, where theology dominated.[42] In reality, this contrast begins to seem less plausible if we read many of the works produced by each of these circles. The chief distinction lies in the more limited production of texts found at Paris, which would seem to suggest a greater preference for action. Beginning in the fourteenth century, the masters of the department of medicine were principally concerned with seeking employment in the service of the king or of the aristocratic households.[43] The most important documentation widely adduced in favor of the existence of a markedly greater degree of intellectualism is the *Conciliator differentiarum philosophorum et praecipue medicorum* by Peter of Abano, a collection of scholastic questions. It is not known whether this work is more greatly influenced by the teachings of the arts or medicine, by the circles of Paris or Italy.[44] The texts written by the masters of the Faculté de Medecine show all the signs of a greater concern for teaching: the late-thirteenth-century *Concordantiae* by Jean de Saint-Amand was continued around 1350 by Pierre de Saint-Flour. This body of work is a collection of quotations of authorities, along with the solutions to a series of questions, arranged in alphabetical order and by key words. It had no counterparts or equivalents in other universities. As for the *Compendium de epidemia*, regarding the plague— the product of a concerted effort by the entire department, drawn up at the king's command in 1348—it was triggered by the solemnly proclaimed desire to work for the "public welfare." Moreover, the consultations of the master Guillaume Boucher, collected at the end of the fourteenth century by a German scholar, show that teaching was done at the patient's bedside. Counter to our received ideas on the subject, medical education as it was known in Paris tended to be more pragmatic than intellectual.[45]

Prior to undertaking medical studies, it was generally necessary to have attended a *cursus artium.*[46] The ideal situation—advocated so many centuries earlier by Isidore of Seville—had thus been attained. An offspring of the venerable *trivium* and *quadrivium,* the education given in the departments of arts had replaced dialectic (the simple initiation into a mastery of discourse) with logic. The other chief innovation was the introduction of natural philosophy. These two modifications can safely be attributed to the enrichment of the Aristotelian corpus known in Latin, as a result of translations. In Bologna, the ties between the arts and medicine were strengthened by the convergence of these disciplines into the context of a single college.

The program of courses was defined less by subjects and more by the list of texts—of Greek and Arabic origin—that the student was expected to have heard the masters read aloud, while providing commentary. After the literal explanation, the *lectio* relied on the *quaestio* to solve semantic difficulties and to compare and contrast the opinion of the author in question with that of other authors. Quite apart from the use of the *lectio,* university education relied on the *disputatio,* an exercise whereby numerous participants, both masters and students, presented conflicting arguments concerning a given problem. We have documentation concerning the *disputatio* dating back to the statutes of 1220 of the university of Montpellier.[47] On the one hand, this custom allowed Western physicians to single out the contradictions to be found in the ideas of their Greek and Arabic predecessors; it also allowed them to establish, in a dialectical manner, their own body of thought. On the other hand, it led to a fragmentation of the general body of knowledge into a multitude of other problems. This created a poor setting for a general review of the overall explanatory system. The pertinence of a problem introduced by the reading of a text was never questioned.

The questions found in the commentaries of Taddeo Alderotti, which date from the second half of the thirteenth century, offer a good example of the potential subjects for discussion.[48] All areas of interest were touched upon, ranging from the fundamentals of physiology and pathology to the matter of *res naturales, non naturales,* and *contra naturam,*[49] and the effects of certain medicines. The considerable number of questions relating to the issue of complexion demonstrates the central importance of that concept in university teaching, much as was the case at Salerno. Learned medieval medicine was not primarily "humoral," as is too often stated; it tended to operate first and foremost on the basis of complexion and, through that Galenic concept, on the idea of quality. One century after the Salernitan discussions, the problem of elements and their mixture remained current. Avicenna's "Canon of Medicine" introduced a number of new questions, for example: "Is the specific form caused by the elements?" In Avicenna's work, "specific form"[50] refers to the property of a substance that could not be deduced from the mixture of first qualities. It was essentially defined by its effects, which could be perceived only through experience. Certain questions posed by Taddeo Alderotti could serve perfectly as grist for the mills of the detractors of scholasticism: "When a finger is cut, is this a disease in number or in quantity?" or else "Are rockfish, if prepared with vinegar, leeks, salt, and oil, good for patients suffering from fever?"

We cannot deny the existence of this aspect of scholasticism, which passed everything through the sieve of logical argumentation. Nonetheless, the matters at stake were generally more important and sometimes involved the very principles of life. Thus, Pietro Torrigiano, one of the students of Taddeo Alderotti, set forth two fundamental problems in his commentary on Galen's *Ars medica:* "Does the spiritual [vital] virtue give life?" and "Is the soul the act of the body that possesses life?"[51] These questions were treated purely in medical and philosophical terms; theology was never called upon in any way. In contrast with what is too often claimed, the physicians of the Middle Ages knew how to make this important distinction. Their knowledge was secular, even when they belonged to institutions supported by the church in which they were clerics.[52] In the Bolognese setting, at the turn of the fourteenth century, the movement of the heart and the origin of the pulse were also the subject of numerous debates. One of the questions disputed by Alberto de Zanchariis concerned this matter: "Is the principle of the arterial and cardiac pulse a virtue of the soul or merely incorporated heat?"[53] In his commentary on *Ars medica,* Torrigiano devoted three long sections to this problem.[54] Torrigiano demonstrated the inadequacy—in philosophical terms—of the position held by most Galenists, who considered the pulse to be a manifestation of the vital virtue, attributing to the dilation and contraction of the vessels the role of purifying the spirit issuing from the heart, regulating its transmission. Increasingly influenced by the interpretation of Aristotle, Torrigiano concluded that the pulse was the result of a mechanical process, due to the heating of the blood.

The questions that have survived for our consideration reflect in some cases true scientific debate—the expression of what we might fairly call "research"—and in other cases, mere scholastic exercises designed to train students in logical reasoning and remind them of fundamental knowledge. We could place the *Quodlibet* of Giacomo da Piacenza in this second category.[55] Presented in Bologna in the 1320s, it contained ten questions, nine on theory and one on practice. The first three concerned "natural things": "Is the virtue of nutrition essentially the same thing as the virtue of growth?" "Can there be a spirit that is radical to, or mixed with, the members that is greater than the heat of the complexion or the spirit that runs?" and "Is it possible to see something that is inside the eye?" Two questions followed on "non-natural things": "Can air temper the heat of our body?" "Can celestial bodies be the cause of a crisis on earth?" Then came four questions on "things against nature," that is, infirmity and disease: "Should a child born with a major malformation of the foot be described as ill *ut nunc* or *simpliciter*?" "Is there such a thing as a sextan fever?" "Is it hard to eliminate the dryness of the liver, or its humidity?" "Can any day be critical?" The *Quodlibet* ended with the question *in practica*: "Should one bleed a patient at the beginning of a sanguinary aposteme?"

Despite its scholastic nature, this set of questions, linked as it was to the reading of Hunayn ibn Ishaq's *Ysagoge*, confronted some fundamental issues, which were at times the subject of harsh debate. Thus, the question about the newborn infant's malformed foot refers back to a complex interpretation of a Galenic text, involving the definitions of the normal and the pathological, in their various degrees. At the beginning of Galen's *Ars medica*, the author distinguishes—with reference to the states of health and disease, and a neutral state—a category of *haplos* (*simpliciter*, meaning "simply" or "absolutely") and another category of *en to nun* (*ut nunc*, or "inasmuch as in the present").[56] Since Galen himself had been fairly unclear, the various medieval interpretations posited a contrast between a congenital state and an acquired state, between nature and accident, between a permanent and a passing state, and so on. In the work of Gentile da Foligno, during the first half of the fourteenth century, this distinction led to a definition of the neutral state as an intermediate state—intermediate, however, between *simpliciter* health and *ut nunc* health, rather than between health and sickness. The *Quodlibet* of Giacomo da Piacenza thus provides documentation of a question that was particularly debated in the Bolognese circle of the fourteenth century.

The Authorities

In the field of medicine, there was no break in the pace of translating—from both Greek and Arabic—between the eleventh and fourteenth centuries.[57] Following the achievements of Constantine of Africa, Gerard of Cremona took up the torch, working in Toledo in the second half of the twelfth century. He considerably enriched the stock of translated texts: numerous works by Rhazes, Avicenna's "Canon of Medicine," *Cyrurgia* by Albucasis (al-Zahrawi), the *Practica* by Serapion (Ibn-Sarabiyun, eleventh century), and the commentary of Ibn Ridwan on Galen's *Ars medica.* These were the works used most widely until the end of the Middle Ages. Their popularity continued even longer, for they were still being published by printers of the Renaissance. At the same time that these writings from the Muslim East and West were being translated, Gerard of Cremona had translated a number of Arabic adaptations of Galenic treatises: *De complexionibus, De simplicium medicamentorum temperamentis et facultatibus, Methodus medendi, De crisibus, De diebus decretoriis,* and so on. This Arabo-Latin corpus was echoed by the Greco-Latin translations being done by Burgundio da Pisa, also during the second half of the twelfth century. At times, he was translating the same texts as Gerard of Cremona. The effort to assemble the authentic and complete works of Galen formed the framework of the concerns of the Middle Ages: at the turn of the fourteenth century, Peter of Abano undertook the completion of the project begun by Burgundio da Pisa, but it was not until Niccolò da Reggio (1308–1345) that the Galenic corpus was truly augmented in any significant fashion. After the thirteenth century, nothing more was translated from Arabic. In 1282, by order of Charles I of Anjou, king of Sicily, Farag ibn Salim translated into Latin the voluminous work by Rhazes, *Continens* [Book that contains all]. Other works with a practical intent had been translated as well: the Taisir that Ibn Zuhr, the great twelfth-century Andalusian physician, had dedicated to Averroës and, most important, a body of treatises attributed to a pseudo-Mesue. These treatises presented a general picture of the chief diseases, with their treatments; it was largely based on Galen, as well as on the Hippocratic tradition.

The progressive arrival of all these translations, up to the middle of the fourteenth century, provided many opportunities to renew university education. At first, oddly enough, university teaching was not based on the more recent translations done during the twelfth century, but rather relied on the corpus of the "Articella," which formed the foundation of the curriculum required of the students. The Parisian statues of 1270–1274 did not mention any texts but these. The university teachers still followed the path blazed by the Salernitan teachings; innovation was put off for some later time, although the works that had been translated more recently were used by the masters to buttress their arguments.[58] The turning point came, simultaneously in Montpellier, Paris, and Bologna, during the years from 1270 to 1320. Avicenna's "Canon of Medicine" made its debut in the study programs, as did the "New Galen,"[59] a reference to the translations by Gerard of Cremona and Burgundio da Pisa. This twofold introduction coincided with the assimilation of Aristotle's zoological corpus, translated for the first time from the Arabic by Michael Scotus in Toledo around 1210, and translated again later, this time from the Greek by Guillaume de Moerbeke around 1260. Aristotle's medical views were reinforced by the interpretation that Averroës gave of them in his *Colliget*, translated by a Jew named Bonacosa, in 1285, and in the commentary on Avicenna's *Poem on Medicine*, translated in Montpellier by Armengaud Blaise in 1284.

The five decades from 1270 to 1320 were marked by this rather rough confrontation between Galenism and Aristotelianism. In the eyes of historians, this has become the prime concern of medical scholasticism. In reality, however, it is necessary to distinguish three levels in the use that physicians made of the work of Aristotle, without counting the study of elementary logic, common to every intellectual of the Middle Ages.

The first level consisted of a reliance on Aristotelian physics to explain natural phenomena and to place the functioning of the human body within an overall interpretation of the universe. As we have already seen, this procedure had been adopted at Salerno.

The second level involved the consideration of Aristotle's theories concerning anatomy and physiology. It was at this level that conflicts with Galenic medicine were most frequent.

The third level involved problems of method and of scientific investigation. It relied not on the texts of natural philosophy but on the *Prior Analytics* and the *Metaphysics*.

On more than one occasion, Galen himself had indicated his differences with Aristotle's anatomy and physiology. Among those differences preserved by scholasticism were, in order of importance, the respective roles of the heart and the brain, the origin of sperm, and the existence of a female seed taking an active part in conception.[60] According to Aristotle, the heart was the source of heat and life; it governed not only the vessels (no distinction being made between veins and arteries), but also sensation and movement.[61] According to the Galenists, by contrast, there were three or four principal organs: the brain, the heart, and the liver. These were respectively the source of the nerves, the arteries, and the veins. The testicles, which might also be counted among the principal organs, completed the development of sperm, which originated from the blood. This disagreement between the two authorities led to different sorts of questions: Is the heart the only principal organ? Is it nobler than the brain? Do the nerves originate from the brain? and so on. The masters answered these questions in many different ways. Taddeo Alderotti maintained an Aristotelian position, while making subtle changes of his own.[62] He held that, in the sense of "principal instrument of an operation," there are four principal organs; in the sense of "principal root," there is but one: the heart. Likewise, the nerves may have their origin in the heart, but it is in the brain that they become perfect transmitters of sensation and movement. The Bolognese students of Taddeo Alderotti put their support behind Galen, for the most part. The celebrated anatomist Mondino de' Liuzzi wasted no time on trying to reconcile the two authorities: "It has been established that the opinion of Aristotle has been the cause of great errors in medicine, and that is why it is better to rely upon Galen than Aristotle."[63] Pietro Torrigiano, however, being a bit more of a philosopher, considered the heart the foremost organ of the body. The heart, he felt, was associated in some way with the soul; it was the origin of the heat and vital spirit that flowed through the body. All the same, he thought that the brain was the source of all sensation and movement, as well as the origin of the nerves.

The turn of the fourteenth century at the university of Montpellier was a period marked by the personality of Arnald of Villanova, who died in 1311. Physician to the king of Aragon and to the pope, translator from the Arabic as well as a heterodox theologian, Arnald of Villanova wrote a great many medical works that revealed a vigorous body of thought, which hearkened back to an "authentic" Galenism.[64] Concerning the issue of cardiocentrism, or the supremacy of the heart, he adopted a position quite close to that held by Pietro Torrigiano.[65] Certainly, the heart was the "prime principle," but an organ is described as "principal" when it is the seat of a faculty (a "virtue") that influences and directs other parts of the body. There are four organs that fit this description: the heart, the liver, the brain, and the testicles. They could be described as "manifest or proximate principles." It was of no particular concern to a physician that the heart should be the prime principle. If some disturbance were to occur in the nutritional virtue, then the instruments of nutrition would require treatment, not the heart. Although he never said so, Arnald of Villanova relied on Avicenna, who stated in his "Canon of Medicine," concerning this disagreement between Aristotle and Galen: "As long as one looks at this problem more as a physician than a philosopher it is immaterial whether all faculties are centred in the heart or each has its own separate centre."[66] Conciliatory with regard to a number of crucial points of disagreement between Aristotle and Galen, Avicenna established boundaries between medicine and philosophy: "Although their [the physicians's] view appears to be superficially more plausible, the philosopher's [Aristotle's] view is really the correct one."[67] Following his lead, the masters of scholasticism distinguished between a *via philosophorum* and a *via medicorum*.[68]

Aside from the influence of Avicenna, we can discern in the work of Arnald of Villanova the influence of the model offered by astronomy.[69] The mathematical system of eccentrics and epicycles was not considered strictly true in terms of cosmology and the science of movement, but it served to do calculations that offered a reliable accounting of phenomena, as we can see from the prediction of eclipses. Likewise, medical science salvages appearances and makes it possible to treat diseases. The disagreements between Aristotle and Galen gave physicians an opportunity to redefine the meaning that they attributed to their art. For some of them, such as Arnald of Villanova, it was therapeutic action that should guide theoretical choice, since the sole purpose of medicine was practice. For others, such as Peter of Abano, since medicine was also a speculative science, it could have no other truth than that of natural philosophy.[70]

Limited as they were to a few general questions, the conflicts between Aristotelianism and Galenism triggered less medical controversy than did certain propositions of Avicenna or Averroës on more specific matters. Although it often served as a source of inspiration to him, Arnald of Villanova did not particularly esteem Avicenna's "Canon of Medicine." He condemned the book's popularity among his contemporaries, who were happy to recite it stolidly, without making the slightest effort to think for themselves. In numerous citations, he pointed out errors made by Avicenna, whom he suspected of having read Galen only superficially. The harshest controversies were in any case triggered by the reading of Averroës's *Colliget*. This work not only defended Aristotelianism but also sparked new debate—over minor points of detail—on a number of commonly accepted ideas. Thus, Averroës's definition of fever, for example—which presupposed a mixture of two types of heat, one natural and innate, the other counter to nature and pathological—led to countless disputes. At the center of this controversy lay the fundamental question of the mixture and alteration of qualities, and their variation in intensity.[71]

The influence of Aristotelian thought went well beyond a few matters of anatomy or physiology. Reading the *Nicomachean Ethics* and *Metaphysics*[72] led to a greater precision in the definition of medicine. Aristotle, in effect, made a distinction between *episteme* and *techne*, translated respectively by the Latin *scientia* and *ars*. "Science" consisted of a judgment of things that are universal and necessary; its conclusions, through demonstration, derive from first principles. "Art" belongs to the domain of doing; its origin derives not from the thing but from the artisan. It has to do with things that are contingent, and not with the necessary. Aristotle himself placed medicine in the realm of *techne*. Although the Salernitan commentators did not hesitate to accord the two parts of medicine—theory and practice—the standing of sciences, that position was no longer wholly tenable after the thirteenth century. While it was true that medicine was a science, given that it was based on universal principles (those of natural philosophy) and that it relied on demonstration, its object was contingent, the specific, which definitely tended to give it the standing of an art. At the heart of the innumerable medieval discussions, we can distinguish a tendency to make theory a science and practice an art. This accomplished nothing more than to shift the problem toward the matter of articulation among these two parts.[73]

Reading Aristotle also served to encourage thinking about method. Despite the adjustments called for in Avicenna's "Canon of Medicine," the system of the four causes set forth in the *Physics* was ill suited to medicine.[74] The material cause, in particular—which Avicenna linked to members, spirits, and humors, subject to health and to disease—could only with great difficulty be integrated into a Galenic system based on a modification of quality identified with the efficient cause. Pietro Torrigiano, for instance, considered only the search for this efficient cause to be of any use to the physician. More fruitful was the comparison that a number of commentators made between the three Galenic paths to knowledge in medicine and the theory of demonstration given in the *Prior Analytics*.[75] Taking inspiration from Ibn Ridwan, a number of authors drew correspondences between Galen's "analysis" (*dissolutio* or *resolutio* in Latin), his "synthesis" (*compositio*), the demonstration of the fact (*demonstratio quia*), and the demonstration of the cause (*demonstratio propter quid*).

In this way, attention shifted from the organization of knowledge, imagined by Galen, to scientific investigation. The discussions of the commentators of the fourteenth and fifteenth centuries tended to show the difficulty of applying the *demonstratio propter quid*—usually proper to the domains of mathematics and physics—to medicine. Their reflection drew equally on the distinction drawn by Averroës between the "demonstration of the sign" and the "demonstration of the cause."[76] This development was sometimes considered a major milestone between the *scientia experimentalis* of Robert Grosseteste and the Galenic method. This is a point of exceeding complexity, and it has given rise among modern critics to controversies worthy of scholasticism.[77] While the transposition of a system of thought proper to one era into another is always a dangerous thing, it remains true, nevertheless, that the confrontation between Galenism and Aristotelianism did not produce impasses only. Rather, it led to an increased depth in Western epistemological thought.

Reason and Experience

Around 1265, the English scientist and philosopher Roger Bacon wrote a treatise entitled *De erroribus medicorum*, translated into English as "On the Errors of Physicians."[78] Among the errors that he condemns in the book are a lack of familiarity with the simples used in medicaments, ignorance of languages other than Latin, and scorn for astrology and alchemy. Bacon's most violent attack, however, was leveled at the excessive penchant of doctors for logical argumentation:

> The generality of physicians give themselves up to disputes about numberless problems and useless arguments, and give no time to experience as they ought. Thirty years ago they used to give all their time to experience, but now by the art of "Topics" and "Elenchi" they multiply infinite casual questions, and still more infinite dialectic and sophistic arguments in which they get absorbed, so that they are ever seeking and never discovering truth. For discovery is by the path of sense, memory and experience especially in the applied sciences of which medicine is one.

This diatribe by Roger Bacon should be understood not as an all-encompassing condemnation of what scholastic medicine had become, but rather as simple historical evidence of a specific era. The period of thirty years to which Bacon refers corresponds to the establishment of medical education in the university of Paris, a town where the English scientist had lived more than once. It is likely that during this time the masters were chiefly concerned with adapting their discipline to the university context. This required that they develop the body of logical reasoning proper to any scholastic exercise. Petrus Hispanus, or Peter of Spain, who became pope in 1276 with the name of John XXI, had studied in Paris during the 1220s, before taking up teaching in Siena between 1246 and 1250. Aside from his commentaries on the "Articella," he wrote a major work of logic.[79] Following the approach delineated by Robert Grosseteste, Bacon worked to lay the foundations of a *scientia experimentais*. His conception of this science conferred on it three objectives: to certify the conclusions of deductive reasoning in the speculative sciences; to add to the ranks of the existing sciences a new body of knowledge, not available solely through reasoning; to succeed in unveiling the secrets of nature, beyond the limitations of existing sciences. With this last-mentioned objective, Roger Bacon's "experimental science" was once again linked with natural magic.

Although Bacon's reproof may well have been justified in a specific time and place, it is wrong to say that medieval physicians took no interest in experience. Indeed, they wrote extensively on the subject. What they rejected en masse, however, was blind empirical procedure, which still seems to have had a few adepts here and there.[80] The masters of the universities—like Galen before them—believed that all experience must be buttressed by reason. The theme of the relationship between reasoning and experience during the Middle Ages is far too vast to be treated in a few lines.[81] I shall limit myself here to indicating the chief questions raised by the commentary on the first aphorism of Hippocrates, where one reads that experience is "deceptive" or "treacherous," depending on which version one prefers of those found in medieval translations.[82] The definition given by the commentators of the term "experience" is Aristotle's definition: experience comes from a multitude of memories of a single thing.[83] While this definition may be better suited to acquired experience, to medical practice born of numerous attempts, when applied to the first aphorism of Hippocrates it serves chiefly to explain experimentation, and more precisely, pharmacological experimentation, which requires the repetition of the same intervention under identical conditions.

The tone had, in fact, been set by Galen; in his commentary, he advanced two fundamental ideas:[84] experimentation cannot be practiced on human beings as it is on other objects, because of the risks involved; interpretation is difficult, because the precise cause of the effect obtained cannot be isolated with certainty. In a fifteenth-century annotation to this last statement, Ugo Benzi insisted on the concept of time: the human body is subject to continuous variations, caused by internal and external factors; an identical effect can be obtained only over a brief lapse of time. This linked up with another idea from the same Hippocratic aphorism: "opportunity [is] fleeting." To conduct a pharmacological experiment successfully, Avicenna—following in the footsteps of Galen and al-'Abbas[85]—had established a list of conditions to follow. Six of those conditions would eventually cast new light on the relation between cause and effect; the seventh ruled out the use of animals, which could not yield results applicable to humans.

In their commentaries, the Italian masters linked the proposition "experience [is] treacherous" with the successive proposition, "judgment [is] difficult." They were then led to evaluate the degree of certainty that could be expected from the medical art, according to whether it was founded on reason, experience, or both together. This is the subject of a question posed by Gentile da Foligno (who died in 1348) in his commentary on Avicenna's "Canon of Medicine": "Can all knowledge in medicine be acquired with certainty?"[86] He devoted a lengthy analysis to its solution. In the course of the reasoning, we find the classic case of a medicament whose effect cannot be determined by any means other than experience, since its action is based on "the specific form," rather than on the interaction of the first qualities. The instance given is that of a rhubarb which attracts bile just as a magnet attracts iron. According to Gentile, only anatomical knowledge, confirmed through dissection, is obtained with certainty through experience. In other fields, this is not the case. In particular, "all knowledge whereby a physician must make a decision on the basis of an intensive or extensive quantity is conjectural or arbitrary." The first obstacle is found in the infinite variations of weights and measures, which make it impossible to interpret correctly the results obtained by another physician, in a different time or place.[87] The principal obstacle, however, is that previously pointed out by Galen: the difficulty of taking into account the various levels of intensity that a quality can attain.[88] The problem of quantifying qualities lay at the heart of numerous debates in the Middle Ages, in philosophy and in physics. Without question, in the field of medicine, it was Arnald of Villanova who took thinking on this subject to its highest level. Drawing on a pamphlet by al-Kindi, translated by Gerard of Cremona, Arnald proposed a mathematical system that would allow one to calculate the degrees of intensity—of heat, cold, dryness, and moisture—of a drug made up of many different simples. Despite the sophisticated technical nature of the calculations called for by Arnald of Villanova, and his laudable efforts in favor of quantification, the whole was based on the supposed division into "degrees" of the qualities of the simples. These degrees had been established by tradition or by an entirely subjective evaluation. In the fifteenth century, the Catalonian physician Antonio Ricart applied this method to the calculation of humoral mass.[89]

Physicians of the fourteenth and fifteenth centuries declared, on countless occasions, that it was impossible to obtain reliable and accurate measurements. Not merely mouthing a Galenic "dogma," they were expressing a growing awareness of a real obstacle. Outside anatomical observation and pharmacological testing, the authors saw no other possible applications for an experimental procedure. When, however, it was no longer a matter of medical knowledge as such, but of practical competence, acquired experience played a much more important role. Gentile da Foligno exhorted his reader: "Be sure that every medical knowledge yields fruit only after extensive habit and long experience. Good practice, subjected to the principles of the art and the ways of demonstration, depends upon a twofold approach: a scientific approach, which is taught, and an experimental approach, i.e., the acquisition of knowledge through exercise on specific cases. This last approach cannot be taught, but can only be acquired through habit."[90]

The New Currents in the Fourteenth and Fifteenth Centuries

From its origins till the end of the fifteenth century, university medicine was never a single, monolithic body of knowledge. Various currents ran through it: some of them were rich in promising innovations, while others tended toward a progressive disintegration. An intense surge in intellectual activity marked the years 1270–1320. The leading authors whom we have already mentioned—Taddeo Alderotti, Pietro Torrigiano, Arnald of Villanova, Jean de Saint-Amand, and Peter of Abano—all lived and worked during this period. In 1316 or 1317, Mondino de' Liuzzi published his *Anathomia*, the first treatise in the Western Middle Ages to describe the dissection of the human body. Looking back at the end of the fourteenth century and the beginning of the fifteenth century, a historian is struck primarily by the reappraisal of practice, a consequence both of the conditions imposed by the demands of society and, at the same time, of epistemological thought. This was also a time of doubt, accentuated by the epidemics of plague.

Reliance on Dissection

The history of dissection in the Middle Ages is difficult to separate from legend. Despite the efforts of medievalists to establish the facts, the phan-

toms that haunt their readers often win over the desire to explore historical reality. There is a subtle thrill that comes from scattering figurative
sulphur around the practice of opening bodies.[91] There is likewise a tendency to turn Mondino de' Liuzzi into either a hero daring to challenge
prohibitions or reticence, or else a symbol of medieval obscurantism.
Mondino did perform dissections, but, blinkered by limitless faith in the
observations of Galen and hindered by the quibbles of scholasticism, he
saw nothing. The problem of dissection thus crystallized the vision that
modern man, after the Renaissance, wished to form of the Middle Ages.

The church never explicitly forbade the dissection of human bodies.[92]
The judicial actions about which we know anything were carried out
against grave robbers and body thieves. This was the case, for example, in
the trial of four physicians, held in 1319 in Bologna. The physicians were
accused of stealing a freshly interred corpse and opening it at the home of
a certain Master Albert.[93] The only text that could be interpreted as a
prohibition of dissection was the papal decree *Detestande feritatis*, promulgated by Pope Boniface VIII, and dated September 27, 1299.[94] This
decree prohibited, on pain of excommunication, the dismembering of a
cadaver or the boiling of pieces of a cadaver to remove the flesh from the
bone. The decree was meant not to prohibit the work of anatomists, but
rather to discourage the custom of cutting up mortal remains to make it
easier to transport them, or else to divide them in different resting places,
in some cases in accordance with the last wishes of the deceased. This
procedure, developed solely to facilitate the long-distance transportation
of cadavers, had become in some sense fashionable by the last decades of
the thirteenth century, and it was against this mode that the pope issued
his decree. The minimal effect that this decree had on the spirit of the
anatomists is evident, considering that it emanated in the same years
during which dissection became increasingly common.

We find no evidence of any earlier regulations. The reluctance attributed to Christians, by certain authors of the Middle Ages, dates back to
well before the establishment of ecclesiastical power.[95] Galen already practiced dissection, working essentially on animals, in accordance with a
custom that was later taken up at Salerno. There, anatomical demonstration was based on the observation of a pig, considered the animal most
similar to humans. The first Salernitan *Anathomia* dates from the end of
the eleventh century and was attributed to a certain master Copho.[96] It is
impossible to determine whether the dissection of animals was practiced
elsewhere. A historian finds evidence of dissections only when they led to

the establishment of regulations or to the writing of an anatomical treatise. The same is true of the dissection of human cadavers.[97] If the *Anathomia* by Mondino de' Liuzzi constitutes the first explicit documentary evidence, it seems quite probable that the practice existed at Bologna during the last years of the thirteenth century.[98] There is no reason not to suppose that a number of physicians or surgeons may have been practicing dissections without publicizing their activity.

The chief innovation at Bologna was the idea of holding public events, intended to illustrate the teaching. The objective was essentially educational. Rather than stemming from problems obtaining whatever papal dispensation may have been required, the true obstacle to the spread of this practice lay in the difficulty of procuring a cadaver and preserving it in adequate conditions. The Parisian surgeon Henri de Mondeville, who held an anatomical demonstration in Montpellier in 1304, resolved this difficulty by making use of figures and an artificial skull. Although the first statute that called for a public session every two years dates from no earlier than 1340, it may well be that, in the period straddling the end of the thirteenth and the beginning of the fourteenth centuries, dissections were practiced at the university of Montpellier. A short time prior to the demonstration of Henri de Mondeville, Arnald of Villanova insisted on the necessity of observing corpses.[99] At Paris, the first anatomy found in the sources dates from as late as 1407.[100] Perhaps we should consider this delay one of the consequences of the corporate rivalries that split physicians and surgeons. Nonetheless, here and elsewhere, we should make a careful distinction between the official version and the actual state of practice.

Anatomical observation was not based merely on the "incision" of a cadaver, accompanied by a ceremony. Ossuaries offered ample opportunity to observe the organization of the skeleton. The surgeon Henri de Mondeville, at the turn of the fourteenth century, and the physician Jacques Despars, in the fifteenth century, explicitly referred to the observations they made in the cemetery of the Saints-Innocents of Paris. De Mondeville cited his observations to rebut Aristotle, who had stated that women's craniums had only one circular suture. Despars did so to refute the number of cranial bones proposed by Albertus Magnus.[101] Other opportunities for observation were provided by medical examinations. The earliest testimony available to historians dates from the turn of the thirteenth century. At the request of Pope Innocent III, physicians examined two victims, without opening their bodies. The custom of the "postmortem" examination—whether or not it resulted in autopsies—developed in settings marked by an extensive deployment of the law, especially in Bologna and in Provence.[102] Generally physicians and surgeons were jointly involved in these medical examinations.

A number of different social and cultural factors may be cited to explain the resurgence of a practice that had been abandoned for many centuries. At Bologna, the presence of the law, with its constant search for manifest evidence, may very well have played a role. The development of surgery certainly offered favorable conditions. Nonetheless, a growing reliance on dissection can be explained, essentially, by the growth of Western anatomical knowledge, based on Galenism. From the eleventh to the fourteenth centuries, Western science acquired a certain degree of precision. After *Pantegni*, Avicenna's "Canon of Medicine" became the principal work of reference. In Avicenna's first book, there is a description of the "similar parts," that is, bones, muscles, arteries, and veins. In the third book, there is an exposition of every disease that could affect the body, from head to foot, preceded by an anatomical description. As available information progressively became more precise, the contrasts among authorities increasingly prompted physicians to verify *de visu*. This prompting was made all the stronger by the fact that Galen's major anatomical works were not yet known, or were just beginning to be. The treatise *De locis affectis*, translated on two separate occasions, oriented the reader toward an awareness of the conformation and location of the various organs. The treatise *De usu partium corporis humani*, however, had not long been in circulation, and then was so only in an Arabo-Latin adaptation that covered only the first nine books. The complete Greco-Latin version, translated by Niccolò da Reggio, did not become available until 1317; this coincided with the publication of Mondino de' Liuzzi's *Anathomia*. The Bolognese master had thus never been able to consult it. The flourishing of Western anatomical science, therefore, can be explained by both the discovery of the Galenic texts and by the reliance—however exceptional—on dissection. The translation of the work *De usu partium corporis humani*, which offered detailed and consistent descriptions, was just as decisive for Europe in the fourteenth century as *Administrationes anatomicae* was in the sixteenth. Before one could criticize Galen, one had to reach his level. This was the long task that awaited medieval translators and physicians.

The debates over the respective roles of reason and experience should likewise be linked to this newfound dependence on observation. When

Gentile da Foligno listed the results of dissection among the reliable evidence that could be acquired through experience, he was probably influenced by Averroës's *Colliget*. The traditional breakdown of medicine into theory and practice gave anatomy an ambiguous status. An integral part of theory in terms of its subject matter (one of the seven *res naturales*), anatomy belonged nonetheless to the realm of practice in terms of the method whereby knowledge was acquired, based as it was on data received through the senses. The Bolognese statutes of 1405 (which basically called for education through the reading of Avicenna's "Canon of Medicine") show some evidence of this difficulty and the solution that was adopted. While the chapters in the first book, concerning the "similar parts," were excluded from the program *in theorica* and were not mentioned anywhere, the descriptions contained in the third book were included in the teaching *in practica*. Averroës's *Colliget* accorded a clear standing to anatomy. It explicitly stated that anatomy depended on an experimental approach, oriented toward practice, much the same as the study of the virtues of medications.[103] Anatomy thus acquired its own methods of teaching. We may well still wonder why the decision was made to cut open human cadavers, rather than pigs, as had been done at Salerno. It may be that the seventh rule stated in Avicenna's "Canon of Medicine," rejecting the reliability of pharmacological experimentation on animals, was taken to be applicable to all forms of experience. Moreover, the social prestige for which the university masters so yearned probably led them to recoil at the idea of imitating the workaday actions of butchers. They required a noble material on which to work. The experience of surgeons also led to a greater understanding of the differences between humans and animals. All the same, none of these reasons alone suffices to explain the lifting of so great a prohibition.

Despite the novelty of its presentation, Mondino de' Liuzzi's *Anathomia* was to a great degree still in thrall to book learning.[104] In *Anathomia*, the division between "similar parts" and "instrumental parts" was maintained, the former requiring a special preparation of the cadaver in order to be studied. The glaring errors made by Greek and Arabic predecessors were not corrected. The organs were described according to their physiological purpose. Lack of an inherited body of medical lore and ignorance of Galen's *Administrationes anatomicae* led to a renewed reliance on the late Alexandrian tradition. Mondino—and, after him, a number of anatomists right up until the sixteenth century—adhered to the descriptive grid set forth for the observation of cadavers in John of Alexandria's commentary on the treatise *Ad secta*.[105] Six characteristics were to be noted: the number of members (two kidneys, one liver, and so on), their nature (osseous, fibrous, and so forth), their location, their relative size, their shape, and their connections. Mondino added two further criteria to this list, which for the Alexandrians had been part of the observation of living bodies: necessity and operation. Lastly, Mondino called for a recitation of all of the diseases that could affect each anatomical element. Thus, the opening of the body made it possible to answer a number of questions established in advance, according to an interpretive scheme. This procedure was similar in method to the way in which books were analyzed according to an *accessus ad auctores*. The body was "read" before it could be "seen." Despite these limitations, anatomical discourse changed considerably from the fourteenth century onward.

Proof through dissection was still no more than a form of rhetorical argument. Even though many errors had been perpetuated, a number of minor details in the descriptions clearly spoke of a shift in the general point of view. For instance, it is well known that Mondino de' Liuzzi held tight to the idea of a division of the uterus. Two traditions were commonly accepted around that time: one, Galenic in origin, stated that the organ was split into two ventricles; the other, handed down from the eleventh century via the pseudo-Galenic treatise *De semine*, argued for seven divisions.[106] Even though the latter solution was not as widely found in the sources, Mondino opted for it. He observed seven cells in the uteri of two female bodies that he had dissected. Nonetheless, he added a restriction: "These cells are simply a sort of hollows in the matrix designed to allow sperm to coagulate with menstrual blood."[107] The purpose that tradition assigned to these cells had been preserved, but they had lost much of their reality. For that matter, one may well wonder whether Mondino had not actually chosen seven on the basis of actual observation. After all, the symbolism of the number seven had lost much of its power over fourteenth-century physicians, who were by this time more inclined to choose the Galenic solution, proffered by most Arabic texts. It must have been easier to "see" numerous crannies than to see a clear two-part division. When, toward the middle of the fourteenth century, Gentile da Foligno commented on the passage in "Canon of Medicine" in which Avicenna described the division into two parts, Gentile noted: "There are no ventricles in the matrix, but there exist certain cells, even though there is no division perceptible by dissection."[108] This sort of observation clearly showed how far anatomical discourse had advanced in the fourteenth century, and how much of a limit was imposed on it by physiological theory.

The Reevaluation of Practice

The distinction between theory and practice underlay medical education from the twelfth century throughout the Renaissance. The meaning that this distinction acquired over the course of the centuries modified in accordance with social and intellectual transitions. Although the educated practitioner continued to claim close ties between his art and natural philosophy, during the fourteenth and fifteenth centuries he was generally more and more anchored to life in the city. The masters of the universities, even the most renowned, could not escape the constraints of everyday practice. These new conditions clearly played a part in the thinking concerning the relations between theory and practice.

The isolation of a purely speculative objective had allowed medicine to attain standing as a university discipline. Avicenna's "Canon of Medicine" offered a number of definitions that were clearer than those found in the *Pantegni,* confirming that each branch of medicine had the status of a science. Theory was a *scientia scientalis,* whose final objective was the knowledge of principles; practice was a *scientia operativa,* whose final objective was the knowledge of "the quality of what one was about to do." At the turn of the fourteenth century, doubts were beginning to be heard about the validity of this division, which was not to be found in Galen. Pietro Torrigiano noted that the distinction was not as sharp as in philosophy. In medicine, practice necessarily depended on theory, but theory had to be based on practice. Even if certain authors tended to insist on a speculative purpose to their art, the prevailing trend in Italy, Montpellier, and Paris was to conceive of medicine as being entirely oriented toward action.[109] Arnald of Villanova felt that a scholar could not qualify as a physician if his knowledge of the principles *(doctrina cognitiva)* did not contribute to his knowledge of practical applications *(doctrina operativa).* He rejected the idea—set forth in Averroës's commentary on Avicenna's *Poem on Medicine*—of an essentially speculative science.[110] Another conception had been presented by Averroës in his work *Colliget:* "The art of medicine is an operative art derived from true principles." This definition was maintained for the most part. For example, in a commentary dating from 1339, the Parisian master Pierre Chauchat declared: "In order to have success in the art of medicine, it is better and more useful to verify principles through operations than to question these principles using a demonstration *propter quid.*" This declaration was not made in a vacuum; in 1335, the Faculté de Medecine of Paris had established a requirement of a practical internship for all of its graduates.[111]

While pointing out the benefits that a practicing physician could draw from his experience, Pierre Chauchat's declaration also established the limitations of that experience. It was a matter of "verifying" the principles, not questioning them, much less inventing them. Still, we should keep in mind that the "principles" in question were not restricted to the universally accepted fundamentals of physiology and pathology. This term also referred to rules of pharmacology and the interpretation of this or that disease, areas that involved numerous discrepancies among the authorities. The experience of the practicing physician, which allowed him to decide and to make choices, constituted an alternative to logical reasoning. To this extent—certainly limited—practice could help in the development of theory.[112] The spread of Ockhamism, beginning in the 1320s, quite likely affected many university teachers and students; Ockhamism considered sensible intuition to be the foundation of scientific knowledge. Its influence can be detected in the work of Pierre Chauchat. It is explicit in the work of the Florentine master Tommaso del Garbo (who died in 1370). Del Garbo makes mention of the *via moderna,* in particular to defend the principle of ontological economy and to reject unneeded categorical distinctions.[113]

Apart from these potential influences—still poorly understood—the development of the practitioner and the passage from the general to the specific both occupied medical thought proper, inaugurated in the last years of the thirteenth century. The introduction of Galen's *Methodus medendi* was of enormous importance in this context. The translation by Gerard of Cremona, based as it was on an Arabic version, was entitled *De ingenio sanitatis.*[114] The expression *ingenium sanitatis* (or *ingenium curativum*) designated during the fourteenth and fifteenth centuries the process whereby the physician passed from thought to action, from general principles to their application in a specific situation. It included the recollection of book knowledge, reasoning, experience, and the virtue of "prudence" that Aristotle attributes to the artisan. In another translation by Gerard of Cremona—the *Enumeratio scientiarum* by Al-Farabi—*ingenium* designates any and all artifices invented by humans, as an application of theoretical principles. This included algebra and the invention of machines. According to Al-Farabi, the *scientia ingeniorum* required a preparation of natural bodies in order to render them suitable to support the desired effect. In the same way, medieval therapeutic procedures were not limited to the prescription of a specific drug for the treatment of a specific disease. They also took into account the patient's personality, age, background, and so forth. In other words, there was reliance on a prior preparation of the body to accept the effect of a medicine. In 1299, the Montpellier master Bernard de Gordon listed the ten *ingenia* necessary in the treatment of diseases. Use of this ambiguous term thus made it possible to describe simultaneously the scientific nature of medical practice and its component of improvisation in accordance with each special case.

The attention paid to practical conditions corresponded to the publication of works intended for the education of physicians in the field. Various types of medicine were described. Most likely influenced by jurists, who tended to write out opinions given regarding specific cases, Bolognese physicians began—around the time of Taddeo Alderotti—to write accounts of examples taken from their practice. These *Consilia*, based on real and on fictitious cases, presented the personality of the patient (sometimes his or her name), social standing, age, complexion, symptoms of the disease, supposed causes of the disease, and diet and treatment prescribed. From Bologna, where it appears to have originated, the habit of drawing up *Consilia* spread throughout Europe during the fourteenth and fifteenth centuries. It became especially popular among the masters of the university of Padua, who devoted themselves to the practice with abundant results. Antonio Cermisone (who died in 1441) wrote more than two hundred of these, meant to illustrate a reading of the third book of Avicenna's "Canon of Medicine."[115] Although they differed radically in terms of conception and objective—being fundamentally educational in purpose—the *Consilia* hearkened back in a certain sense to the *Epidemiae* of Hippocrates, which the medieval West never knew directly. The *Epidemiae* reached the West in a partial echo through the works of Rhazes: the *Secreta medicinae* and *Continens*, both translated during the second half of the thirteenth century, demonstrated the lessons to be learned from the description of concrete cases. Possibly influenced by Rhazes, whom he so admired, Arnald of Villanova insisted on the physician's responsibility to inform others of the results of his own experience. Arnald put this advice into practice with the composition of *Experimenta*.[116] Although it was not as elaborate in form as the Italian *Consilia*, it still fulfilled the same concern of recording the *particularia*.

Alongside these works, which presented specific cases, the fourteenth and fifteenth centuries brought forth the renewal of the genre of the *Practica*.[117] From the *Lilium medicinae,* by Bernard de Gordon, completed in 1305, all the way to Michele Savonarola's *Practica maior,* written from 1440 to 1446, this sort of encyclopedia collected and presented everything that was needed to practice the art of medicine. Despite the title of *Practica,* these works integrated the fundamental theoretical information, concerning the concept of complexion, for instance. They also offered the author an opportunity to present a number of *casus,* accounts of his own personal successes, as well as the failures in some cases of his colleagues. The obligation to write out the procedure followed in a concrete case inevitably led to a justification of its application. This often meant supporting one authority against another. As reliance on the scholastic question *(quaestio)* fell from favor in the *Practicae,* it became common practice in the fifteenth century to ridicule the sophisticated refinements that one gladly attributed to one's colleagues. Michele Savonarola, paraphrasing Galen, mocked the long beards of the partisans of disputation; Antonio Guaineri abandoned to his rest in heaven his predecessor, Bernard de Gordon, who disagreed with the pseudo-Mesue; Ugolino da Montecatini pretended that his work was based primarily on his own experience.[118] I could continue citing examples at length. With this removal at arm's length of the authorities and scholastic reasoning, the authors found themselves facing the harsh reality of their inefficacy. The ordeal of experience was a cruel one, though numerous excuses—ranging from the patient's disobedience to the apothecary's dishonesty, and the incompetence of a colleague, cited just above—could be adduced to explain these failures. The *Practicae* of the fifteenth century spoke eloquently of a certain disarray. The plague was certainly the chief indication of this state of confusion: the physician's impotence was displayed for all of society to see. The proliferation of *Regimina* and *Consilia,* which every master felt called upon to write, did little or no good. The growing attention focused on *particularia,* which were meant to "verify" the principles, did nothing but assist in their progressive disintegration. If practitioners of the fifteenth century still managed to maintain the unstable balance between theory and practice, by Molière's time, the break was complete.[119]

At the dawn of the Renaissance, the part of medicine designated as "practical" was strangely overgrown. The intellectual subdivision of medicine had taken a direct toll on the organization of university learning, which was split between *theorica* and *practica.* This partition of medical knowledge began with the Parisian statues of 1270 and 1274. At Bologna, the earliest evidence of it appears during the 1320s, while at Padua, it dates from the end of the fourteenth century. It gave rise in Italian universities to two distinct types of professors. The masters *in practica* were still fairly few in number and of lesser prestige in the fourteenth century, but they became preponderant at the end of the Middle Ages and in the Renaissance. After the middle of the fifteenth century, the greatest Paduan masters taught *in practica*. The teaching of theory tended to dwindle to a sort of preparatory pursuit.[120]

The Temptation of Astrology

Because of the bond that linked it to natural philosophy, medicine could not entirely escape the temptation of astrology. Aristotelian cosmology—which described a hierarchy of movements transmitted from the primum mobile down to the sphere of Earth—offered a unitary vision of the world in which the human microcosm mirrored the macrocosm. Moreover, respectable authors in the field of astronomy, such as Ptolemy, considered medical astrology worthy of a place of its own. The Arabo-Latin translations of the twelfth century had yielded a great deal of information in this field.[121] A corresponding explicative system buttressed both disciplines: much of astrological theory was based on the interaction of first qualities. To each planet and to each sign of the zodiac a twofold characteristic was assigned, indicating heat and cold, dryness and moisture. The author of the pseudo-Galenic treatise *De semine* even stated that the intensity of these qualities varied through four degrees, much as was the case with medications.[122] The moon was the mistress of flows par excellence. A subtle combinative mechanism could be adapted to the theory of complexions and the theory of humors.

Because of its previous passage through the *cursus artium*, all university medicine had received at least a dusting of rudimentary astronomy; the application, therefore, of astrology to medicine was a fairly natural development. All the same, it was by no means an obligatory one, and many practicing physicians saw no need for astrology at all. In the thirteenth century, Roger Bacon deplored this disinterest: "the fourth defect is that they do not take into consideration the celestial events, on which depend every alteration of the lower bodies . . . , now the physician who does not know how to observe the places of the planets and their aspects, operates purely by chance."[123] During the first decade of the fourteenth century, Peter of Abano wrote of the same resistance to astrology. He pointed out the absurdity of thus rejecting the help of a science that made it possible to adjust regimen and treatment, to predict the precise moment in which a disease would develop toward the crisis, and to foresee major epidemics.[124]

It is true that Greek and Arabic medical sources offered only infrequent encouragement. The most important advocate of astrology was Galen, in his treatise *De diebus decretoriis;* in the third book, he wrote that chronic illnesses follow the course of the sun, and that acute illnesses follow that of the moon. In the same book, Galen also proposed calculating a "medical month," based on astronomical data. This calculation would help to predict the critical days of an illness.[125] On the one hand, the presence of astrology in the Galenic corpus provided a weighty argument in its favor. On the other hand, Avicenna—who had written, among other things, a refutation of astrology that was not translated into Latin—expressed considerable reservations in his "Canon of Medicine." He rejected the soundness of Galen's calculations and, as a general rule, upheld the autonomy of medicine. A practitioner should not be at all concerned with first causes, about which he could do nothing.[126] A practicing physician should care only about proximate and manifest causes. Medieval authors split, some taking the attitude of Avicenna, while others did not. Some authors made extensive use of astrology; others used it not at all. Most authors opted for a moderate use, in connection with the prescription of bloodletting and purges and the determination of critical days. Epilepsy and menstruation were two areas in which mention was often made of the moon's action.

The Black Death of 1348 drove physicians to take clearer positions on the subject, as it had become traditional to attribute the outbreak of the epidemic to the conjunction in 1345 of Mars, Saturn, and Jupiter. Approximately twenty years later, the adversaries of astrology in turn found grounds for reinforcing their ideas through the virulent and scientifically based critique written by Nicole Oresme. One of the most outspoken of these adversaries of astrology was the Parisian master Jacques Despars (who died in 1458). While rejecting any scientific basis for making use of astrology, he conceded that a physician might well pretend to rely on it to mollify his patient.[127] Astrology had become fashionable, at every level of society. Medical discourse had been profoundly affected, especially where the plague was concerned: Pietro da Tossignano advocated isolating patients considered to be bearers of infection; nonetheless, in the advice that he addressed to the duke of Milan in 1398, he mentioned the idea of a predisposition of places in accordance with their astrological ascendants, or rising signs.[128] Rather than being a consequence of philosophical postulates—which could be discarded entirely if one relied on Avicenna's "Canon of Medicine"—the use of astrology was an indicator of the growing interest in medical practice. Subjected to the pressures of society and faced with the inefficacy of their art in the face of major epidemics, physicians saw astrology as a potential source of aid. Some physicians accompanied the use of astrology with a return to natural magic, with the attribution of a specific virtue to one heavenly body or another.[129]

Despite the natural resistance that the modern mind may have, the astrological component—though not universally accepted, even in the Middle Ages—is an integral part of the history of medical thought and contributed to its enrichment. A barber, for example, limited his use of astrology to the consultation of an almanac to determine the best time for letting blood. A physician who made use of astrology, by contrast, was required to take more complex factors into consideration and would have to establish a patient's horoscope. Unless he received help from an astrologer colleague, the physician himself would have to work with astronomical charts that allowed him to calculate the positions of stars and planets, and with instruments such as the astrolabe and its forerunners. This gave physicians occasion to work with problems and techniques of measurement.[130] Many renowned medieval builders of astronomical instruments and various other machines were astrologers and physicians. Among the better known of these was Giovanni Dondi (who died in 1389), who conceived and built a planetary clock. Himself the son of a physician (Jacopo Dondi, author of a repertory of medicaments), Giovanni Dondi taught medicine at the university of Padua. There he disputed a number of scholastic questions, some of which have survived. The Paduan milieu around the turn of the fifteenth century was one in which astrology and medicine were closely linked; it later became one of the most innovative schools of the sixteenth century. The astrological mode that swept medicine at the end of the Middle Ages thus had a twofold influence. It encouraged some doctors to turn their attention away from the true essentials of their art and toward magic; and it helped other doctors to develop the habit of observation, calculation, and the use of complex instruments.

Medicine's Place in Western Medieval Culture

Medieval knowledge was marked in particular by its unitary character: the absence of airtight compartments separating disciplines meant that when one discipline progressed, others were thereby affected. Subject to the influence of philosophical thought, logic, astrology, or such other arts as alchemy, medicine in turn managed to permeate the rest of culture, as a whole. Without doubt it was in the first half of the twelfth century that medicine exerted its most deep-rooted influence, thereby contributing to the emergence of a new concept of nature. Medicine in this period was seen as the most advanced discipline. By virtue of the translations done by Constantine of Africa, medicine was the first discipline to gain access to the Arabic body of knowledge. A few scattered and tangled items of information had been transmitted through Catalonian culture in the fields of mathematics and astronomy, at the end of the tenth century, but it was not until the years 1130–1150 that these sciences underwent a major renewal, through a series of important translations.[131]

The work of Constantine of Africa revealed an ambition that went well beyond the mere education of practicing physicians. In his prologue to the *Viaticum* of Ibn al-Gazzar, the translator distinguished among three categories of readers: those who were interested in medicine to enrich their general area of knowledge, those who wished to practice medicine, and those who wished to attain both objectives.[132] For the first and the last category of readers, he suggested the *Pantegni.* This suggestion, which surely corresponded to a precise need, was widely adopted. Beginning in the early twelfth century, the *Ysagoge* of Hunayn ibn Ishaq and the *Pantegni* were both widely read and used by laymen; the same was true of the treatise *De natura hominis* by Nemesius, bishop of Emesa, translated by Alphanus, archbishop of Salerno.

A product of the circle that formed around the cathedral school of Chartres—where the texts of the "Articella" were read and analyzed—the natural philosopher William of Conches made reference to these medieval sources in his *Philosophia* (1125), and in the adaptation of the same in the form of a dialogue, titled *Dragmaticon philosophiae* (1144–1149).[133] He preserved their definition of the elements, concept of complexion, and location of the mental faculties in the cerebral ventricles. The influence of medical thought was not limited to scattered information gleaned here and there; it was also felt in the interpretation of matters extraneous to it. Thus, for William of Conches, the four forces—attractive, retentive, digestive, and expulsive—administered by the "natural virtues" served as a model for his description of meteorological and cosmological phenomena. The naturalist vision of things conveyed by medical texts seems to have disturbed a number of theologians. The doctrine of spirits, or *pneumata*, and the location of mental faculties in the brain threatened to engender confusion of a materialist sort.

An adversary of William of Conches, the theologian Guillaume de Saint-Thierry himself wrote a treatise entitled *De natura corporis et animae*, between 1138 and 1145.[134] The description of the body and its functions was based on new translations, especially of the *Pantegni*. Still, the author insisted that the spiritual soul was not corporeal in nature, and that the beauty of the body was not the basis of the dignity of man. Guillaume de Saint-Thierry established bounds beyond which it was not possible to venture.

The admission of medicine into the university could hardly help fostering new and closer ties with other disciplines, principally with natural philosophy, taught in the course of arts. In the thirteenth century, attention was inevitably focused on the physics of the elements and the concept of complexion, as well as on the psychophysiology suggested by the theory of cerebral faculties. This latter field had been enriched by the translations of the works of Avicenna. The "Canon of Medicine" and the treatise *De anima* introduced a number of new concepts, such as that of "common sense," the intermediate faculty between imagination—which apprehends the impressions of the senses—and the estimative virtue, which makes distinctions.[135] Because Avicenna very clearly placed the cerebral faculties, or internal senses, in the field of the experience of the senses, and not in the intellective order, this theory did not clash with the requirements of theology. The principle of thought remained on a transcendental level. Avicenna's "Canon of Medicine" gave philosophers a number of other new topics for thought, particularly the nature of scientific knowledge. The concept of specific form was taken up by Robert Grosseteste (who died in 1153) to promote the reliance on experience. Moreover, the Galenic methods of "resolution" and "composition," as they were defined in a number of Arabic medical works, served to encourage the thoughts of this philosopher on inductive reasoning in the context of *scientia experimentalis*.[136] As we have seen, Roger Bacon—who carried on the work of Robert Grosseteste on certain points—took close interest in medicine, without ever actually practicing it himself.

Every philosopher of nature in the thirteenth century had opportunities to engage in medical interpretation. In the second half of the century, one of the chief subjects of thought was surely the theory of generation. Since everyone knew that Galen and Aristotle had stated radically differing points of view, simply reading the treatises could not suffice. It was necessary to complete one's reading with the Arabic medical texts that presented the Galenic view. From Albertus Magnus to Gilles of Rome and Thomas Aquinas, medical sources helped to define the nature of sperm, the respective roles of men and women in conception, and the process of formation of the embryo.[137] In Dante's *Convivio*, three forces were distinguished in the sperm: complexion, the formative virtue, and the virtue derived from heavenly bodies.[138] The first two concepts came directly from medical theories. All discussion of the nature and origin of the soul included a debate on the process of generation.

Medicine's influence on natural philosophy reached its apex in the twelfth and thirteenth centuries. There were contacts in later centuries, of course, but they were sporadic; the two bodies of thought fed less on each other with the passage of time. We should view this as a result of the overall development of philosophy, which progressed from a speculative stage—in which cosmogony and man's place in the universe were at the center of all concerns—to an analytic and critical phase. Natural philosophy in the fourteenth century concentrated on problems of measurement and its language.[139] As we have seen in the examples of Arnald of Villanova and Gentile da Foligno, medicine did not escape this current. Physics and mathematics had replaced medicine as the beacon disciplines; the breadth of forms, the quantification of qualitative intensities, and the definition of movement were among the chief subjects of thought. Astronomy was the principal beneficiary of this development as the Middle Ages gave way to the Renaissance.

As for medical learning, it remained sharply oriented toward the training of professionals, as society demanded. The time of amateurs, of the first category of readers described by Constantine of Africa, had in part come to an end. With a few rare exceptions, people studied medicine in order to practice it. By virtue of this greater openness to society at large—and no longer just to intellectuals—medicine became of interest to the average educated person. An encyclopedic movement had marked the thirteenth century in France. Bartholomaeus Anglicus, Thomas de Cantimpré, Vincent de Beauvais, and the anonymous author of *Placides et Timeo* had all assembled the fundamental knowledge of every field.[140] Medicine played a major role in each case.

In the fourteenth and fifteenth centuries, literature took inspiration from medical models, far more than did philosophy; the encyclopedias of the thirteenth century served in some cases as popularizing bridges. Medical inspiration was certainly not a new feature in medieval literature: as early as the end of the eleventh century, the poet Baudry de Bourgueil cited the names of Hippocrates and Galen, while listing a number of issues that emerged from the problems posed by the Peripatetics. Around

1200, the enigmatic André la Chapelain—long thought to have codified the courtly ideal—made use of a medical description of the sexual act to provide certain definitions of love. The translations by Constantine of Africa included a *De coitu*, which inspired a number of medieval treatises on the subject.[141] A medical concept introduced by the same translator was to enjoy a long life in literature. Just at the time when the concept of courtly love was developing, a chapter of *Breviarium dictum viaticum* introduced the concept of *amor ereos*.[142] The concept of lovesickness, invented in antiquity, entered Western nosology and poetry. Shortly after the first publication of Constantine of Africa's version, this same chapter from *Breviarium dictum viaticum* was translated again, this time separately. In all likelihood, this subject was of interest to the Norman court of southern Italy. Marked by physical perturbations and psychological states of obsession, the sickness was transformed from "erotic" to "heroic" under the dual influence of Ovid and courtly love. As one anonymous commentator put it in a thirteenth-century commentary on the *Breviarium dictum viaticum*, echoed by Arnald of Villanova in his short work *De amore heroico*, lovesickness chiefly affected gentlefolk. Much as physicians drew on Avicenna's "Canon of Medicine," and enriched their descriptions with a psychophysiological interpretation that was bound up with the theory of the internal senses, conversely poets rediscovered the Ovidian tradition and the Arab medical tradition in a theme that was unflaggingly evoked and amplified—the theme of "heroic love." The philosophical background thus gained in depth.

Although at first this notion had been separate, it gradually linked up with the concept of melancholy, as the latter theme invaded late-medieval literature.[143] Arab authors still played a decisive role, providing long and detailed explanations concerning both melancholy the humor and melancholy the disease. A reflection of a current that also affected medicine, astrological interpretations were increasingly popular. Suddenly the melancholic temperament, long deplored and subject to Saturn, acquired new worth. Under the influence of a number of factors—among them Aristotle's *Problemata*, 30.1, first translated into Latin before 1210 by David de Dinant—melancholy became an attribute of creators and exceptional men. In the fifteenth century, time itself lay in the shadow of melancholy. At the same time, the word "melancholy" came to mean a state of sadness without cause. Even if they only rarely treated the bonds between body and soul directly, these physicians of the Middle Ages examined in depth—in correspondence with their reading—the concept of physiological causes of psychological states and madness. The interaction of the primary qualities in the system of complexions, the role played by the spirits, and the idea of humoral inflammation that is found in the concept of "scorched melancholy"—all these offered, with the cerebral localizations, an exceedingly nuanced range of possible explications. The interpretation was sufficiently coherent to offer a convincing model.

The objects of eternal ridicule (as ineffectual practitioners), the physicians of the Middle Ages nonetheless managed to transmit certain of their ideas to philosophers and poets.

～ 8 ～

The Concept of Disease

MIRKO D. GRMEK

Since the earliest civilizations, human thought has been profoundly affected by the idea of disease. This concept is, in fact, a family of ideas that has developed throughout history; in modern societies, ideas tend to differ according to social class and level of education. Their study is equally the domain of the historian of medicine and the social anthropologist. In popular systems of representation of health and disease, we find even today manifestations of the ideas that dominated the medical theories of the past.[1]

The etymologies of various terms that designate disease, in Indo-European languages, show certain fundamental characteristics of the original conceptualization.[2] One point strikes us immediately: there is no term common to all the languages of the Indo-European group. In some languages, moreover, there is a notable profusion of synonyms. Their meaning derives from four different semantic fields: (1) weakness, lack of strength, loss of capacity to perform work; (2) deformity, unsightliness; (3) discomfort, feeling of unease, malaise; (4) suffering, pain.

The initial conceptualization of the diseased state entails an objective criterion, as for instance the inability to perform work, for oneself and for the community, as well as a subjective criterion, which ranges from discomfort to sharp pain. Cognate terms designate disease, on the one hand, and evil, wickedness, and ugliness, on the other. The concept of disease is not socially neutral: it entails a judgment in moral and aesthetic terms. A man is diseased when he is unable to work as hard as before, when he suffers physically, and when certain changes in his body lower his social worth and alter the everyday rhythms of his life, at times to the point of threatening his survival.

Defining Disease

At first glance, it would seem a simple matter to offer a practical definition of disease. And yet the attempt is soon met with insurmountable difficulties. First of all, there is a fundamental difference between "being sick" and "having a sickness." The terms used in ordinary language fail to reflect this difference. Those writing in English have established a subtle and fundamental distinction between "illness" and "disease"; certain German authors make the same distinction between *Erkrankung* and *Krankheit*. French, Spanish, and Italian fail to supply this discrete terminology.

The term "illness" should be used to describe the immediate experience of a sick person, the "experience" of disease, while the term "disease" should be reserved for the conceptualization of disease by physicians.[3] There is a further distinction, however, expressed well in French, between *être malade* (to feel sick) and *être un malade* (to be acknowledged as sick), hence the need of introducing a third term, "sickness," to indicate the perception of disease by the nonphysicians who come into contact with the person in question. When dealing with the state conceived as "disease," it is possible to distinguish between the anatomical and physical perturbations suffered by the patient and "objectively" detected by the physician (the *pathos*), on the one hand, and the medical interpretation of the same, in the form of clinical or anatomophysiological entities (the *nosos*), on the other.[4]

A complete definition of disease would have to take into account all the aspects mentioned above, as well as integrate them, a task which has clearly proved impossible. Definitions of disease tend to be caught in the vicious circle of stating that disease is the opposite of health or else based on specific hypotheses concerning the essential nature of morbid phenomena. Unfortunately, these hypotheses not only are specific but tend to be incomplete as well.

A further difficulty can be found in the confusion between "disease" and "diseases," which is to say between the conceptualization of disease in general (definition of the pathological in the context of the physiological) and the conceptualization of specific diseases (definition of nosological entities). In the first case, the basic problem lies in the ambiguity of the concept of biological and social "norms"; in the second case, the difficulties derive from the "ontological status" of the diseases.[5]

Are diseases entities or processes? Do the definitions of diseases themselves reflect an objective reality, or are they merely a convenient way of mastering intellectually a complex and inconstant reality? In other words, do we "discover" nosological entities, or do we "invent" them? These questions sum up a debate that, ever since the dawn of Western medicine, has opposed supporters of a dynamic "nominalist" pathology and those who follow a "realist" ontological nosology.

According to the ontological conceptualization, it is possible to distinguish two historical phases: at first, the existence of a disease—the *ens morbi*—was conceived as a concrete entity; later, in a philosophically more refined version, it was developed into a logical type, an idea. While admitting that diseases exist, in the strong sense of the term, only in the world of ideas, one could nonetheless attribute a sort of potential existence to diseases (according to interpretations deriving from Platonic tradition), a potential existence that determined their manifestation in the form of actual pathological states. Over against these "ontological" interpretations, others held that nosological entities were merely concepts with arbitrary outlines, not derived as such directly from our physical existence, and varying over space (cultural differences) and time (historical differences). Thus, diseases should be considered as models for the explication of reality, rather than constituent parts of reality.[6] In modern Western medicine, such conceptualization entails fuzzy boundaries and internal contradictions whose extent and meaning can be grasped only through study of the vicissitudes of a long and complex historical process.[7]

The Primitive Ontological Conceptualization

In the primitive ontological conceptualization, disease was identified as an inanimate material object that penetrated an organism from without ("corpuscular theory," or *Fremdkörpertheorie*), or as a material living being ("parasitic theory"), or as an immaterial being ("demon theory").

Primitive thought did not clearly distinguish between the cause of a phenomenon and the phenomenon itself. An arrow or a poison that entered the human body was not merely the cause of sickness but the sickness itself.[8] Often, witch doctors would attempt to remove a disease from a patient in the concrete form of a pebble or other object. In scientific medicine, we still find extensions of this conceptualization in the idea of intoxication.[9] Corpuscular theory underlies a great many therapeutic procedures used today.

In archaic medicine, it was common to imagine disease as a parasitic animal, most often a worm, that either made its way into the human body or developed there spontaneously. Despite certain similarities with modern concepts of pathogenic microbial parasitism, primitive parasite theory historically played no role in the foundation of medical bacteriology.[10]

"Savage thought" reveals an understanding of the causal link between phenomena that is profoundly different from that found in the Western scientific conception of the world. Not only is there confusion between cause and effect, but there is also intermingling of natural and supernatural phenomena. While, in some cases, the "cause," or we should say the "essence," of a disease is quite evident (trauma, cold, heat, poisoning, starvation), more frequently disease strikes invisibly, and a man "falls ill" without direct experience offering the slightest hint as to the why or the wherefore. Thus, there is a tendency to personify the disease: it is conceived as a malevolent spirit that causes disease in a human being by penetrating the body. This theory of demonic possession is strongly buttressed by the subjective experience of the patient, who feels transformed, as if he has been invaded by an alien will.[11] Ancient peoples believed they were able to distinguish among and even classify the disease-causing deities or demons. The personification of disease has left traces in our language. Even when the conceptualization of disease had become perfectly rational, we continue to say, in medical texts and in literature, that disease "strikes" a person, that it ravages like a "savage beast," that it "devours" the flesh.[12]

As a rule, when disease was conceived as an entity, it was "added" to a healthy organism, but in ancient medical folklore there are instances of the opposite explanation: it was believed that certain pathological states were caused by the absence of an essential component of the organism, especially following a "theft of the soul."

In archaic medicine, the power of efficient causes was attributed to factors of an ethical nature. It was thus more important to establish the reason "why" someone fell sick than it was to discover "how." Disease had a moral meaning: at times it might be a way of testing (as in the Bible story of Job, for example); more commonly, it was thought to be revenge taken through the evil acts of a person endowed with magical power; in most cases, however, it was considered a punishment from the gods, or retribution for the violation of a taboo. Divine punishment is exemplary in cases of terrible plagues: Apollo unleashed a pestilence upon the Achaeans, as did Jehovah with the Philistines. Crushed by forces that are beyond their understanding and against which it is impossible to impose their will, humans in savage and archaic societies simply lived in a state of resigned submission and continual fear.

The earliest Western literary documents—such as the Homeric epics, the Holy Scriptures, and archaic myths—reveal the existence of concepts of infirmity (permanent alteration of an anatomical structure or a physiological function without there being a pathological process underway), trauma, intoxication, mental illness, sudden death, and plague *(loimos)*. The three last-named categories of pathological phenomena were thought to be instances of divine intervention.[13] The same is true of disease in the strictest sense *(nosos)*. As the other Cyclopes said to Polyphemus, after he fell for the ruse of Ulysses: "If no man hurt thee, and thyself alone,/That which is done to thee by Jove is done;/And what great Jove inflicts no man can fly."[14] In the worlds of Homer and Greek classical tragedy, the exemplary disease is chronic wasting away: it is a "terrifying demon" that causes pain and melts the flesh.

The Boeotian poet Hesiod (ca. eighth century B.C.) recounted the myth of a Golden Age, when men lived "safe from suffering, hard labor, and painful diseases that carry them to death's door"; he explained the origin of all evils through the myth of Pandora. Supposedly, diseases *(hoi nousoi)* emerged from a magic box; they then "wander[ed] uncountable among the places of men" and visited men "in their guise" *(automatoi)*, some by day, others by night, "bringing suffering to mortals, in silence, for Zeus in his wisdom has denied them speech."[15] Hesiod spoke of diseases in the plural, and not of disease, in the singular, as did Homer before him. Diseases had become numerous and—another new development in comparison with earlier texts—they struck men spontaneously, through a type of causality all their own, without any personal fault or direct divine intervention.[16]

For Homer, disease was not part of nature: it came from outside nature; sent at the whim of the gods, it overrode human nature. A major step forward in Greek medical thought came when disease was made part of the natural order. The text of Hesiod offers a glimpse of the beginning of this restoration of nosology to the context of physiology: however they might disrupt harmony and disturb natural equilibrium, diseases were here conceived as being part of nature and, as a consequence, were subject to certain rules. This naturalistic recovery of diseases was undertaken in the context of a magical and religious prescientific conceptualization that grouped magical causality with natural causality.[17]

Dynamic Conceptualization

The Beginnings

Over the course of the sixth and fifth centuries B.C., the subtle logic of the Greek "physiologist" philosophers and the clinical experience of the founders of a new "medical art" introduced a dynamic interpretation of disease in place of, or at least alongside of, the ancient ontological concept.

A physician and philosopher from southern Italy, Alcmaeon of Croton, set forth the earliest known definition of natural disease, around 500 B.C., a definition free of any magical or religious interpretations. According to the doxography of Aetius:

> Alcmaeon says that health is preserved through the equality of rights [*isonomia*] of the qualities of humidity, dryness, heat, bitterness, sweetness, etc., while the exclusive rule of one of these [*monarchia*] produces disease. Disease develops, as for its causative agent, because of an excess of heat or dryness; as for its origin, because of an excess or a lack of food; as for its location, in the blood, in the marrow, and in the brain. He says that in some cases diseases arise from external causes, such as waters, places, exhaustion, anguish, or such things. Health is a [good] mixture.[18]

This text, of enormous importance to the history of medical ideas, is chiefly known in the version provided by H. Diels and W. Kranz in their edition of the pre-Socratics.[19] Now, the version in question is, in fact, a reconstruction of Aetius's citation, taken from two different sources, a text by Johannes Stobaeus and a passage from Plutarch; the latter, in turn, is a reconstruction taken from a number of different manuscripts. The "long" version, which is usually quoted, contains a number of sections that are clearly later interpolations; these alter its meaning. The list of qualities offered is completed so as to create an orderly series of pairs; there is a comment that states that "the monarchy of one or the other of the opposites is the source of corruption," concluding that the definition of health is the "blend of the qualities in proper proportions."

Alcmaeon used a political metaphor whose meaning is clear: "monarchy" indicates the dominance of a single quality over all the others, and not the dominance of one member of a pair over the other. The *isonomia* that characterizes a state of health is a balance involving, in equal measure, all of the elementary qualities of the human body. Alcmaeon's definition not only expresses the Pythagorean idea that sickness is essentially a disharmony or an imbalance; it also summarizes the concrete observations of the physicians of his time concerning the sites of pathological perturbations and their perceptible causes. The concept of health was linked to the concepts of beauty and the golden mean. A new "medical art" was established with the precise goal of assisting human nature to preserve and rediscover proper proportions and harmony, both within the body and in relation to the outside world.

The analogy between organism and society was a commonplace of ancient thought. Its corollary was the analogy between disease and war. The medical concept of disease was always to be profoundly influenced by the metaphor of combat: disease attacks the organism, which defends itself by its "nature" *(physis)* and through the intervention of the physician; the forces of the organism combat the forces of food; and, finally, disease itself is nothing more than the expression of a struggle between the various component parts of an organism. While Hippocratic physicians were able to depersonalize the concept of disease, they could not eliminate the metaphor of combat. Hippocrates did not hesitate to say that "the art consists of three terms: the disease [*nosema*], the patient, and the physician . . . The patient must cooperate with the physician in combatting the disease."[20] If physicians used such metaphors, statesmen and historians— for example, Thucydides—turned the tables, using the medical model of disease to explain political events.[21]

Humoral Pathology

Alcmaeon's terminology found no echo in subsequent medical literature. Hippocratic physicians gave the name *dyskrasia* (in place of *monarchia*) to the fundamental disorder that constitutes disease (*nosos* or *nosema*);[22] they called the healthful equilibrium either *eukrasia* or *symmetria* (in place of *isonomia*). In fact, they conceived of disease as a complaint of the body characterized by a "disturbance in the mixture" of the fundamental humors, triggered by a loss of the "proper proportion" in the relations between hot and cold or between wet and dry. Galen was to write in the second century: "Almost all of my predecessors have defined health as a good mixture [*eukrasia*] and proportion [*symmetria*] of the elements."[23]

The idea of the golden mean was a dominant one throughout antiquity. The *Problemata*, a composite work that is at least partly attributed to Aristotle, begins with a rhetorical question that already contains the answer: "Why do great excesses cause disease? Is it because they produce either excess [*hyperbole*] or defect [*elleipsis*]? And after all these constitute disease [*nosos*]."[24] But an excess or a lack of what? To answer this fundamental question, classical Greek thinkers developed humoral pathology and the quaternary scheme.

According to Plato and Aristotle, who probably based themselves on Empedocles or some other pre-Socratic philosopher-physician, diseases were the result of perturbations in the mixture of elementary qualities, or rather of their "hypostases," primary constituents that are the "roots" of all bodies.[25] A text from the Hippocratic corpus, the treatise *De diaeta* [*Regimen*], also states: "Now all animals, including man, are composed of two things, different in power but working together in their use, namely, fire and water."[26] Disease is the loss of equilibrium between these two elements. To prevent it, one must be vigilant in maintaining the proper balance of nourishing foods and exercise. The other Hippocratic physicians opposed these ideas, holding that the chief cause of disease is found in substances more immediately accessible to our senses, that is, the humors. The author of *De prisca medicina* forcefully attacked those who approach medicine based on "a postulate, such as heat, or cold, or dryness, or moistness, or any other postulate that they may choose," and not observable reality: "For there is in man salt and bitter, sweet and acid, astringent and insipid, and a vast number of other things, possessing properties of all sorts, both in number and in strength. These, when mixed and compounded with one another are neither apparent nor do they hurt a man; but when one of them is separated off, and stands alone, then it is apparent and hurts a man."[27]

In other passages of this treatise, the author states that these substances are "humors" *(chymos)* and that disease results from their "intemperate" state *(akrasia)*.

For nearly all the Hippocratic authors, disease was the expression of a disorder—not in the primary constituents, but in the fluid components of the human body. It would seem that at first the number of fundamental humors was indeterminate; later, it was limited to two (bile and phlegm) or three (bile, phlegm, and blood). The existence of a pair allowed for the idea of a struggle between two opposite principles, while the concept of a triad derived from an ancient Indo-European tradition. All the same, it is clear that the adoption of the quaternary scheme as an explicatory system had a notable advantage, in that it allowed the cross-linking of a double set of opposed principles. This is an ideal scheme for speculation based on binary logic. Empedocles showed how useful it was with his model of four elements and four primary qualities.[28] And so a fourth humor was added to the three already established, just as spring was added to the traditional tripartite scheme of the year, and adolescence was added to the three traditional ages of man. In the fifth century the fourth humor had not yet been determined: it was water, or else black bile. The latter first appeared in medical literature as a variety of bile and later became a humor *sui generis*.[29]

Classical humoral pathology, traditionally presented as the most authentic creation of Hippocrates, was first explicitly formulated in a treatise written by his son-in-law Polybius, *De natura hominis*, written on Kos around 410 B.C.:

> The body of man has in itself blood, phlegm, yellow bile and black bile; these make up the nature of his body, and through these he feels pain or enjoys health. Now he enjoys the most perfect health when these elements are duly proportioned to one another in respect of compounding, power and bulk, and when they are perfectly mingled. Pain is felt when one of these elements is in defect or excess, or is isolated in the body without being compounded with all the others. For when an element is isolated and stands by itself, not only must the place which it left become diseased, but the place where it stands in a flood must, because of the excess, cause pain and distress.[30]

After this text, and for more than two millennia, most physicians in the Western world were firmly persuaded that, save for the case of trauma, disease was general or a local perturbation of the mix of the four humors.[31]

Hippocratic physicians already distinguished, at least implicitly, between the etiology of disease and what modern physicians call the pathogenesis. Hippocratic physicians believed that the latter was essentially a humoral disorder, and that it constituted, as much as clinical symptoms, the essence of disease. The treatises *De morbis*, *De affectionibus*, and *De affectionibus interioribus* particularly addressed this aspect of disease. According to certain Hippocratic texts, and especially the treatise *De flatibus*, disease was a defective flow of air through the body, and its causes were a poor diet and anomalies in the surrounding air. We should note that, according to the Aristotelian text transmitted in the papyrus entitled *Anonymus Londinensis*, this pneumatic pathology was in accordance with the authentic teachings of Hippocrates himself.

In any case, Hippocratic physicians did consider external air, especially wind, to play a major role in the etiology of internal pathological states. The imbalances of humors that manifest themselves as diseases are caused by interactions between an internal factor—the constitution of the individual—and external factors, such as climate, diet, exercise, and traumas. Hippocratic medicine, then, took its inspiration in this matter from the tradition of "pedotribes" (athletic trainers of the young) and dietitians, clearly rejecting both the speculations of the pre-Socratic philosophers and their efforts to reduce medical reality to a series of abstract principles. They likewise rejected sacral medicine and magical and religious explanations of disease.

For Hippocrates, there was no actual sacred disease.[32] He refused to accord that attribute even to the disease that in his time was still called the "sacred disease" *(hiere nousos)*. This name was used to describe epileptic seizures, which struck brutally and suddenly, affecting the entire human being, twisting the body and driving out the soul, starkly appearing as the work of a supernatural power. "It is not, in my opinion, any more divine or more sacred than other diseases, but has a natural cause, and its supposed divine origin is due to men's inexperience, and to their wonder at its peculiar character," wrote the author of the treatise *De morbo sacro*.

According to Greek physicians, there was no true sharp division between health and disease.[33] Linking *eukrasia* and *dyskrasia* was an endless array of intermediate states. There were mixtures of humors that, while remaining within the domain of health, lay the groundwork for disease. The external appearance may hint at the existence of such weakness (apoplectic habitus, phthisic habitus, and so on). These ideas, clearly present in the Hippocratic corpus, were to be developed further, particularly in the Galenic theory of the temperaments, idiosyncrasies, and diatheses.

The Spatial and Temporal Aspects of Disease

According to Aristotle's *Problemata*, "Disease implies motion, while health is a state of rest."[34] In fact, Greek physicians in the classical age believed that disease was neither an entity nor a state, but rather a process: it had a temporal dimension. According to Hippocrates, disease was not merely a "bad mixture of humors." Rather, it was the entire set of events whereby this imbalance was engendered, and the work—compared metaphorically with coction—with which the "nature" of the organism brings about healing or, if this effort of the body is insufficient, either allows the disease to persist or ends in death. Disease was a process punctuated by crises that manifested themselves, at regular intervals, either by the evacuation or the deposit of the perturbed humors. As Emile Littré put it, in the view of Hippocrates: "disease, independent of the organ that it attacks and the form that it takes, is something that has its own course, its development, and its end; in this system, what diseases have in common is more important to consider than what is specific to them."[35]

Disease then, for a Hippocratic physician, was an event that extended over time; one had to grasp its diachronic regularity in all its phases through an intellectual operation, called prognosis. The manifestations of disease—the symptoms—had no medical meaning unless put into a historical context.[36]

While all of the authors of the Hippocratic corpus agreed on the temporal dimension of disease, they differed on the subject of the spatial structure of pathological events. Does disease always concern the entire organism, or can it be localized? Is it the whole man who is sick, with the disease manifesting itself secondarily through local symptoms? Or, rather, is one specific part of the body affected, while the suffering spreads only secondarily to the rest of the body? Medical historians traditionally distinguish two opposing schools of thought among the Hippocratic authors. One opinion, known as the doctrine of the school of Kos, favored a global view of disease; the other, linked to the school of Cnidus, was interested primarily in location and nosological entities.[37] Charles Daremberg offers an admirable summary of these two schools of thought: "It is in the writings of Cos that we find the *organism* and the *disease;* it is in the writings of the Cnideans that we should search for the *organs* and the *diseases.*"[38] Recent criticism tends to revise the importance of this distinction; it is now considered to be an artifact introduced by historians who projected into the past a conflict of modern times.[39]

From Alexandrian Anatomy to Galenic Synthesis

The chief weakness of the Hippocratic conceptualization of disease is the absence of any anatomical criteria. By constantly making reference to fluid components, it tended to overlook the exact location of pathological phenomena, hidden within the body. During the Hellenistic era, the anatomical research done by the school of Alexandria helped to enrich the concept of disease: to the *dyskrasia* of the humors was added the lesion of the solid structures. In the medical doctrine of Herophilus, we still find humoral pathology, coexisting with new concepts of anatomophysiology; in the doctrine of Erasistratus, by contrast, solidist pathology entirely supplants Hippocratic humoralism. For the Erasistrateans—influenced by the atomism of Democritus, the axioms of Euclid, and the art of Alexandrian engineers—disease was essentially a "mechanical" disorder, or, to be more specific, a "hydromechanical" disorder, affecting the function of the three systems of vessels.[40] It is true that certain treatises in the Hippocratic corpus offer an explanation of pathological phenomena involving the blockage of the movement of air and humors through the vessels, but this explanation is subordinated to an essentially nonsolidist pathology. Alexandrian physicians gave the concept a new epistemological standing.

The mechanical conception of disease attained a peak of glory with the work in Rome of Asclepiades of Bithynia. But the Empirics had proffered exceedingly persuasive arguments to demonstrate that it was probably impossible to know what really went on inside the human body, whether healthy or sick. As a result, many physicians simply renounced both the fundamental concepts of humoral pathology and the mechanical explanations of disease. These physicians reverted to the ontological conception of disease, which was thus nothing more than an "ideal type" of the clinical symptoms.[41]

A new path had been blazed by the methodic sect. Themison of Laodicea revised the teachings of Asclepiades by replacing the anatomical concept of localized disease with a global anatomical concept. Thus, disease was nothing more than a disorder in the movement of particles inside the body's conduits, which were either too taut or too loose.

The general concept of disease that, in the final analysis, antiquity was to bequeath to the Middle Ages, is a synthesis of Hippocratic humoral pathology and the discoveries made through anatomical dissection. The main paladin of this synthesis was Galen. Following the work of Quintus and Numesianus, he succeeded in integrating the results of the anatomophysiological research of the Alexandrians with an apparently faithful exegesis of the Hippocratic treatises.

According to Galen, disease could be either a general *dyskrasia* of the four humors[42] or a local affection of the tissues (due either to excessive relaxation or to tension, or else to an excessive presence of one of the four elementary qualities) or of the organs (caused either by a lesion or by a change in the composition, size, or position).[43] The Galenic concept of disease is at once humoral, pneumatic, and solidist. There is an innate nature, upon which occasional external factors act, triggering functional disorders *(pathos);* the set of these disorders, and their continuation, constitute disease in the more general sense *(nousos).* Disease is a dysfunction. Disease is part of nature to the extent that it derives from natural causes, but it is also in a certain sense *para physin,* contrary to the "natural" development of life.[44]

Clinical Entities and Their Classification

The subdivision of the clinical landscape, of observable pathological events, poses a number of practical and logical problems. To begin with, there is confusion between symptoms and diseases, a confusion that is easy to understand—and even justified—in a medical system that defines nosological entities by their prime symptoms or through a syndrome varying in makeup.

From the earliest origins of the Latin and Greek languages, we find names of diseases, a clear indication of just how ancient the establishment of certain nosological categories must have been.[45] The Hippocratic corpus made use of an existing nosological vocabulary; it also made use of radically new ideas, such as "clinical files," with precise descriptions of cases. To "explain" disease*s* (in the plural, no longer merely "disease"), it became necessary to make minute observations of the natural signs that mark their development. As the modifications of humors could not be immediately detected, the physician was forced to guess at those modifications by observing and interpreting symptoms. If the Hippocratic authors were not actually breaking new ground with their concepts of imbalance of elementary properties and *dyskrasia* of the humors, in comparison with ancient Indian and Chinese physicians, they were certainly superior to all their predecessors in terms of the methodological principles on which they based their clinical observations. In their logical structure, in the codification of their analytical procedures, and in their efforts to break free of their doctrinal foundations as much as possible, the clinical observations recorded in the seven books of the *Epidemiae* remain even now a model of how Western physicians approach a patient and record their observations.[46]

Hippocratic physicians studied and treated patients, not diseases. They were well aware that diseases had no autonomous existence; they knew that a disease was only an intellectual tool allowing them to establish certain constants. From the multitude of symptoms, a few fairly clearly defined groupings emerged: these were the nosological species called diseases. Their actual number was indeterminate, or even infinite, for there was an infinite range of possible mixtures of the humors. Diseases could change and turn from one disease into another. These nosological entities, then, correspond—at least in that part of the Hippocratic treatises traditionally attributed to the school of Kos—to what modern physicians describe as clinical syndromes.

A physician should be able to reach a diagnosis, which is to say, he or she should be able to recognize a syndrome and guess the disease in the sharper sense, the fundamental disorder that lies hidden behind the symptoms.[47] The Hippocratic authors of *Prognosticon, Prorrheticon, Praenotiones Coacae,* and the seven books titled *Epidemiae* wanted to dispense with the idea of nosological specificity and, by means of prognosis and concrete clinical observations, delineate a set of general rules concerning the course of the symptoms, without implying a specific diagnosis.[48] They did not attain this goal, however.

Hippocratic prognosis, in fact, was a sort of disguised diagnosis. The practical value of such a procedure is sharply inferior to that of reliance on nosological entities. Criticism expressed by the Empirics from the third century onward forced physicians to recognize the usefulness of morbid entities and to assign to syndromes a privileged epistemological standing that, for certain authors, might be that of ideas existing separately from the human spirit. "Certain symptoms," pointed out Stephen of Alexandria in his commentary on the therapeutic treatises by Galen, "constitute the species [idea] of a disease, and always characterize them. The empirics describe them as *pathognomonic,* because they characterize the nature of the morbid species, such as for example, coughing, fever, dyspnea, and the pain in the thigh of pleuritis."[49]

Medicine at this time was more and more clearly demonstrating Aristotle's remark that there is no science of the individual or the unique: while it may be true that a physician observes and cares for individuals, the medical art as such can conceive only of general rules. Medicine during the Hellenistic and Roman eras, therefore, tended to rely on the Hippocratic treatises that described diseases. It was in this spirit—close to what modern historians consider to be the heritage of the school of Cnidus—

that Celsus, Soranos of Ephesus and his Latin translator Caelius Aurelianus, Aretaeus the Cappadocian, Rufus of Ephesus, and Galen drew up synthetic charts of numerous diseases.

In their didactic writings, medical authors had to classify diseases. Efforts to assemble nosological entities into large groups culminated in results that were at once highly satisfactory in practice and inconsistent and arbitrary in theoretical terms. The most ancient classification recorded in literary form is the threefold division indicated in a poem by Pindar: diseases that develop spontaneously in the body, traumas, and diseases caused by the external influence of the seasons.[50] In accordance with the transition from the tripartite Indo-European tradition to the Greek binary mode, this classification reappears in the Hippocratic treatise *De morbis I* in the form of a twofold division: diseases triggered by an internal cause are distinguished from those due to an external cause; in turn, the latter diseases are divided into injuries and sicknesses caused by excessive heat, cold, dryness, or wetness.[51]

Plato attempted a philosophical classification of nosological entities but reached a dead end. An Athenian physician of the fourth century B.C., Mnesitheus, applied the Platonic method of diaeresis to the medical art and to disease; he established—on the basis of the division into quality/quantity, breaths/humors, pairs of elementary properties, innate elements/acquired elements, seasons, and body/soul—a hierarchic system of genus, subgenus, and species.[52]

In educational accounts, the principle of classification is most often topical, by location: arranged by regions affected from head to heel *(a capite ad calcem)*. Diseases were also classified in terms of their final prognosis (mortal, dangerous, and benign; incurable, difficult to cure, and easy to cure). Of particular importance was the distinction between acute diseases and chronic diseases, a distinction that dated back to the classical period (Hippocratic treatises already mentioned acute diseases as a distinct group), but that was not fully developed until Roman times, particularly in the work of Aretaeus the Cappadocian, Soranos of Ephesus, and Galen.

The Concept of Disease in Medieval Medicine

The explanations of the concept of disease in the scholarly literature of the Middle Ages are based, essentially, on the texts by Galen. In some cases, these explanations summarize those texts or offer commentary with direct reference to them, but more commonly they are based on those texts through the medium of an exceedingly complex tradition, which had become impoverished during the monastic period of Latin medicine and was later replenished and contaminated by Byzantine and Arab authors and by the scholastics.

According to Isidore of Seville—an author writing in the seventh century who was always on the lookout for the deeper meanings of words, and who is a perfect illustration of the scholarship of his time—"health is the integrity of the body and the proper mixture of human nature, inasmuch as heat and moisture are concerned." The word "disease [*morbus*] in the general sense indicates all sufferings of the body," and, he believed, originated from "the power of death [*mortis vis*]." All diseases, as this author points out, "originate from the four humors."[53]

Simplified Galenic humoral pathology dominated all Latin medical literature prior to the school of Salerno, as well as the earliest writings of that school.[54]

If Arab authors, such as Avicenna, accepted as a sort of medical dogma the theory of the four humors, they nonetheless subjected it to an exceedingly rigorous logical analysis and distinguished between the equilibrium of humors and the equilibrium of primary qualities. This work of interpretation would later be continued by the physicians who taught in the universities of medieval Europe. Emphasis was thus laid on the concept of *complexio* (Latin) or *krasis* (Greek); this state was thought to determine either health or disease, which was fundamentally a mixture of the four primary qualities, and not of four humors. If this was actually the opinion of Aristotle,[55] Galen defended in his works on pathology a point of view that was much closer to the Hippocratic tradition. While claiming to be Galenic, the scholastics posited an idea of disease that was, in fact, a sort of compromise between the teachings of Galen and those of Aristotle. The system in question was, as Per-Gunnar Ottosson put it, a "qualitative pathology" and not a "humoral pathology,"[56] as is commonly thought.

The diagnostic procedures of medieval physicians represented a step backward with respect to ancient clinical practice.[57] The examination of pulse and urine had been refined to the point of having no relationship to pathological reality. Likewise, astrological diagnosis developed as a practical consequence of the idea that events in the human body corresponded to the locations of the celestial bodies.

The fundamental question of the ontological standing of nosological entities was necessarily dealt with in the context of the great scholastic debate concerning the nature of universals in language. Whereas "nominalists" felt that nothing really existed besides the patient himself and that diseases were only so many names, the "realists" believed that diseases possessed a real existence and that the sick were only particular contingent manifestations of that existence. The context of this debate was essentially theological, but the success of the realist thesis encouraged a return to the ontological idea of disease.

In the popular depiction of disease, the belief in magical factors—such as demonic possession and divine punishment—had never disappeared. Despite the vigorous criticism of scholarly physicians or rationalist philosophers, most of the common folk—and indeed probably the majority of those working in the healing arts—refused to abandon the archaic belief that disease was the result of moral stains or the breaking of a taboo. This belief incorporated the idea of infection and encouraged purificatory practices. No wonder the learned physicians of the classical and Hellenistic ages rejected those practices.[58] Expiatory inscriptions *(tituli piaculares)*, particularly numerous in the second and third centuries A.D., show that disease was often experienced and conceived of as the punishment of some shame.

The fathers of the church revived the ancient magical ideas. The concept of shame as a nonmaterial cause of disease was replaced by that of sin. More blame was thus put on the sick themselves, and confession was added to the ancient purificatory rites and exorcisms.[59]

For physicians of antiquity, all diseases were somatic. Diseases of the soul, they felt, were nothing but an invention of the moralists. The result of that particular point of view was the division of the field of psychic illnesses between physicians and philosophers.[60] For the men of the Middle Ages, however—in both Christendom and in the Islamic world—it was impossible to separate bodily events from their spiritual significance. The relationship between body and soul was so intricate and so multifaceted that disease was necessarily a psychosomatic entity. Avicenna, for example, wrote that passions formed part of the pathogenetic process. Christian physicians felt that disease was, first and foremost, a moral disorder. If Christian physicians and philosophers thought of disease as a disorder, they did so in a world in which—in their view—disorder was the rule. Disease supposedly made its first appearance on earth immediately following the original sin and the loss of corporal immortality, in the wake of expulsion from the earthly paradise. After that fatal fall, disease became, so to speak, the normal state of the human race.

To the primitive archaic mentality, a sick man was a sinner: you would only fall sick because you had done something wrong. Certain Greek and Roman rationalist physicians upended this concept; they thought that the sinner was a sick man. He behaved badly because disease deprived him of healthy free judgment. Christian doctrine took its inspiration from these two contradictory sources: it wished to conciliate the Semitic conception of the disease-causing role of sin with the Greco-Roman naturalistic conception and arrived at a twofold treatment, at once moral and physical. Christ, "the first physician," healed bodies to show that his curative powers extended to the soul, as well.[61]

If the Middle Ages contributed little to the development of the medical model of disease, it did give a new value to experience. By linking the etiology of disease with sin, it turned that etiology into a path to redemption.

In the Christian world, *infirmitas,* the diminished social capacity experienced by the sick and perceived by those around the sick, became a moral test for the sick and an opportunity to exercise one's virtues for those around the sick. Opposed to *sanitas, infirmitas* was nonetheless a path toward *salus.*

~ 9 ~

Therapeutic Strategies: Drugs

ALAIN TOUWAIDE

Between the "fire and iron" of the archaic period[1] and Hippocratic helleborism,[2] there yawns an abyss; the same abyss stretches between helleborism and Nero's theriac. Each of these therapeutic methods corresponded, in all likelihood, to a different theory.[3] We say "probably" because little has survived that is either explicit or intact. A veritable "therapeutic archaeology" is needed to discover the concepts that underlay medication—or *pharmakon*—and its use, both in antiquity and in Byzantium.[4]

In a passage from the *Republic*, dating from the fifth century B.C.,[5] Plato criticizes the use of *pharmaka* and states that reliance on "fire and iron" is preferable. Scholars have used this statement to deduce that *pharmaka* had been added to the traditional therapy that used "fire and iron" in some period not long prior to the time when the philosopher wrote.[6] Actually, mention had already been made of *pharmaka* as early as the *Iliad* and the *Odyssey;* in that context, the term was used to describe both healthful and harmful products,[7] a clear demonstration that *pharmakon* indicated a unitary idea, that of a substance introduced into the body to modify its state.[8] The ambiguity of the concept made it necessary to apply an adjective to the term *pharmakon* when using it to describe a poison. The purpose of the adjective was to specify the nature of the modification thus being induced.[9] This usage lasted for some time: we find instances of it as late as Galen, a further indication of the ambiguous connotation inherent to the very concept of *pharmakon*.[10]

From Evacuation to the Modification of Pathogenic Material

During Plato's time the question of therapy arose because the "scientific" medicine of the period—namely, that of Hippocrates and his contemporaries—had begun to delve into the matter of how *pharmaka* worked, particularly following the development of dietetics; this scientific medicine made use of *pharmaka*, probably in the context of traditional practice.[11] Physicians made an effort to establish a rational foundation for pharmacology and to integrate it into the general context of nosology, in accordance with the principle of opposites: this principle held that the action of a medication should be opposed in nature to that of the specific pathological process.[12]

An overall evaluation of the pharmacology of the Hippocratic corpus has already been carried out, and emphasis has been duly laid on the attribution to the *pharmaka* of qualities corresponding to those of the humors (hot, cold, dry, and wet).[13] It has also been pointed out that the Hippocratic use of the *pharmaka* corresponded to the mechanism that underlay therapy based on "fire and iron," although it took a different form. That mechanism involved the expulsion of pathogenic material from the body, and it has been hypothesized that Hippocratic medication-based therapy presupposed the theory of the *pharmakon* found in Aristotle's *Problemata*.[14]

Actually, the problem posed by *pharmaka* for Hippocratic physicians was that of physiological modifications: both those that caused diseases and those that restored a state of health. Hippocratic physicians were aware of these questions, at least beginning in a certain period, that of the treatise *De locis in homine* (especially chapter 45), believed to date from the fourth century B.C.

In the context of humoral physiology, the Hippocratic treatises of the fifth and fourth centuries B.C. described these modifications in material terms: disease or a state of health derived from the presence or absence of a nosological material—a humor. This point of view was not new, and can be detected as early as the *Iliad* (4.217–219), where a physician sucks a wound to extract the harmful substance or even potential evil influences from it, and in the therapy based on "fire and iron." In the case we are examining, however, this material was eliminated not through surgery but rather through the use of *pharmaka*, administered for a purgative, emetic, or diuretic purpose.[15] This was a twofold quantitative conception of solid and void; to explain the movement of humors induced by *pharmaka*, it made reference to a dynamic of attraction not unlike that of plant sap, prompted by the qualitative analogy between humors and *pharmaka*.[16]

In the Aristotelian corpus, the question of *pharmaka* was addressed in the *Problemata*,[17] attributed in part to Aristotle, with further additions by members of his school.[18] The *pharmaka* play a role here, alongside "fire and iron." As in the Hippocratic corpus, they are examined in the context of the issue of change and, albeit with a differing approach, still with a view to a therapy based on opposites.[19]

The Aristotelian analysis relies on the logic of the process of digestion:[20] the *pharmakon* is not assimilated, even though it is introduced into the body in the same way as foods. This *pharmakon*, because it is not digested, and in all likelihood because it is constituted by a compact mass, drives before it all that hinders its progress,[21] specifically, the pathogenic material. It is finally evacuated from the body, along with the material in question. The *pharmakon* thus causes a movement, comparable with the movement caused by exercise, which prompts expulsion of extraneous substances.[22]

In this context, two different pharmacological dynamics are suggested. The first—as in the Hippocratic corpus—is that of attraction. This attraction, however, is not exerted between identical qualities, as was the case in the Hippocratic corpus; rather, it occurs between substances on the one hand and organs on the other: the bladder attracts liquids and the stomach attracts solid and earthy substances.[23] The second dynamic is based on the action of gravity—in the meaning the word was given then, and not in the modern technical sense. Thus hot (and therefore light) substances caused a movement upward, while cold (and therefore heavy) substances caused a movement downward.[24]

Although they differ from the Hippocratic theory in their overall approach and dynamics, these concepts hearken back to the same general body of thought, which is based on quantitative considerations and on the mechanical movement of the *pharmaka*. All the same, with respect to the Hippocratic corpus, the conceptual system of the *Problemata* ventures further, suggesting dynamics that are more concrete than mere vegetal attraction, both with the idea—or perhaps we should say, depiction—of undigested material that moves obstacles, and with the principle of gravity, or weight.

In the *Problemata* we also glimpse another mode of action of the *pharmaka*, of an entirely opposite sort: the "dissolution" of pathogenic materials.[25] This is a significant difference: while remaining within the bounds of a conception of quantitative evacuation, there emerges a theory of a "qualitative" modification of the pathogenic material, which, under the action of the solvent, changes its form and is dragged away by the digestive flow, disappearing to all intents and purposes, even if it is not quantitatively suppressed. Here we can recognize the Aristotelian theory of change, conceived in terms of continuity of the material substrate, subject to modifications of form.

This sort of concept was adopted by Diocles of Carystos (in the fourth century B.C.)[26] in his toxicology of poisoning of animal origin. According to the introduction of the treatise *De venenatis animalibus* (wrongly attributed to Dioscorides), Diocles of Carystos, in his *Epistula de tuenda valetudine,* had proposed the following syllogism: in the major premise we find the general principle taken from *opinio communis,* according to which "to great effects, great causes should be attributed." Diocles maintained in the minor premise, that animal poisonings are great effects, since they cause serious physiological alterations and, in some cases, death. Therefore, he concluded, they should be attributed to great causes, and hence to large animals. And yet, Diocles continued, such a conclusion is contradicted by reality, since venomous animals are, for the most part, small, in some cases too small to see. To resolve this contradiction, inherent in the syllogism, Diocles introduced the idea of *dynamis,* in the Aristotelian sense, that is, of a potential capable of transforming itself and deploying all of its effects, to the point of bringing about consequences markedly greater than its original state. This concept contradicted the major premise of the syllogism, to some extent, because small causes could thus provoke effects that were greater than their cause. When applied to the problem of poisonings of animal origin, this concept made it possible to escape the vicious circle that derived from the syllogism: venomous animals, negligible in size, can still cause great effects, by transmitting a *dynamis.* To be precise, venomous animals inject a venom, which therefore contains the *dynamis.*

The term *dynamis* appears—both in the Hippocratic corpus and in the *Problemata*—in reference to *pharmaka,*[27] but it does not seem to have the specific meaning attributed to it by Diocles. We see, for example, in the *Problemata* competition from the term *arete,* which means, chiefly, "quality."[28]

With this theory, the phenomenon of corporeal change, which follows on the introduction of a substance, was transported definitively from the quantitative realm to the qualitative realm: in quantitative terms, the organism remained unchanged yet was subject to a modification in its own intrinsic quality. The dynamic of the material introduced into the body changed, too: it was no longer a matter of mechanistic physics, however it functioned, but rather—as Diocles explicitly stated—a matter of a progressive propagation of the *dynamis,* beginning at the point of inoculation.[29]

The theory was taken up again by Erasistratus and presented in more explicit terms.[30] From animal venoms it was then extended to cover plant toxins and *pharmaka,* as we find in Dioscorides's treatise *De materia medica,* where the term *dynamis* is used in a sense that, while not clearly defined, recalls the meaning employed by Aristotle and Diocles.[31] Although we cannot be sure exactly when this transposition occurred, let us emphasize that the term *dynamis* appears in the title of a treatise by Mantias (of the second or first century B.C.), taken as an equivalent to *pharmakon.* This was probably in accordance with a practice that was common and ancient even then.[32]

The earliest work on medicinal plants that has survived intact, book 9 of Theophrastus's *Historia plantarum,* of questionable authenticity,[33] summarized the information then available on the subject,[34] and in particular reported a number of practices that were in all likelihood traditional. This work attests to a body of knowledge concerning *pharmaka* and their actions that was already quite extensive.[35] Although Theophrastus made use of the term *dynamis,* he does not seem to have been familiar with the theory of the *dynamis* of the *pharmaka,* even if it is generally held that he took the contents of his work from Diocles.

Toward an All-Encompassing Theory

With Herophilus, it would seem, came a return to a certain degree of pragmatism. This shift certainly did not rule out extensive reliance on *pharmaka,* especially since, with Alexander's expedition and the discovery of biotypes unlike those found in the Mediterranean region, the number of plants known to the Greek world had greatly increased.[36]

In connection with therapy, Herophilus had written that "medications are the hands of the gods."[37] Some have considered this statement an allusion to another therapeutic "approach" (alongside dietetics, *pharmaka,* and surgery), perhaps a reference to incubation or magic.[38] Perhaps, however, the phrase should be considered as a statement of a theory of *pharmaka.* According to Galen's interpretation, in fact, Herophilus meant to say that, in order for *pharmaka* to attain their effects, one must manipulate them properly.[39] This consideration constitutes a theory of medication, which is moreover not at odds with the concept of *dynamis*. In order for *dynamis* to work, it required a properly prepared medical material. In any case, Herophilus's statement supplied a theoretical foundation for the pharmaceutical art, since the preparer had to be a specialist and could no longer be identified with the physician—if we accept that this ever happened, as has been hypothesized[40]—who carried with him the medical materials required by his practice. The expression may have been an allusion to a divine providence toward men, which had endowed them with health-giving knowledge. This view of affairs, confirmed by Dioscorides, constituted a "genealogy," if not a "theology" of the *pharmaka*.

Toxicology, on which he relied for the formulation of his theory of *dynamis*, was used by the empirical school, founded by Philinus of Kos in the third century B.C.,[41] among other things to refute that very theory. One of the arguments used was that rabies, then considered to be a form of poisoning, required a period of incubation: the Empirics, who accepted only the evidence of the senses, rejected the idea that the poison inoculated by the bite of a rabid dog could be a *dynamis*, as the injection was not followed by any direct effects.[42] The rejection of speculation concerning the invisible probably forced the Empirics to reject any theories on the mode in which *pharmaka* acted. As far as medication-based therapy was concerned, they stuck to their theory, known as the "theory of the tripod," which involved transferring from one syndrome to another syndrome, with similar exterior manifestations, the remedies that had proven effective in the treatment of the first syndrome.

Empiricism, which by principle rejected the sort of thought on which the theory of *dynamis* rested, could have undercut that theory. Such was not the case: empiricism in fact enriched the field of rationalist pharmacology with a new experimental dimension—though not in the modern sense of the term—as we learn from the writings of Dioscorides, who cited experiments certainly conducted in an effort to establish the *dynameis* of medical materials.[43]

The concept of qualitative propagation of *dynamis* met with redoubtable competition from the corpuscular materialism set forth by Asclepiades of Bithynia. He explained physiological change as exchanges of particles, in the context of a materialism that was more refined than the earlier version, of hollows and solids.[44] In this way, the corpuscular idea was used in the context of pharmacology for the first time, ancient though it may have been, and attested as early as Leucippus. When applied to a broad range of medical materials, this was without doubt a seductive theory, at least to judge from the list of "Asclepiadian" pharmacologists mentioned by Dioscorides, though he was highly critical of them.[45] Among their number was Sextius Niger (first century A.D.), whose treatise on medical materials is considered to have been a source for Dioscorides and Pliny. This fact indicates just how fertile the corpuscular concept had been in the field of *pharmaka*, given that Dioscorides appropriated the contents while condemning the theory as "pointless chatter."

In an extension of the theory of Asclepiades that appeared during the first century B.C., known as methodism and based on an elementary physiology of tension *(status strictus)* and relaxation *(status laxus)*, the *pharmaka* were supposed to counter those states by inducing, respectively, states of relaxation or tensions, according to the principle of opposites. Despite this intentionally simple scheme, methodism made use of a broad array of medical materials from the outset and possessed considerable knowledge of the properties of *pharmaka*, with subtle gradations.[46] The various currents of pharmacology at the dawn of the Christian era were drawn together—with the exception of methodism—in the treatise *De materia medica* by Dioscorides. Dioscorides, in effect, based his work on the theory of *dynamis*, enriching that theory with the empirical standards of a certain body of experimentation and with information taken from Sextius Niger.[47] Dioscorides added to this synthesis of methods a further synthesis of concrete information, with the objective of being exhaustive, as he pointed out himself.[48] Thus, he presented a complete and veritable file on each medical material; in particular these files contained all the information needed to recognize the medical materials in the field and to understand their properties and actions. This constituted an extension of the theory of Diocles, with *dynameis*, both general[49] and specific.[50] These descriptions were completed by instructions on how to prepare and administer the medications.

Dioscorides offered, along with this body of practical information, a speculative dimension, expressed implicitly by the structure of the treatise. For example, he clearly shared Herophilus's view of the divine origin of the *pharmaka;* we find an indication of this view in the presence of the iris, in the opening section of the book. In Greek, "Iris" indicates the plant in question; but it also refers to the rainbow and to a mythological messenger of the gods, the goddess of the rainbow. Therefore, the treatise opens with an evocation of a link between heaven and earth, both material (rainbow) and divine (Iris, the messenger of the gods).[51]

Moreover, Dioscorides suggested an explanation of the origin of the *dynameis* of the *pharmaka*, thereby filling a gap. Once again, he did so through allusion; he used the treatise structure, in which the medical materials were organized according to their *dynamis*.[52] Here, too, we can detect a reference to the toxicological model, in which this procedure is essential. Now, this grouping overlaps the grouping whereby the simples are arrayed according to one or another of their natural characteristics. From this parallelism between action and nature—*dynamis* and *physis*—it was considered possible to deduce a linkage of effect to cause, that is, an explanation of the origin of the *dynamis* of the *pharmaka* and, at the same time, an explanation of the differences among the various *dynameis*, since different properties obviously corresponded to different natures.

This link between *dynamis* and *physis* introduced a certain historical aspect to the field of *pharmakon;* according to Greek thought, *physis* was a history, the history of the creation of the *kosmos*, taken not merely as a narrative, but first and foremost as the foundation of reality. Therefore, to the archaic mind-set, materials partake of all the phases of creation of the *kosmos* to which they are linked. Thus, perfumes, which are specific to the gods, were—by this reasoning—warm and airy. Minerals, by contrast, belonging as they do to the age of iron, are cold and heavy. The uses to which *pharmaka* were put derived from the *dynamis* that each possessed in virtue of this cosmogony: perfumes, since they are hot, were used to treat gynecological problems, assumed to be caused by an excess of humidity, while minerals, being cold, were used to treat skin disorders, believed to result from excess heat.

The relationships between *pharmaka* and the cosmos thus introduced a hierarchy of medications. That hierarchy can be detected in the structure of Dioscorides' work, which the author states is original, without explaining in what way. The medical materials are arranged in groups, in a succession—historical or hierarchical, mingled together—that corresponds to the phases of the cosmogony linked with these *pharmaka* (perfumes and scents come first; mineral products conclude the work).

Thus, with Dioscorides, the theory of *pharmaka* attained completion. First, the theory called itself complete, both in method and in the body of information assembled, which was based moreover on a theory that could account for the actions of all *pharmaka*. Furthermore, the theory took a global form, integrating the *pharmaka* into the general context of the universe.

In certain manuscripts, the text by Dioscorides is accompanied by illustrations of the medical materials under study.[53] And although it has been ventured that these figures date back to the Greek herbalist Cratevas (of the second or first century B.C.), believed to be the author of the first illustrated herbarium,[54] it is not known whether they illustrated the original version of the treatise of Dioscorides.

In Search of a Universal Medication

The current that culminated in the treatise of Dioscorides—therapy through simple medications—at that time faced sharp competition from another current, that of therapy through compound medications, which associated a number of simples. Already practiced by Herophilus, this therapy developed primarily with Mantias.[55]

Toxicology once again played a part in this development, especially with the sovereigns of the realms that emerged from the dismemberment of the empire of Alexander the Great. This may already have been the case with Antigonus Gonatas (ca. 320–239 B.C.), king of Macedon; Antioch III (ca. 242–187 B.C.), king of Syria; and Ptolomy IV (ca. 244–2059 B.C.), king of Egypt. It definitely was the case with Attalus III of Pergamum, who reigned from 138 to 133 B.C., and who was reputed to have tested the effects of poisons on his slaves.[56] His contact with Nicander, the second-century B.C. author of the earliest known works of toxicology, is certainly an indicative datum.

In the *Theriaka* and *Alexipharmaka*,[57] which may have been written on the basis of the work of Apollodorus (third century B.C.),[58] Nicander treated intoxication from both animal venoms and plant poisons. If the toxicology of poisons demonstrated a clear understanding of the specific action of toxins, with remedies offered for each, the toxicology of venoms was still quite vague, for the actions of the venoms were not clearly differentiated, and the remedies were even less so.[59]

The most renowned of Hellenistic sovereigns in the field of poisons was Mithridates VI Eupator (132–63 B.C.), the king of Pontus, who gave a new direction to toxicology—that of compound *pharmakon* and habituation. The development of this *pharmakon*, even though it was based on experimentation,[60] could not have failed to involve theoretical speculation. The principle that would have informed such speculation must have been the specific action of each poison and the consequential specificity of the remedies for each. Therefore, Mithridates mixed together all of the remedies for all possible cases of poisoning, hoping to use a single *pharmakon* to treat every possible sort of accident. This must have been the underlying reasoning[61] (and not that of an interaction of the *pharmaka* that made up the compound, which would have resulted in new properties).[62] It is not possible, therefore, to speak of a universal *pharmakon*, capable of acting on any pathology whatsoever. Progressively, Mithridates habituated himself so well, with small doses of poisons, that, when he was defeated by the Romans, he was unable to take his life by poison and was forced to have his throat cut. He was not the inventor of the principle of habituation, however. It had already been set forth by Aristotle[63] and Theophrastus.[64] Rather, Mithridates first applied these principles to compound *pharmaka*, making them into a preventive preparation.

Compositions with multiple ingredients and antidotes abounded in that period; they spread through Rome following the defeat of Mithridates by Pompeii in 63 B.C., the conquest of Egypt in 48–47 B.C.,[65] and, a little later, the Arabian expedition of Aelius Gallus.[66] The last two events encouraged the import of exotic Eastern drugs to Rome.[67] Toxicology and pharmacology, both simple and compound, were quite fashionable in this period, leading to the writing—during the first century A.D.—of syntheses like that of Celsus,[68] the more specific collection by Scribonius Largus,[69] and the vast fresco of the *Historia naturalis* by Pliny the Elder.[70] In this same period Dioscorides wrote a treatise in which the *pharmaka* were presented, according to disease, likewise classified *a capite ad calcem*. Also dating from this period was the information contained in the two treatises of toxicology attributed to Dioscorides.[71] The toxicology of poisons was then attaining its highest point of development, with a diagnostic method based on the typology of toxic actions; the toxicology of venoms did not attain a similar level until Philomenos (second century A.D.) and his treatise *De venenatis animalibus eorumque remediis*.

The pharmacology of compounds was also verging on its highest stage of development and was about to make a decisive step: that of passing from the multiple-ingredient preparations of toxicology toward nontoxicological pathologies.[72] And it was certainly not the presence of opium alone that led to this transition. More likely, it derived from experiences and speculations like those explored by Mithridates.

Pharmaka had become so fashionable that even the imperial powers did not hesitate to make use of poison in settling dynastic squabbles. It was, again, the imperial power that ordered the creation of the most important *pharmakon* of the period, theriac. Nero (A.D. 37–68) had the Cretan physician Andromachus prepare this preventive *pharmakon*. The preparation was based on a formula of Mithridates, modified by the addition of viper flesh.[73] All of this was done in accordance with the principle of preventive habituation through regular consumption of small doses. In fact, the head was cut off the viper, since the head was believed to contain the venom. Then the small amount of venom contained in the body was weakened by cooking and by the addition of many other ingredients. Thus, from the sum of medical materials, an effect was obtained that was greater than the sum of the individual components.

Syntheses

The encyclopedism of the first century A.D. and the development of compound *pharmaka* are found again in the pharmacology of Galen, in which a broad collection of materials was analyzed, requiring a systematic reorganization by the author.[74] In an early treatise, Galen studied the simple *pharmaka*, beginning with a vast theoretical section, and then proceeded to analyze the *pharmaka* themselves, classifying them by type—vegetable, animal, or mineral—and then, within each type, in alphabetical order.[75] An enormous project, it demanded personal checking. It took twenty years, beginning around A.D. 170. Later, Galen went on to deal with the compound *pharmaka*, beginning with the nontoxic ones. Here, too, given the vastness of the subject, Galen adopted a number of subdivisions, first grouping the *pharmaka* according to typology[76] and then, toward A.D. 190, reorganizing them by the part of the body they were meant to affect.[77] Finally, in the last years of his life, Galen dedicated himself to the systematic presentation of the toxic *pharmaka*.[78] Based on the chronology of these treatises, we can deduce that Galen did not turn to the problem of *pharmaka* only in later life. As he tells us himself, beginning in his apprenticeship, he found himself dealing with a case in which, to find an explanation of the pathology in question, he was forced to rely on the toxicological model and on the idea of diffusion by progressive propagation.[79] Indeed, it is likely that Galen used the varied pharmacological experience of an entire lifetime in writing these treatises.

These lengthy treatises are testimony to the many—presumably complementary—facets of Galen's thought. On the one hand, he applied the theory of the *dynamis* to both toxins and remedies.[80] Although this theory was of Aristotelian origin, in Galen it took on Platonic connotations. Indeed, Galen never states that a certain *pharmakon* possesses a certain *dynamis*, saying instead that it partakes of this *dynamis*.[81] On the other hand, he integrated *pharmaka* and animal venoms and plant toxins into the theory of the four humors: the *dynameis*, theoretically limitless in Dioscorides, were reduced in Galen's work to four basic "qualities" (*poiotes*—hot, cold, dry, and wet), to which moreover degrees were assigned, giving rise to as many different properties.[82] Since the qualities were those of the humors, it became possible to fit the action of the *pharmaka* into Galen's physiology and nosology. Moreover, the *qualities*, like the humors, for that matter, were made to correspond with the fundamental constituent elements of the world (air, water, fire, earth), the seasons, and the ages of life. Lastly, poisons and venoms were conceived in terms of *physis*, or essence. Nonetheless, underlying each of these definitions we find the Aristotelian concept of *dynamis*, as we can clearly see in a passage in which Galen, although he is speaking of essence, adopts the reasoning of Diocles, according to which noteworthy effects are produced despite a modest amount of material inoculated.[83]

All these different aspects may well be more complementary than opposite, and they serve to conciliate the dynamic theory with humoral materialism: indeed, *dynamis* and its system of qualitative modifications fits into the logic of the system of humors, which are material entities. The identification of the concept of *dynamis* with the qualities of the humors, moreover, made it possible to establish an all-encompassing system, like that of Dioscorides, which established a link between pharmacology and the macrocosm. Unlike Dioscorides' system, which can be described as medication-based, or pharmacocentric, Galen's system can be called physician-based, or medicocentric. He did not analyze the *pharmaka* per se, but rather placed them in a broader medical theory.

The ancient world had thus reached the height of its potential, as far as the theory of *pharmaka* was concerned, as we shall see from succeeding events. In the Byzantine world, in fact, the treatises of Dioscorides and Galen were often reproduced and almost as often paired, beginning with the first Byzantine medical work, that of Oribasius.[84] This attempt to integrate the two theories extended over time, as we can see from a manuscript of Dioscorides, copied around A.D. 512, or from the books devoted to pharmacology in the context of treatises by Aetius of Amida and Paul of Aegina.

Possibly influenced by Galen's work, an alphabetical reorganization of

Dioscorides' treatise was completed. It was designed to make it possible to find a substance immediately, and basically transformed the treatise into a dictionary of medication-based therapy. Beginning from this reorganization, an alphabetical herbarium was written, documented by the manuscript dating from 512, mentioned above. A third reorganization was carried out; this one was attributed to Stephen of Alexandria, although we have no way of knowing whether he really was the author: the indications of the *pharmaka* reappear in alphabetical order. These three reelaborations transformed the treatise so that it served practical purposes, without any concern for theory, possibly in the context of professional teaching.[85]

The progressive disenchantment with theory was later confirmed, with a renaissance in the context of Byzantine culture; first the prominent and outstanding works of the past were recovered in each discipline, followed by the production of new treatises.[86] In the field of pharmacology, the treatises of Dioscorides and Galen were thus rediscovered and, once again, associated and confused, to the point that the title of a tenth-century manuscript announced that it contained Galen's treatise *De simplicium medicamentorum temperamentis et facultatibus*, whereas it actually contained the text by Dioscorides, reorganized in accordance with Galen's structure and completed with fragments of Galen's text.[87] The implicit structure-based theoretical information found in the treatise by Dioscorides was thus lost, along with all the explicit theoretical information that constituted the introduction to Galen's great work. As for the original production of this period, the treatise by Theophanes Chrysobalantes (tenth century) presents an entire series of prescriptions for diseases *a capite ad calcem*, without any theoretical concepts.[88]

We do not find the appearance of any new theories in the field of *pharmaka* until the Arab world—which had adopted the scientific heritage of Byzantium through translations—encountered a problem that had been of little or no concern to the ancient world and to Byzantium: that of the terminology of medical materials. This problem, in short, referred to the relationship between "words" and "things." The Arab physicians, moreover, developed new theories in the field of pharmacology. Al-Kindi, for instance, formulated the Galenic degrees of the properties of *pharmaka* in accordance with a mathematical model. There was also the invention of a new system of presentation of pharmacological information, the "tables" (in Arabic, *taqwim*, which became in Latin, *tacuinum*). These were used by Ibn Butlan.

The Latin West showed less creativity,[89] and relied on the spread of

Alexandrian knowledge and Latin translations of the ancient treatises,[90] at first in North Africa in the fifth century, and then in Ravenna in the sixth century.[91] In an eminently practical context, Galen's treatise *Ad secta* may have represented the only theoretical reference.[92] Then, beginning in the eleventh century, the West adopted the ancient theories along with their Arabic versions, through the translation into Latin of the Arabic treatises. This work of translation was begun by Constantine of Africa, in southern Italy. It was later carried forward in Toledo, in France, and in northern Italy. Among these works were the *Antidotarium* by Niccolò di Salerno; *Circa instans* by Matthaeus Platearius; and a treatise on poisons by Peter of Abano. It was thus possible to restore to pharmacological practice—which had never ceased—the theoretical foundations that had originally distinguished it.

~ 10 ~

Therapeutic Strategies: Surgery

MICHAEL MCVAUGH

Skeletal specimens from the Bronze Age (and earlier) preserve for us the evidence that well before the first Greek surgical writings some development of practical knowledge had already taken place. The occasional well-set and -healed fracture is one indication, but even more striking, in part for what it implies about underlying assumptions, is the evidence for trepanation: though this seems to have originated as a ritual act, by Mycenean times the technique and instrumentation were well advanced. Bony remains thus let us glimpse a small part of the historical background to the surgical texts that suddenly appear in the Hippocratic corpus.[1]

Three of these texts are particularly noteworthy: *De fracturis, De articulis,* and *De capitis vulneribus.* They deal carefully with a restricted range of physical conditions, and they have been much admired for the precision of their treatments.[2] Some would see the first two of these, which overlap in subject matter and which seem to suggest an emergent medical ethic,[3] as works of the historical Hippocrates himself. *De fracturis* deals with fracture of the forearm in detail as an exemplar, before turning to dislocations of the foot and ankle, leg fractures, compound fractures, and dislocations of the elbow. Similarly, *De articulis* begins with an exemplary case—dislocation of the shoulder—before taking up fracture or dislocation of the collarbone, fractures of nose and jaw, injuries to the spine, dislocation of the hip, and gangrene and amputation. Hippocrates' techniques for reduction were generally effective (though some passages seem impossible anatomically) and were passed on virtually unchanged through our period: of the shoulder, by suspension over a rung of a ladder or over the operator's shoulder; of the hip, by suspension or by traction on "the Hippocratic bench," a device that Hippocrates used in certain spinal injuries as well. Fractures, simple or compound, were bandaged in a wax ointment, splinted when desirable, and covered with another pressure bandage. *De capitis vulneribus* describes the skull and its sutures carefully and distinguishes among a number of different head injuries—contusions, fissure fractures, depressed fractures—so as to explain their different consequences and treatment; fissure fractures (determined by staining with a black ink) and contusions, the author suggests, should often be treated by trepanation.

From the period of the Hippocratic corpus to the time of Celsus (the Roman encyclopedist of the first century A.D.), no surgical texts of any importance survive. Yet when we look at the seventh and eighth books of Celsus's *De medicina* we cannot help but recognize that by now the field had achieved a much wider range of technical proficiency—particularly in the area of operative surgery, which Hippocrates had left essentially untouched. This proficiency is the result of the achievements of a long line of practitioners at Alexandria in Egypt, after 300 B.C.: Celsus himself praised Philoxenos (before 100 B.C.?), but Alexandrian surgery goes back at least a century and a half before that date. What made these surgical developments possible were the anatomical discoveries of Herophilus and Erasistratus, combined with improved instruments and a greater willingness to interpret human physiology mechanistically. These developments led to innovations of considerable significance—among them, apparently, the new (at the time) recognition that the ligaturing of veins and arteries will stop the flow of blood, which made not only therapeutic bloodletting but also more extensive operations much safer. Yet there was no single surgical program: we have evidence of various traditions coming out of Alexandria—one developing an operative surgery in conjunction perhaps with wound treatment, another pursuing the "mechanical" surgery of the Hippocratics, yet another turning to obstetric and gynecological problems.[4]

In a sense, that variety is visible in the organization of Celsus's work, which deliberately treats of wounds and operative surgery in one book, marking off fractures and dislocations into a second.[5] The former, book 7, while covering its subject broadly, cannot really be called systematic, and it singles out certain topics for particular attention. Its discussions of couching for cataract and of paracentesis for ascites, and its even fuller accounts of surgical intervention for hernia (where Celsus explains the use of ligatures to prevent bleeding) and for bladder stone by perineal incision, all reveal the extent to which the progress of anatomy had given surgeons the ability to interpret or visualize the conditions they were tackling. Celsus here also describes instances of what must be acknowledged as plastic surgery (though nothing as advanced as the roughly contemporary reconstruction of the nose by Indian surgeons is in question): reshaping the eyelids, repairing a perforated earlobe, covering a large gap in the skin. Book 7 also discusses the repair of abscesses and wounds, including the use of pins as sutures; here we approach a Hippocratic subject, but Celsus's account of techniques for the removal from the body of missiles, barbs, and projectiles has no counterpart in the Hippocratic corpus. Book 8, however, has little to add to Hippocrates' *De fracturis* and *De articulis* (though it is perhaps more cautious about the general advisability of trepanation). Unsystematic though it may be, *De medicina* still testifies to the remarkable advances made in surgery during the Hellenistic period.

Confirmation that such operations were indeed performed is provided by the many surgical instruments that have survived from Roman times, often of a revealingly specialized form. Among those that have been identified are forceps with roughened tips, required in lithotomy for grasping the stone through the incision; the needles used to depress or couch a cataractous lens; and the vaginal dilator often alluded to by classical writers on obstetrics and gynecology. In addition to such tools designed for specific purposes, a full range of lancets and scalpels, hooks and forceps, probes, scoops, chisels, saws, catheters, and specula has been classified by archaeologists and corresponds well to the instruments that a surgeon would have required for general practice by the first century A.D.[6]

No survey of early medicine, whatever the branch, can pass over the contribution of Galen, both because his writings constitute so much of what has been preserved from classical antiquity and because his authority bulked so large in the Middle Ages. Yet Galen has long been recognized as an equivocal figure in the history of surgery. He agreed with Hippocrates that surgery was, after diet and pharmacy, the third of the avenues to treatment open to the practitioner, yet critics point out that he paid less attention to surgery than to any other branch of medicine, and that none of his major works is devoted entirely to the subject—it is really only in *De methodo medendi* (especially books 13–14) that he treats it at any length.[7] It seems feeble to retort, as some do, that his early role as physician to the gladiators of Pergamum is sufficient guarantee of his surgical expertise.

Two things in particular help explain the reduced importance of surgery to Galen. First, he, like Hippocrates, believed in the unity of medicine and was struggling to combat its fragmentation in a number of different directions: to emphasize one particular aspect, whether exercise of pharmacy or surgery, would be to weaken that unity and make it less able to deal with the health of the whole man. He did not consider the specialist a true physician.[8] Second, for him the health at which the physician aims was an expression of the essential nature or natural state of his client, and therefore medicine properly must either preserve or restore nature. Yet much of surgery does neither. Galen's obvious interest in the discoveries of the Alexandrian anatomists is in this sense misleading, because it is not for the contribution they can make to surgical technique that he valued them. A surgery used to cut away what is natural or to impede the natural expulsive faculties of the body is misguided; Galen really wanted to see only unnatural, foreign substances cut from the body—bladder stones, for example, and cancers. And in the latter case, surgery was not the procedure of first resort, for, Galen believed, cancers in their earliest stages can and should be eliminated by the natural powers of the body, assisted by conservative use of diet and medication. In the surgery for which he did make a place in medicine, Galen was not inclined to innovate, and in at least two instances he chose deliberately to return to Hippocratic techniques in preference to more recent ones: amputation at joints, rather than through healthy bone (as recommended by Celsus), and a tendency to treat hemorrhage by pressure rather than by ligature of the vessels.

It was thus not through Galen that the detailed operative surgery of the classical world was transmitted to later times, nor was it through Celsus, whose work was virtually unknown in the Middle Ages. The critical work was instead the seven-book *Epitomae* of Paul of Aegina, composed in the seventh century as a synopsis of earlier medical writings. It moves from regimen to fevers to internal medicine to toxicology and at last, in its sixth book, surveys surgery, which is thus portrayed—as Galen would have wished—as simply a part of a much broader medical practice.[9] The contents of book 6 are a good résumé of the surgical accomplishments of the Greco-Roman world, but they are in no sense original, and indeed many of them can already be found alluded to in *De medicina*.

Paul (like Celsus) divides the subject into operative surgery and the treatment of dislocations and fractures. The former is given much more attention and is discussed in head-to-toe order. Much attention is given to conditions of the eye: trichiasis, ectropion, chalazia, cataract. Paul describes treatment of an aneurism (in the head or limbs) by ligaturing the vessel above and below the site. He makes wide use of the cautery, not only to prevent the recurrence of dislocations (a Hippocratic technique), or to treat empyema, but to produce eschars supposed to stimulate the liver, spleen, or stomach; he acknowledges its use for dropsy too, though he seems to favor a cautious paracentesis. Operation for bladder stone, hernias, vaginal abscess, fistulas, and varices are among those that follow. Paul's brief discussion of amputation describes cutting through the bone rather than dividing the limb at the joint. He has almost nothing to say about wound treatment in the section on operative surgery, merely a chapter on the repair of wounds of the peritoneum taken from Galen and another, considerable chapter on the extraction of weapons; but toward the end of book 6 he describes trepanation in certain injuries to the skull. The treatment of simple and compound fractures and of dislocations, still essentially Hippocratic, concludes his discussion. Paul's *Epitomae* was translated into Arabic in the ninth century and became the principal surgical source for the medical encyclopedists of Islam, notably 'Ali ibn al-'Abbas and Abu'l-Qasim (Albucasis).

In Latin-speaking Europe, however, where for a thousand years after Celsus there was no important medical writer, nothing comparable was available. The Roman West was in any case transformed by the Germanic invasions of the fifth century and thereafter, and the tradition of medical learning was lost: Celsus himself was rarely copied and never cited, and indeed was "rediscovered" only in the fifteenth century. Only scraps of Greek medicine were available in Latin translation, and they included nothing of importance on surgery. Western Europe thus had to rediscover surgical techniques while redefining what place surgical knowledge should have in the realm of learning. This reawakening of surgery began at the end of the eleventh century, as part of the general European renaissance, and is manifest in a remarkable continuum of Latin surgical writings that can be followed through the fourteenth century. The surgery of the high Middle Ages has left a much greater literature than that of classical antiquity.

Yet because the medieval texts served to justify as well as communicate, we cannot take them simply as factual records of practice. Medieval surgeons soon came to understand that writing itself could set them apart in a society that gave high status to learning and came to see that the fact of participation in an authorial tradition was more important than criticizing or adding to the texts they had inherited;[10] hence medieval surgical literature is often disappointingly derivative or repetitive, and for this reason it allows us to trace the evolving conceptualization of surgical practice in the Middle Ages more easily than it does the acquisition and application of technical skills.

It is superficially convenient to see the revival of surgery—like that of so much of medicine generally—as originating in the translations made by Constantine of Africa in southern Italy (after 1075). Constantine was interested enough in surgery to select the surgical book of al-'Abbas's *Pantegni* as one of the few parts he would translate from its second, practical half; his translation was completed by Johannes Afflacius, and it is apparently this to which Peter the Deacon refers as Constantine's *Liber de chirurgia*. Al-'Abbas's surgery—in the order of its chapters, which it only occasionally rearranges, keeping three-quarters of its contents and adding only a little (including more material on the use of the cautery)[11]— follows the sixth book of Paul of Aegina, and in this way the Greek surgical tradition began to enter the Latin tradition.

Yet Constantine's surgery apparently did not have the immediate impact enjoyed by his more focused medical translations, for surgery seems not to have been an important element of the teaching program, exposition, and commentary, encouraged in twelfth-century Salerno by the Constantinian material. This influence has been detected only in the so-called Bamberg surgery, a surgical compilation apparently produced at Salerno in the first half of the twelfth century. The text mixes some confused anatomical and theoretical passages drawn from pre-Constantinian sources with extended borrowings from the *Pantegni* on matters of practical surgery, and seems also to contain material based on a practical tradition: for example, the application to surgery of the suppos-edly anaesthetic "soporific sponge" (soaked in juice of henbane and poppy), the description of a leaden truss for inguinal hernia, and the treatment of goiter with sponge ashes (which contain a high concentration of iodine).[12]

A more decisive impulse behind a text-based surgical tradition came, a half-century later, from the towns of northern Italy, stimulated by both warfare and economic development; the differentiation of surgery as a craft was in a sense only one aspect of the specialization of trades that began to take place generally after 1100. The book that would have the most influence on thirteenth-century surgeons was the *Cyrurgia* of Rug-gero di Parma: the Latin text we have was polished and structured by Guido d'Arezzo (who taught logic in the Parma *studium*) about 1180, to prepare it for publication, but a Lombard vernacular lies close beneath the surface.[13] The *Cyrurgia* kept the traditional head-to-toe organization of subject matter but divided the work into four books explicitly to correspond with body parts—head, neck and throat, thorax and genitals, legs and feet—the first sign of the search for an organizing principle that would preoccupy surgeons for the next hundred years. There is no formal anatomy in Ruggero's works, however, and (in sharp contrast with the Bamberg surgery) virtually no indication of direct acquaintance with earlier medical literature, not even with Constantine's surgery. Scholars have tried to see traces of the Greco-Arabic tradition in Ruggero's work, but his only direct reference is to Hippocrates' *Aphorismi*, though some of his prescriptions are near-duplicates of ones in the Bamberg surgery (for example, the use of sponge ash for goiter) and his reference to the *siphac* reveals an acquaintance with the new Arabic terminology.

Standing as it does at the beginning of medieval surgery, Ruggero's *Cyrurgia* seems more spontaneous than most of the works that followed it. The general impression it gives is one of practical experience speaking—in its reiterated injunctions not to intervene in visceral wounds, for instance. Its author's willingness to attempt the repair of a wounded intestine by suturing the wall around a cannula is remarkable.[14] Occasionally, indeed, as in its description of methods for reducing dislocations or for treating anal fistula, we seem to hear echoes of the Greco-Arab tradition, but a tradition simplified and confused in the process of handing down. Nevertheless, Ruggero's explicit recommendation to adopt the so-called Trendelenburg position in operating for hernia is much more detailed than the similar hints to be found in a writer like Paul of Aegina.

What undoubtedly *was* an innovation—the conscious use of a textbook for surgical instruction—was due to the generation of surgeons following Ruggero. His text was being used at Salerno by about 1200, glossed with material from a humoral pathology and therapeutics. His pupil, Rolando, who left Parma for Bologna early in the thirteenth century, first appended a set of *additiones* to the *Cyrurgia* (drawing on the Salernitan glosses) and then in effect reedited the work by incorporating these and other materials directly into the text: the product, often known as the *Rolandina*, was influential in its own right, though it is overwhelmingly faithful to its source. Rolando's remark at the end—"the great variety of treatments shows that we must follow the advice of earlier authors"[15]—indicates the power that a written surgical tradition was coming to hold, for better or for worse.

In only two respects does Rolando display any truly new preoccupations of his own. One is his incorporation (at 1.20 and 3.27 of the *Rolandina*) of long passages on cancer that lay great emphasis on explaining the pathology of the disease's various forms in terms of humoral physiology; his explanation is based on Avicenna (and Galen). He does not introduce any new surgical procedures (what therapeutic measures he takes over from his sources are medical), but his very appeal to Avicennan theory at an early stage in its assimilation by European medicine hints at the surgeons' growing interest in fitting their practice into a wider context of medical theory.[16] The other passage where Rolando himself speaks out is 3.25, where he suddenly attacks surgeons who claim that a damaged lung cannot be treated and describes in circumstantial detail a case that others had abandoned but in which he operated successfully.[17] The personal voice is a new feature of thirteenth-century surgery: a written tradition was making possible self-advertisement at the expense of one's competitors in the craft.

The *Rolandina* is not the only testimony to the attractiveness of Ruggero's *Cyrurgia*. Its influence is obvious, too, in the other Latin texts, like that of Johannes Jamatus or William of Conches (in its turn translated into Hebrew!), and Latin glosses based on it in the thirteenth century; in its rapid translation into European vernaculars—Anglo-Norman, Occitan; and in its incorporation into vernacular European surgeries of the fourteenth century.[18]

Toward the middle of the thirteenth century the new Latin surgical literature was altered in its development by its confrontation with the *Surgery* of Albucasis; this work was the last of the thirty treatises composing his *Kitab al-tasrif*. Albucasis's principal source was Paul of Aegina, and thus his work at last made an encyclopedia of Greek surgical practice generally available in the West, but his modern editor has called attention to a number of instruments and procedures that apparently originated with him (or at least in the Arab world): the tonsil guillotine; the trocar for paracentesis; the syringe; the lithotrite; the use of animal gut for sutures; and an anticipation of the plaster cast (among other things).[19] Albucasis's teachings are missing from the *Rolandina*, but they appear in the work of Rolando's slightly younger contemporaries, Bruno de Longoburgo and Teodorico Borgognoni.

Bruno and Teodorico were the first writers in what might be called a new north Italian surgical school. Bruno's *Cyrurgia magna* was completed in Padua in 1252; a draft of Teodorico's *Cyrurgia* was available in 1248, but the revised version that eventually circulated was finished in 1267. The two texts are often identical, though Teodorico's is much the longer, and ever since the fourteenth century it has been assumed that Teodorico borrowed from Bruno; until the various versions of the former's work have been carefully studied, however, the question of priority cannot be resolved. To some extent the works can be treated as one.[20]

In the cities where these two men were professionally formed, Padua and Bologna, a tradition of medical education was beginning to take shape, one that was assimilating the recently recovered achievements of the Greco-Arab tradition. Bruno and Teodorico tried to incorporate these same authorities into surgical literature, though with slightly different purposes: Bruno brought together their various opinions for comparison's sake, while Teodorico used the ancient authorities to authenticate current practice—especially that of his Bolognese master (and perhaps father), Ugo of Lucca. Their sources are Albucasis's *Surgery*, the surgical portions of Avicenna's "Canon of Medicine," and Rhazes' *Book for the Salih al-Mansur*, and Galen's *Methodus medendi* (in Constantine's paraphrase, known as the *Megategni*). All are drawn on extensively, both for physiological explanations and for therapeutic procedures—in their thorough discussions of dislocations, for example.[21] Thus while Teodorico has been credited with anticipating the use of "Dugas's sign" to diagnose shoulder dislocation (and the same sign is quoted by Bruno), both authors have in fact taken this passage directly from Albucasis. They did not accept their authorities unquestioningly, however; Teodorico in particular took occasional advantage of the opportunities of a written tradition to portray his master—and himself—as superior to the ancients as well as to contemporary practitioners. The *Rolandina* had once or twice openly corrected Ruggero's *Cyrurgia* (2.1–3), but Teodorico challenged Avicenna (2.1), Albucasis (2.19), and even Galen (2.17) in Ugo's name and his own. As for Rolando, Teodorico accused him of having stolen from Ugo's practice his boasted cure of a lung wound, a cure to which Rolando had merely been a witness.[22]

The career of Guglielmo da Saliceto (or Piacenza) demonstrates even more clearly how the north Italian surgeons of the later thirteenth century were trying to bring surgery and learned medicine together. Guglielmo practiced both subjects, in Cremona, Pavia, Milan, and above all Bologna; and he wrote texts on both as well, a medical *Summa conservationis et curationis corporis* and a *Cirurgia* whose revised version he completed in 1276. More directly than his contemporaries, Guglielmo tried to associate surgery with the status of the academic *studium*. Bruno and Teodorico both defined surgery as a tool *(instrumentum)* of medicine, and by repeating a traditional etymology that can be traced back to the Bamberg surgery (and, before that, to Isidore of Seville)—"surgery comes from *cyros* which is hand and *agia* which is action"—emphasized the artisanal character of the subject. Guglielmo broke with tradition by omitting this etymology, insisting instead on the rationality of surgery: "surgery," he declared, "is one of the sciences contained within medicine, and it is possible to acquire this science [through reason], without ever having practiced, confirming it by testing it on particular cases."[23] In this way surgeons could hope to share the prestige of the learned physicians in the new universities.

The belief of these northern Italian surgeons that surgical practice required an understanding of medicine is further illustrated by their experimentation with new ways to organize their treatises. Ruggero (and to a degree Rolando) gave his work what might be called a topographical structure: conditions were arranged under parts of the body concerned, listed from head to toe. Bruno and Teodorico broke with this pattern and instead used pathological criteria as organizing principles, first distinguishing conditions marked by *solutio continuitatis* (wounds, fractures) and discussing them, then proceeding to other complaints appropriate to the surgeon. Guglielmo appealed to a different taxonomic principle (but still one based on pathology), bringing together in book 1 conditions produced by internal causes (goiter, scrofula, hemorrhoids), then those produced by external causes (wounds in book 2, fractures in book 3). In all these works it is the broader medical framework that gives structure to the surgeon's practice.

Guglielmo's *Cirurgia* is distinctive in one other organizational respect: it is the first medieval surgical text to present a separate section on anatomy, though this is quite short and comes curiously late in the work (book 4), almost appearing as an afterthought. The importance of anatomy to the healing arts had long been recognized (in principle) by the Middle Ages: Salernitan writers produced brief texts on the subject in the twelfth century, intended to be illustrated by the dissection of a pig. The discussion of anatomy found in new Arabic works like Rhazes' *al-Mansur* no doubt reinforced the growing interest in anatomy that is obvious by the midthirteenth century. Guglielmo's concerns, however, were by no means merely academic. He explained to his readers that he would not be exhaustive in his treatment or try to speak of parts not apparent to the senses but would instead describe the number, position, and arrangement of members of which the surgeon would need to be aware as he used the knife of the cautery. Earlier surgical writers had certainly shown an intermittent awareness of the importance of anatomical considerations to their practice, but Guglielmo was the first to emphasize it to this extent.

From the manner in which Guglielmo described wound treatment in book 2 it is obvious that for him a knowledge of anatomy was not simply a theoretical necessity but something that he kept constantly in mind in his practice. His account of throat wounds (2.7), for example, begins with a description of the throat's internal structure—arteries, veins, esophagus, trachea—and the consequences of damage to each, explaining the varying outcome in four cases he had observed personally.[24] Although such allusions to personal practice can also be found in Rolando and Teodorico, the regularity with which Guglielmo presented brief case histories to illustrate or justify his methods is another distinctive feature of his *Cirurgia,* and gives the reader a certain confidence that the work is more than a synthesis of earlier surgical literature. No doubt such narratives were inserted as much for self-advertisement as for instruction, and it is not unreasonable to imagine that they were selected or even embellished for publication; yet even so Guglielmo manages to evoke a surgeon's clinical encounter as vividly as anyone since Galen. Clinical experience comes through, too, in his corrections of earlier techniques: "don't listen to those [surgeons in the tradition of Ruggero] who advise suturing the intestine around a cannula placed within," he warns, "because a cannula is unyielding and cannot be expelled by nature, and it can pierce the intestine almost immediately."[25]

Yet the newer surgical writings, especially those of Bruno and Guglielmo, did not have the success enjoyed by the Ruggero-Rolando tradition. Teodorico's work had somewhat better luck and was incorporated into later Latin surgery as well as translated into many vernaculars; in late-medieval Spain it was for a long time the dominant surgical text. The real European impact of this northern Italian surgery, however, came in a different way, when it was brought in person to northern Europe by the Milanese Lanfranchi, who had studied in Bologna with Guglielmo da Saliceto and practiced in Milan before political turmoil there forced him to flee to France in 1290; he practiced in Lyons for a few years before coming to Paris in 1295. There, in what he hailed enthusiastically as "a land of peace and scholarship," he finished his *Chirurgia magna* in 1296. Though we have no solid contemporary evidence for Lanfranchi's professional associations in Paris, he may have had some ties to the faculty of medicine there, for in certain respects—the scholastic flavor of its first chapters, for example, or the frequency with which it appeals to Greek and Arabic authorities—his great work appears to have been composed with an academic audience in mind, which is consistent with thirteenth-century surgery's persistent attempts to assimilate itself to learned medicine. Although Lanfranchi alludes to personal experience much less often than his master Guglielmo, significantly one of his few case histories is designed to contrast his practice favorably, not with a professional colleague's, but with that of an unlearned empiric, a *laicus*.

True to his master's model for organizing surgical knowledge, Lanfranchi included a separate exposition of anatomy in his textbook, and even placed it at the beginning of his work, immediately after his discussion of the nature and purpose of surgery—which, again like Guglielmo, he represented vigorously as a science grounded in theory, not as a mere manual craft. However, the *Chirurgia magna* introduced one organizational feature that is not to be found in any of the Latin surgeries we have so far considered but would subsequently become routine. The book's final section is an *antidotarium*, a compendium of the drugs that a surgeon may use to cleanse, to eat away, to soften, or to regenerate the flesh: their general function, preparation, and specific applications are all explained. It is difficult not to suspect that this new focusing of attention on pharmacy may have been yet another way in which surgeons were attempting to draw their discipline closer to medicine.

Lanfranchi was the means by which much of Europe became acquainted with the new Italian surgery. Not only his textbook but his teaching activity in Paris communicated the ideal of a scientific discipline to French surgeons. Henri de Mondeville, writing in the French capital only ten years later, proclaimed that his "Surgery" would be based on Avicenna, Teodorico, and Lanfranchi. His indebtedness to the last may have been more than literary, for Mondeville tells us that he studied medicine at Montpellier and then taught surgery at both Montpellier and Paris, where he became surgeon to King Phillipe IV le Bel; and he could thus have followed Lanfranchi's instruction in person.[26] Certainly in a great many respects Mondeville's work embodied and developed the tendencies already clear in his Parisian predecessor's. The specific debt he announced was to Lanfranchi's treatment of ulcers and other diseases (for wound treatment, Mondeville followed Teodorico; he was prevented by death from writing on the treatment of fractures). But he also adopted the new practice of concluding a surgical textbook with a pharmaceutical section, discussing drugs and their preparation; he placed his discussion of anatomy at the very beginning of his work, before even his explanation of the nature and function of surgery; and throughout he vigorously promoted surgery as a scholastic science. Even more explicitly than Lanfranchi, perhaps, Mondeville chose to blur the distinction between physician and surgeon and to stress instead the gulf between the intelligent surgeon, literate and grounded in the general principles of medical theory, and the rude, illiterate, empiric craftsman—Lanfranchi's *laicus*. Nor was this merely rhetoric: he quoted widely and accurately from medical as well as surgical sources, including many works less than twenty years old.

The strengths and weaknesses of the new orientation adopted by these surgical writers are particularly apparent in what is certainly the most famous episode in all medieval surgery, the controversy over wound treatment recorded by Mondeville in book 2 of his surgery. It is his report, in fact, that has set the terms in which modern historians have understood the episode. Yet we might wonder about the objectivity of Mondeville's presentation, for it is explicitly cast as a reenactment of Galen's account in the *Methodus medendi* of the competition among three ancient sects: the Methodists, the Empirics, and the Dogmatists. Today, says Mondeville, there are again three sects among practicing surgeons, distinguished by their treatment of wounds: Ruggero, Rolando, and their disciplines enforce a strict diet, excluding all wine, and probe and dress the wound with medicines and ointments so as to evoke a hot abscess in response; the school of Guglielmo of Saliceto and Lanfranchi is less strict, occasionally allowing a broader diet and dressing the wound less violently; but Ugo of Lucca, Teodorico, and their modern adherents give a broad diet, with wine and no water, and intervene little in dressing certain wounds. This new method of Teodorico, which Mondeville advocates vigorously, consists in cleansing the wound as gently as possible, bathing it with hot wine, suturing it if necessary, and bandaging it with cloths again moistened with hot wine.[27]

Mondeville's manifesto has often been interpreted as an anticipation of antisepsis and as a triumph of objectivity and empiricism, but this reading makes him a modern and misinterprets the purpose of the medieval text. For there is nothing dispassionate about Mondeville's "Surgery," whose attacks on those he considers unqualified are particularly cruel. Though he is more sympathetic to his professional colleagues, his discussion of wound treatment has obviously been cast so as to put him (and his master, Jean Pitart) at a competitive advantage vis-à-vis everyone else.

Moreover, Mondeville does not lay claim to a universal principle, for his treatment is only for fresh, clean wounds and cuts, and he is careful to justify it, not merely because it works, but because it is rational in terms of scholastic medical theory: simple wounds require drying agents to heal; wine is a drying agent; and so forth. But Mondeville agrees with earlier writers that a wound involving seriously bruised or lost flesh requires medicines that will break down the damaged material and expel it, and will then help build up new flesh from the bottom of the wound; these must be treated in the time-honored way, with tents to keep the wound open and unguents to provoke suppuration. Such theoretical reasoning provides the force behind Mondeville's argument, for a demonstration of dialectic skill was another way to acquire a competitive edge in the new academic environment that surgeons were hoping to enter.[28]

The successful transplantation of the new Italian surgery into a Parisian setting, represented by Lanfranchi and Mondeville, gave it a new instructional center from which to spread. One of Lanfranchi's students at Paris, Jan Yperman, returned home to Flanders and there published his own account of his master's teachings in the 1320s, diffusing them into the Low Countries. And in the following generation there appeared what is arguably the most accomplished surgical text of the Middle Ages, one that thereafter was the predominant authority for European surgeons for a hundred years and more: the *Cirurgia magna* or *Inventarium* of Guy de Chauliac, sometimes known as the *Ars chirurgica* and finished at Avignon in 1363.

The *Inventarium* is a fascinating work on many counts, embodying as it does the culmination of several intellectual trends we have already observed in medieval surgery. Writers from Rolando to Henri de Mondeville had shown an increasing awareness that the work of their predecessors was the technical setting for their own: Guy's sensitivity to the importance of the past gave rise to a remarkable historical introduction to surgery, one that offers a developmental interpretation of the medieval tradition and roots it, not in the Arabs, but in Paul of Aegina and especially Galen, whom Guy cites repeatedly throughout the *Inventarium*. He shows a remarkable familiarity with the whole Galenic corpus and expresses great admiration for the new translation (from the Greek) made by Niccolò da Reggio in the previous generation.

Guy's praise of Galen demands explanation, since as we have seen the latter did not pay great attention to surgery. What Guy found in the

Galenic writing was not so much surgical technique as an intellectual rationale for surgery. Guy, like Mondeville, had had both medical and surgical training (at Montpellier and Bologna, respectively), and he too argued for the necessary connection between the two disciplines; Niccolò's translation of Galen's *De usu partium*, a work that systematically explains the link between form and function, is quoted repeatedly in the book on anatomy with which—in the now traditional manner—the *Inventarium* begins.

As its title suggests, Guy's work was written to assimilate and coordinate the opinions of earlier writers, from Galen to Mondeville, and the passages it inserts from those authors function as part of the text itself. Again we must remember that textual consistency had emerged, for medieval surgeons, as no less a guarantee of truth than empirical results, which could often be equivocal. Guy is suspicious of innovations, such as Teodorico's method of wound treatment, especially when they seem founded on mistaken scholarship: he rejects (3.1.1) the doctrine of Teodorico and Mondeville that wine should be given to the wounded internally as well as externally, arguing specifically that these authors' dependence on the older translations from the Arabic had led them to misunderstand Galen's meaning.[29]

Hence the *Inventarium* is not simply a mechanical pastiche. Guy not only tries to judge between conflicting authorities, he occasionally introduces something new into the discussion: he treats of tracheotomy and intubation for the first time since Avicenna (2.2.3); against Guglielmo, Lanfranchi, and others, he advocates the immediate closure of chest wounds if there is no damage to internal organs (3.2.5); he agrees with Lanfranchi against their Latin predecessors that internal wounds should be sewn up directly, without introducing any sort of cannula into the lumen (3.2.6); he introduces the use of a weight and pulley for traction in treating a fracture of the thigh (5.2.7); and he describes a new instrument for extracting teeth, the "pelican" (6.2.2)—characteristically, Guy insists that doctors are more to be trusted with dentistry than the barbers who increasingly are taking it over.

The steady evolution of a tradition of surgical writing makes it possible for us to form some judgments about the growth of surgical knowledge by the fourteenth century. We can feel most confident in our assessment when an author questions earlier opinions, or when the originality of what he says compels us to believe that he is describing his own experience: Guy de Chauliac's vivid account of the plague of 1348 (which he himself contracted) is the best contemporary clinical account we have of the epidemic.[30]

Yet in general it remains difficult to assess the practice, the technical ("modern") accomplishments, of medieval surgeons: the details of their actual practice are obscured as much as they are revealed by the demands of the textual form they were so eager to adopt. Their writings are not neutral objective records but weapons in an occupational competition, weapons adapted from a different professional tradition with its own standards. Because literary tradition encouraged authors to incorporate verbatim passages from earlier texts, we may well be doubtful that surgical writers who continued to quote procedures from Albucasis or Galen ever understood them. The haphazard anecdotal content of some surgical textbooks may seem to offer a narrow window into contemporary practice, but even these occasional anecdotes have been seen to be far from straightforward in their interpretation.[31]

The illustrations found in surgical textbooks, though they may seem promising, are equally problematic when we try to use them as guides to actual practice. For example, one particular group of illustrations representing three surgical operations—couching of cataract, excision of nasal polyps, and excision of hemorrhoids—was recopied several times as a unit in the twelfth century, but their detail was often simplified or meaningless, and they could not have functioned as models for instruction; it seems likely that they were simply the last stage of an iconographic tradition going back centuries, perhaps as far as Alexandria. These three operations could have been performed in the twelfth century, but the series is not evidence that they actually were.[32] A similar debasement is evident in Latin manuscripts of Albucasis's *Surgery:* the original Arabic illustrations of instruments were formalized and given decorative touches by successive Western copyists until their construction and function were no longer evident. The new European surgical texts, beginning with Ruggero's, gave rise to their own illustrations, although, curiously, not until the late thirteenth century. These new images did often illustrate their texts closely, yet from the beginning they too possessed an element of stylization that makes them unsatisfactory as a guide to detail; but fidelity to the text still leaves unanswered the question, how far do these texts represent what medieval surgeons did?

To give an example, couching for cataract may have been depicted in twelfth-century illustrations, yet apparently the first medieval surgical text

to describe the operation is Bruno's (the description is missing in Teodorico's), and Bruno's account is based closely on Arab authorities
(Rhazes, al-'Abbas, and Albucasis); Lanfranchi's discussion is similar, and
both write as though they had never seen the operation performed.
Guglielmo da Saliceto, as is so often the case, is more instructive about the
clinical realm—not in what he says but in what he leaves unsaid. His
account of the cataract operation is far more succinct than the others, and
he concludes, "truly, this treatment cannot be taught unless the student
sees the operation with his own eyes; and because the operation is such an
important one, no one should attempt it unless he has already watched
someone else perform it."[33] This does not suggest that surgeons felt
confident about performing the operation, and indeed contemporaries
commented on how rarely it was successful. For the most part, then,
surgical texts of the Middle Ages give an idea of the operations some
surgeons knew, in a general way, how to perform; how often and how
successfully (or indeed whether) they performed them is quite another
matter.

Yet of course there are exceptions to this rule, and one is the operation for anal fistula for which the English surgeon John Arderne (1307–
1378?) was famous. Though not university-trained, Arderne composed
his works in Latin and could draw on scholastic authorities, and in this
sense was comparable to a Lanfranchi or a Guy de Chauliac; indeed, of
these three Arderne was clearly the most influential and authoritative
surgeon for fifteenth-century England, though the other two were more
successful on the Continent. But he is a very different author in that his
great work is a *practica*—that is, it is addressed to a limited number of
quite specific conditions whose treatment he describes with great circumstantial detail, usually with reference to particular cases he has treated;
indeed, the account of *fistula in ano* opens with the names of two dozen
Englishmen he has cured of the ailment. Earlier medieval surgeons had
shown no confidence in their ability to cure anal fistula, yet Arderne's
procedure was not radically new, being a development of one proposed by
Albucasis (and by Paul of Aegina); perhaps his conservative postoperative
treatment helps explain his announced successes. Arderne's verbal account
of the operation is reinforced by a series of illustrations, keyed to the text,
which make the procedural details crystal clear and themselves represent a
significant innovation in the communication of technique. Here is one of
the few cases where we can be quite sure that written knowledge stemmed
from actual surgical practice.[34]

Arderne provides something of a transition to a new kind of surgeon beginning to be seen in the fifteenth century: a man reporting on his own practical experience—often gained in contemporary warfare—while capable of drawing on the background of learned tradition, but writing in the vernacular, and no longer aiming at an academic audience. An English *Fayre Book of Surgery* composed in 1446, which fuses its author's battlefield experience with citations from Guy de Chauliac (who could now be read in more than one English translation), is thought to be the work of Thomas Morstede, who had gone to France in 1415 with the army of Henry V.[35] More impressive still is the first German surgery, composed about 1460 by Heinrich von Pfalzpaint, which describes a procedure for rhinoplasty using skin from the arm (introduced by the Brancas of southern Italy shortly before) and which was perhaps the first surgery to discuss wounds caused by firearms—a new age was presenting surgeons with new problems.[36] Yet there were new opportunities as well. Fifty years or so after the invention of printing, books were for sale containing the works of Guy de Chauliac and Ruggero di Parma, of Teodorico Borgognoni and Guglielmo de Saliceto—not just in Latin but often also in vernacular translations. Writers like Morstede and Pfalzpaint might still be outnumbered by the perpetuators of the older academic line, but the introduction of printing meant that both the learned and the practical traditions could anticipate a greatly enlarged audience in the sixteenth century.

～ 11 ～

The Regimens of Health

PEDRO GIL SOTRES

Even as the medical art came into being, physicians were already concerned with hygiene. In Greece during the fifth century B.C., we find clear expression, in the context of religious and magical concepts, of a series of precepts on diet meant to ensure health. These precepts were based on experience. Overeating, exposure to the cold, and insufficient sleep, for example, were all actions with obvious links to a person's state of health. For that matter, in all cultures, hygiene is a product of the level of technology, and it reflects what we describe as a society's creature comforts. Insulating oneself from the cold directly relates to building houses and solving problems of waterproofing, lighting, and ventilation. Similarly, clothing requires fabric-weaving and other technologies. Greek hygiene incorporated—in addition to the factors of experience and technology—norms based on Pythagoreanism, a religious and philosophical system that codified a specific way of life as a means to attaining ritual purity.

Hygienic Works from Hippocrates to Galen

Diet is the topic found most frequently in the works that make up the Hippocratic corpus. *De prisca medicina* treats the medical art as a step in the progressive discovery of a regimen of life, which came on the heels of the discovery of the rules of cooking. Another treatise, *De diaeta* [*Regimen*],[1] constitutes the culmination of dietetic learning in the classical period. Dating from the end of the fifth century B.C., it declares that health is dependent on the balance between what one eats and what one's body consumes. The intake of food may lead to a plethoric state, which should be counterbalanced by physical exercise. Attention to physical activity and nourishment, however, does not rule out the importance of other hygienic factors, such as sex, age, and place of residence. The factors that determine a state of health are analyzed in detail. For example, a list is drawn up of the traditional staples of the Greek diet: grains (wheat, barley, and spelt), dried and green vegetables, meat, fish, eggs, dairy products, and fruit. Among the beverages, mention is made of wine, vinegar, and water. Also mentioned for their influence on health are baths, sexual activity, and physical exercise, as well as the natural methods of evacuation and vomiting. The treatise reveals a regimen planned in accordance with the four seasons; there is also a description of fifteen diseases caused by dietary imbalance. Last of all, the author of this treatise explores the importance of dreams. The historical importance of this treatise was considerable, and a number of specialists believe that the concept of hygiene developed from its postulates.[2]

A century after *De diaeta* [*Regimen*] was written, another hygienic text appeared, which was to have a lasting influence on medieval medicine. This was the *Epistula de tuende valetudine*, written by the physician Diocles of Carystos, working in a Peripatetic milieu. This treatise is a sort of catechism in how to prevent disease. Diocles' "Epistle"—following a tradition common to ancient and medieval writing on hygiene—is addressed to a specific person, a member of the higher ranks of society. The treatise recommends a way of life that revolves around the care of the body. It calls for sessions of exercise in the morning and afternoon, in accordance with a program that follows the cycle of the day. Dietetics thus becomes a full-fledged Peripatetic *bios*, with rules for an ethics of the body.[3] The underlying idea is that since bad habits cause diseases, certain diseases are the result of individual behavior. Medicine acquires a pedagogic attitude, in accordance with the postulate that it is possible to maintain one's health through specific education, as long as one learns to make proper use of morally neutral objects.

The "Epistle" by Diocles of Carystos is structured along two separate thematic axes. On one hand, the hygienic treatments are arranged in accordance with the seasons, as was the case in *De diaeta* [*Regimen*]. On the other hand, the author describes the treatments on the basis of the various parts of the human body: head, thorax, stomach, and bladder.

These two structures, barely sketched out here, are the origin of a tradition that was to flourish during the Middle Ages.

In the context of Greek philosophy, another work devoted to hygiene was written after the year A.D. 81: Plutarch's *De tuenda sanitate praecepta*.[4] Men of culture, who were not physicians, were led to explore the field of medicine because of the parallels between the study of the body and ethical philosophy, which was the study of the care of the soul. The link between philosophy and medicine was anything but fortuitous, indeed, it was necessary. A philosopher is a physician of the soul, and his task is to procure the well-being of the soul through *paideia*, or education. Plutarch was concerned with the preservation of health, as a preliminary condition of a spiritual life. He rejected out of hand both a life of excess and that Stoic rigor that aimed at the elimination of all pleasure, through a strict and uniform regimen of life, based on artificial and constraining remedies. In this and in other fields, Plutarch was a supporter of a life lived according to the golden mean, deeply rooted in Aristotle's *mesotes*.

The very structure of this work—which takes the form of a dialogue—reveals that its author was not a physician. The text does not present a catalog of the healthiest foods and beverages, nor does it offer systematic references to what would in time become known as the *sex res non naturales*, or "six nonnatural things." Rather, it offers recommendations on what is good to eat and drink, on exercises appropriate to intellectuals, and references to bathing. What predominates, however, is the goal of attaining harmony between body and soul, fundamental both to the preservation of health and to a virtuous life.

With Galen, hygiene acquired its titles of nobility; this was chiefly by virtue of the synthesis that he carried out among the Hippocratic ideas, Aristotelianism, and the discoveries of Hellenistic science. Galen's treatise *Hygieina*[5] is a work of great importance and was known to the Middle Ages through two translations done in Italy. The older of these two translations was completed by Burgundio da Pisa in the thirteenth century; it was a condensation of the original. In texts of the same period, it was known by two different titles, *De regimine sanitatis* or *De custodia sanitatis*. Later, in the fourteenth century, Niccolò da Reggio completed a new translation of this work; he dedicated the text to King Robert of Sicily. It was a complete translation of the original.[6]

Galen's treatise was not systematic. Nonetheless, we must recognize its remarkable originality. It is organized around a central fulcrum: the study of individual complexion as the subject of hygienic treatments. One should devote individual attention to each patient, he argued, because the preservation of health differs in accordance with the complexion. The body of a patient with a warm complexion requires different treatment from that of a patient with a cold complexion. Likewise, the way of life of a corpulent person will not be the same as that of a thin person.

Galen's conception of health postulates the existence of an ideal equilibrium, a perfect harmony. Alteration of this harmony is the cause of disease. Midway between the two extremes—equilibrium and imbalance—we find individuals who are, so to speak, "neutral," who neither enjoy perfect health nor suffer from disease. Galen's work was not intended for those who enjoy excellent health; it was directed at those whose health is imperfect or feeble, a mixed state that covers a vast array of nuances and variants. A state of health can be altered in two ways: through internal causes, or through external causes, the most important of which is the action of the surrounding air. To guard against these dangers, and to attain an advanced age, it is necessary to follow rules of hygiene. This means, essentially, that one must attend to one's periods of sleeping and waking, exercise and rest, hunger and thirst, the food and drink one consumes, states of repletion, baths, and emotions. These ideas were to become canonic in later Galenism, as the six nonnatural things.[7]

Since the complexion of an individual changes with the passing years, Galen was moved to structure his discourse around the ages of man. The first steps, which correspond to what we call childhood, are marked by the predominance of warm and moist humors, which is explained by the vigor of innate heat and the abundance of radical moisture, two factors underlying the exceptional rate of growth of a child. At the other extremity of this chain of life, old age is characterized by cold and by dryness; this is the season marked by the almost total disappearance of innate warmth and moisture.

From birth, a child must be surrounded with care, of the soul as well as of the body. Galen recommends feeding the infant on mother's milk, to assure continuity with what the baby received in the uterus. The paid wet nurse is viewed unfavorably, but if used, she must follow strict rules of living, unlike the mother. The wet nurse must adhere to a preordained diet, abstain from sexual relations, and engage in moderate physical exercise. This advice from Galen was to pass unchanged into the cultural heritage of the Middle Ages. We find it in medical texts as well as in manuals of pedagogy. The child is not to be weaned until the age of three, although he should receive other food as well, such as bread. The regimen is completed with baths and games, corresponding to the nature of the child. Once the child is seven years old, he will be entrusted to masters who will teach him to read, to have proper morals, and to exercise the body.

Between the ages of fourteen and twenty-one, the chief hygienic measures concern physical exercise, nourishment, sleep, and sexual activity. All these activities should be practiced in moderation. Galen emphasizes the importance of physical exercise as a means for the preservation of health. He establishes the best times to exercise (before meals) and lays particular emphasis on massages, strictly linked to an athletic context. He then presents a vast repertory of forms of physical exercise: running, jumping, wrestling, hiking, and horseback riding. Galen also turns his attention to baths, examining their function and their various forms, according to water temperature. Lastly, he lists a number of rules for the proper use of various dietetic and therapeutic substances (oxymel, vinous compounds).

As for old age, all possible means should be used to provide heat and moisture to correct the subject's complexion. Galen recommends baths in hot water, and moist warm foods like wine. Physical exercise, practiced in moderation, is necessary to prevent the extinction of natural heat.

In Byzantine circles, physicians had begun to attribute health to the six nonnatural things: air/environment, exercise/rest, food/beverages, sleeping/waking, evacuation/repletion, and passions. Of course, this set of elements was already present in Galen's work, but their canonic structure dates from late antiquity.

A typical example of the dietetic literature of late antiquity was the pamphlet titled *Epistula Anthimi ad gloriosissimum Theodoricum regem Francorum*, also known by the title *De observatione ciborum*. We know nothing about the author, a physician named Anthimus; we know only that the work was dedicated to Theodoric, king of the Franks from 495 to 525, and thus dates from a period beginning at the turn of the sixth century A.D. The philosophy contained in this short work is quite simple: health derives from the food that man eats. When the food is good in quality and is prepared properly, it is digested properly and gives strength to the body. The same is true of drink, which must be suited to the food and should not be abused. Improper consumption of cold beverages, for example, provokes an alteration of the stomach. In hygienic terms, the chief points of interest in Anthimus's work lie in the list of foods that it contains, in the way in which these foods are assorted and combined, and in the observations concerning their preparation. Surprisingly, wine is indicated as proper accompaniment to only a few dishes.

Writings on Hygiene in the Middle Ages

Medical literature circulating in the Christian West between the ninth and eleventh centuries was quite scanty. Among the texts that have survived, most belong to a genre that dated from antiquity: the genre of short treatises, eminently practical in content, devoid of all theory, and often drawn up in epistolary form. Most of these texts, attributed to Hippocrates at the time, tend to concentrate on two matters: hygiene and bloodletting. Among the hygienic texts, we find a number of translations from the Greek of the "Epistle" by Diocles of Carystos,[8] with numerous variants. These versions are all based on the opening outline of the Peripatetic philosopher: first, advice concerning the care of the body, gauged to the different seasons; next, rules for preserving the health of the organs. In manuscripts from the high Middle Ages, there are numerous fragments of the treatise by Anthimus, often failing to mention his name.[9]

During the high Middle Ages, culture retreated to the monasteries, and we can find evidence in monastic rules of the existence of hygienic rules. We have an example of this in Saint Benedict of Nursia's monastic rule, which served as a model for many others: it established the times for the monks to sleep, their dietary rules, and so on. In another type of source, however, the *Consuetudines,* we find information in greater detail. For example, specific advice is given concerning the frequency with which monks should practice bloodletting, as well as the manner in which they should do so.

Hygiene in Works of Arabic Origin

Knowledge of Greek medicine in the Latin world was made possible in part through its transmission via Arab authors. This knowledge was funneled to the medieval West through two quite specific geographic sites: southern Italy and, later, Castile. By the end of the twelfth century, Latin medicine could make use of a series of works that were to prove fundamental in the scientific development of medical knowledge within the universities. Hygiene lay at the heart of this process of transmission. The presence of Arabic works in Latin circles prompted the development of new genres of writing.

The most important texts, in terms of influence on medieval hygiene, were four works translated in southern Italy by Constantine of Africa: the

Ysagoge, the *Pantegni,* the *Liber dietarum particularium,* and the *Liber die-tarum universalium.*

The *Ysagoge* (a Latin translation of fragments of the "Questions about Medicine" by Hunayn ibn Ishaq, or Johannitius) set forth in a concise and often cryptic style the chief definitions of Galenic medicine, adapted to the context of a philosophy of nature. Hygiene was treated in terms of the six nonnatural things. This work was, in part due to its very brevity, the subject of a considerable body of commentary, especially in the circles of the school of Salerno.

Through the commentaries written by university professors, many of the theoretical features connected with hygiene to be found in the *Ysagoge* later acquired a permanent place amid the "rules for a healthy life" of the Middle Ages. The chief exceptions were the status attributed to bathing and sexual activity, which were not well integrated into the system of the six nonnatural things. Certain authors considered bathing to be comple-mentary to physical exercise; others linked it to the elimination of prod-ucts of the third digestion, which takes place in the limbs, and therefore with the pair of evacuation/repletion.

A second text translated by Constantine of Africa was even more important to the development of ideas on hygiene. This was al-'Abbas's *Pantegni,* a vast synthesis of all medicine. Despite the relatively low esteem in which this work was held when scholastic medicine was at its height—Avicenna was esteemed more highly—the *Pantegni* exerted great influence in the field of hygiene, as evidenced by the presence of its expository scheme in most *regimina sanitatis* ("rules of health"). The fifth book of the theoretical part, entirely devoted to hygiene, was based on the six non-natural things. The author commented on the various alimentary sub-stances, broken down into homogeneous groups: grains, fresh and dried vegetables, fruit, meat, dairy products, eggs, honey, and beverages.

The other port of entry—as it were—for medical science in the West was the Castilian city of Toledo. In the middle of the twelfth century, this was the point of convergence for the three great medieval cultures: Chris-tian, Hebrew, and Arabic. Here many Arabic texts, which later served as inspiration to Latin physicians, were translated. The leading figure in this intellectual adventure was Gerard of Cremona, canon in the cathedral from 1157 to 1187 and quite probably the head of a full-fledged school of translators of Arabic works. Among those works, the two chief texts on hygiene were Avicenna's "Canon of Medicine" and Rhazes' *Continens.*

Throughout the fourteenth century, the "Canon of Medicine," one of the most widely read books in medieval universities, served as the basic manual for students of medicine. Evidently, its concepts of hygiene greatly influenced the rules of health of the Middle Ages. Avicenna held that hygiene and medicine were two complementary practices. The former teaches one how to care for one's body and to maintain it in good health. The latter, by contrast, is devoted to the care of the sick body. There was nothing new in all this, at least thus far. The truly new idea lay in the way that one could preserve good health, something quite different from what could be read in the books translated in southern Italy:

> The art of preserving the health lies in an equilibrium among the things that we have described. There are seven things that should in particular be kept in mind: the equilibrium of the complexion, the selection of food and drink, the elimination of that which is superfluous, care for the composition [of the body], the rectification of that which is breathed in through the nostrils, a moderate exercise of the body and the spirit, which in a certain sense also involves sleeping and waking.[10]

Here again are the six nonnatural things, with the addition of a preliminary mention of the equilibrium of the complexions. Avicenna considered hygiene from a number of standpoints: the age of the individual (childhood, maturity, or old age), deviance from the norm, the seasons, and certain special circumstances, such as voyages. It was the medical concept of complexion, however, that served as the central axis of the hygiene of "Canon of Medicine," giving the text a greater depth than that of the *Pantegni*. Avicenna structured hygiene around a "natural thing," that is, a reality "made necessary by the nature of the body," and no longer around one of the nonnatural things, alien to human nature.

Another medical encyclopedia translated at Toledo was *Continens*, by the Persian physician Rhazes. This author advocated simple rules, bordering on ordinary good sense, devoid of verbose theory. Eminently practical in inspiration, Rhazes' sound recommendations were widely incorporated into the *regimina sanitatis*, intended for a nonspecialist public.

Two additional texts of Arabic origin, translated later, played minor roles in the development of medieval hygiene. The first of the two, known as *Secreta secretorum*, was wrongly attributed to Aristotle.[11] The second was known to the Latin world as the *Colliget* and was a medical encyclopedia written by Averroës, a physician of Cordoba.

Entirely different in character was another text, known to the Latin West by the title *Tacuinum sanitatis*. Written by the Christian physician Ibn Butlan, who practiced in Damascus around the first half of the eleventh century, this text focused solely on hygiene. The structure of the *Tacuinum sanitatis* adheres to the model of the six nonnatural things, which had previously been used by al-'Abbas. The originality of this work, however, lies in the presentation of its body of hygienic knowledge in the form of forty tables *(taqwim)*. The author's intention was to provide a work that could easily be consulted by a broad public. We do not know the name of the translator who turned *Tacuinum sanitatis* into Latin. We know, on the basis of a notation on a manuscript, only that it was done at the court of Manfred, who reigned as king of Sicily from 1257 to 1266.[12] In the West, this work circulated in two different versions. One was complete,[13] while the other was abridged but had handsome illuminated illustrations.[14] For each of the six nonnatural things, but especially for the components that make up the diet, the following aspects were presented: the complexion *(complexio)*; the conditions and characteristics that must be joined in the substance in question *(electio)*; its usefulness in terms of health *(iuvamentum)*; the harmful effects that it can cause *(nocumentum)*; the way in which such harmful effects can be avoided *(remotio nocumentum)*; the type of humor that it generates *(quid generat)*; and the concrete applications of the substance under consideration. There can be no doubt that the *Tacuinum sanitatis* marked the debut in the Latin world of a series of texts devoted solely to hygiene, even though the presence of its hygienic precepts in medieval monastic rules remains difficult to indicate. This is probably due to the extreme simplification of the advice given, meant to suit the cultural level of its readers.

From the end of the thirteenth to the beginning of the fourteenth century, in clearly defined geographic areas, there was a general reawakening of interest in Arab hygiene; this interest took the form of hygienic writings addressed to specific individuals. In 1299, at Montpellier, Jacob ben Makir, of the family of the Tibbonides, translated into Latin the regimen of Albuali Avenzoar, father of Avenzoar, the author of the *Taysir*. Three years later, also at Montpellier, Armengaud Blaise translated the regimen written by Maimonides for the sultan Saladin. The regimen of Avenzoar[15] was structured around the six nonnatural things and the care required by the various organs of the body. The regimen of Maimonides[16] added to these concerns a series of items of practical advice for the sick who cannot consult a doctor, as well as a number of considerations having to do with the individual health of the sultan himself and an attempt to provide an etiological explanation of his symptoms. The influence of these two dietetic works on the *regimina sanitatis* remained quite limited.

The Regimina Sanitatis

The medieval rules of health constitute a genre marked by orientation toward individual hygiene. Incorporating the Greek and Arabic tradition, these works began to appear during the course of the second half of the thirteenth century and attained their greatest degree of diffusion and popularity at the end of the Middle Ages.

These rules of health were intended for the use of men of high social rank and were meant to provide them with advice designed to reduce the danger of disease. Solidly rooted in Greek individualism, they were generally dedicated to actual individuals, although there are writings dedicated to the public at large. While the former sort of texts abound with individually tailored comments (references to the complexion of the person in question, references to his diseases, allusions to the social class to which he belongs or the religion that he practices), the latter, or "university" regimens, so called because they were frequently linked to the teaching activity of their authors, tended to take into consideration all of the possibilities of human life (the many different ages, the complexions, and certain situations, such as travel or convalescence). They are largely written in Latin. Beginning in the second half of the fourteenth century, however, we begin to see them either translated into—or even written directly in—the various vernacular languages. Although they are written for the most part in prose, there are examples of regimens written in verse, thus taking advantage of the memory aids offered by rhythm. The most distinctive instance of this latter type is the popular *Regimen sanitatis salernitanum*. As Karl Sudhoff[17] has clearly demonstrated, this work is not old enough to have been written in the setting of the medical school of Salerno. Moreover, it was far less popular in the Middle Ages than in later centuries.

To understand the specific features of this genre, we can make use of another criterion, that of the "descriptive idea of the author."[18] From this point of view, we can discern a second tradition, separate from the medieval hygienic writings in the tradition of the school of Salerno that followed the organizational criterion of the six nonnatural things. This second approach was linked to the city of Toledo and focused on complexion as the leading feature of hygiene. A third descriptive idea was based on the scheme of treatments that could be applied to the various limbs of the organism. The origin of this third family of *regimina* is not clear. Although this scheme is present in part of the treatise by Avenzoar, that work cannot be considered the prototype, since its translation was done after the appearance of many texts on hygiene that follow this order of presentation. Suffice it to consider the tradition of texts in the manuscripts that are titled *De conferentibus et nocentibus* (anthologies of various prescriptions, meant to protect each limb of the body from disease).[19] There was a fourth type of hygienic writing, in which the prevailing consideration was the age of the patient, independently of the descriptive idea employed. Consider, for example, the regimen written for the young princes of Burgundy, composed in French in the fifteenth century,[20] or the regimen written by the physician Guido da Vigevano for the French king, Philip VI of Valois.[21] Lastly, there is a vast array of medieval writings that present no particular systematic order. This group includes the *Regimen sanitatis salernitanum*, mentioned above, whose bulk increased progressively over the years through the addition of new verses. The absence of an organizational scheme was often accompanied by another characteristic—anonymity—especially in the fifteenth century.

In chronological terms, the first period, which corresponds to the debut of this literary genre, covers the second half of the thirteenth century. Its most distinctive examples are the two regimens, quite different one from the other, by Johannes de Toleto[22] and Aldobrandino of Siena.[23]

The second period was the time of the most brilliant production of regimens, the first half of the fourteenth century. During this time, university physicians wrote regimens, including some classics, in which profundity of content was matched by simplicity of form. Arnald of Villanova,[24] Bernard de Gordon,[25] and Maynus de Mayneriis[26] took the genre to a level unrivaled in later years.

The last period extends from the middle of the fourteenth century to the end of the fifteenth century. Distinctive features of this period were, first of all, the abundance of writings of the genre, the result of a growing demand caused in turn by the development of those urban classes which constituted the audience. Another characteristic of this period was the increase in popularity and accessibility, indicated by the growth in the number of regimens in the vernacular and by the appearance of anonymous regimens. The latter *regimina* were probably anonymous because they were written by obscure physicians of no particular renown; the names of these, adding nothing to the prestige of the work, were often

overlooked entirely and, in time, forgotten. A third distinctive feature—
production in verse—assisted the spread of these increasingly popular
texts.

In these late hygienic writings, the chief authority invoked was that
of Avicenna. The Salernitan tradition had provided the framework, but it
was by this point in Avicenna's "Canon of Medicine" that readers sought
ideas concerning hygiene. One significant example is offered by an analysis of the quotations introduced into the *Regimen sanitatis* by Chunrardus
Erstensis,[27] written in the fifteenth century: seventy quotes from Avicenna
as opposed to ten quotes from Galen. Clearly, the work of the Persian
physician had acquired remarkable influence through the universities.

The Principles of Medieval Hygiene

The Environment

The *regimina sanitatis* usually began by examining the effect on man of his
environment. This set of factors was termed *aer*, but this term encom-
passed a vast content. Aside from the qualities of the surrounding air, the
term extended to include the prevailing winds, the physical geography, the
influence of the seasons, one's home, and one's clothing. Arnald of Villanova described this set of factors with the more suitable term *operimenta*.

For medieval medicine, air was the element most indispensable to the
preservation of life. The vital root of human life was innate or natural heat,
located in the heart. Just like a flame, innate heat could not continue to
yield warmth in the absence of air. The air breathed in was thought to
penetrate to the heart, cooling it and preventing its radical moisture from
being consumed. Respiration also served as the route whereby smoke
produced in physiological combustion was expelled toward the exterior.
With diastole, the heart drew to itself the air required to cool it; with
systole, it expelled its own smoke.[28] The relation between air and heart,
therefore, was exceedingly close. Any change in the quality of the air
directly affected the heart, and thus the entire organism. It was modification of the air that provided the explanation of the so-called pestilential
diseases, so devastatingly important in the Middle Ages.

It was thus necessary to look for places where the air was pure, in the
meaning given by Avicenna's "Canon of Medicine." Avicenna's work was
the common source, on this point, of all the *regimina sanitatis*. Air was
considered to be pure when it was not mixed with any extraneous vapors,

any type of smoke, or any harmful substance.[29] There were other identifying conditions: clarity or luminosity, as opposed to murky or dark *(nebulosus)* air; movement, as opposed to stillness, with open air preferred to the air contained by the four walls of a house or beneath a roof.[30] Also, air was supposed to be "thin," not dense. When possessed of all these qualities, air was seen to have positive effects on the health of the individual: "it clarifies the blood, making it thin and pure; it also does the heart good and calms the spirit, it does the body good and speeds the third digestion in the limbs."[31] Finally, it was advisable to make use of temperate air, which is to say, air in which the four complexional qualities were well balanced. This, it seems, was true of air in the springtime.[32]

The conditions of the air could be modified by other factors as well. Some of these affected the qualities and substance of the air, while others instead had an extrinsic nature and could be provoked by celestial bodies, minerals, plants, or animals.[33] The surprising absence of astrological references[34]—with the corresponding lack of theoretical elements—may well have been a result of the audience to which the *regimina* were addressed, an audience that usually had no medical or scientific knowledge. There was a wide array of opinions concerning the factors that could modify the quality of the air. Certain authors stated that air improved near a stream, a sunny meadow, or a forest.[35] Others claimed that one should avoid the woods or fields planted with certain vegetables.[36] Most of these contraindications had to do with the intense odor found in the places in question. For the same reason, it was recommended that one stay away from animals, including such domesticated animals as cows, oxen, or pigeons. Lastly, it was considered unhealthy to live near sewers, latrines, cemeteries, and so forth, because the processes of putrefaction could alter the air.

Physicians considered the city a far more hygienic place to live than the unhealthy countryside. This may be explained by their residence in the cities, which were becoming increasingly important throughout the Middle Ages. Only Maimonides, writing for the sultan Saladin, praised country air as better than city air.[37]

As for the prevailing winds, one was encouraged to live in places where the wind blows from the north or the east. This was the orientation suggested for windows. Many texts recommended against living in newly built houses.[38] Other texts, fewer in number, claimed that excessively old houses were not hygienic.[39] As far as materials were concerned, houses built of rough-hewn stone or plaster were deemed unhealthy, especially if the roof was made of the same materials.[40] Large, tall houses allowed one to enjoy purer air but were also colder than small, low houses. It was believed to be harmful to the health to live on the ground floor or, worse still, in the basement, where the air was heavier and denser. The ideal thing was to live on the second floor of a house *(inter duo sollaria)*, with a ceiling of some height.[41]

It was in any case always possible to modify the composition of the air with artificial means to attenuate its harmful effects. Chill and damp could be modified by lighting a wood fire in a room, as long as one did not get too close to the fire, lest it dry the body out. Coal was frowned on because it burns badly and emits fumes. The air could be improved even more rapidly if one added some salt, incense, or aromatic herbs to the fire. If, however, the air was too hot and dry, the remedy was to sprinkle the room with water and vinegar, or hang wet cloths along the walls. It was also possible to place plants that were considered cold, such as roses and violets, or grape leaves, around the room. When the air was corrupt, or when there was danger of an epidemic, it was best to close the windows and to make use of such aromatic substances as aloe, amber, or incense.

Clothing, too, offered another means of protecting oneself from the immediate environment. Except for the occasional precious and perfumed outfit,[42] and save for other clothing described as "fine and green,"[43] the *regimina sanitatis* went no further than to offer limited information on the materials used, without examining the various elements of clothing in any detail. Clothing protects humans from bad weather, from heat and from cold. It was also held to create a temperate environment by reflecting the vapor emanated by the skin. Finally, clothing transmitted to the body the qualities it possesses both in potential and in actuality. The warmest clothing is that made of animal hide, followed by wool, cotton, silk, and linen, which was considered the coolest fabric.[44]

Physical Exercise

The second nonnatural thing was the pair of movement and rest *(motus et quies)*. A healthy life involved alternation between exercise and rest. Under the heading *motus,* physicians assembled a number of different factors. The most important of these were, on the one hand, the work and the profession done by the patient and, on the other hand, the physical exercises the patient engaged in for pleasure (called *exercitia,* in the narrow sense). As Bernard de Gordon emphasized, the latter practice was absolutely necessary to the maintenance of a good state of health: "Exercise is one of the best things that can be imposed upon the human body."[45] Given its importance, we should examine the way in which these authors conceptualized *exercita*.

Avicenna, in his "Canon of Medicine," offered an illuminating definition: physical exercise "is a voluntary movement that demands deeper and faster respiration."[46] Bernard de Gordon later specified the concept of voluntary movement as follows:

> the work of carpenters, farmers, merchants, et al., is not a physical exercise, since we do not observe voluntary movement, speaking properly, but rather forced movement. Moreover, merchants, bourgeois, and their like, walk a great deal, for long periods and over long distances; but here too we are not dealing with a genuine physical exercise. In order to have this, one must walk at one's own initiative, without doing anything else, at a fast pace, until one feels tired, and one's breathing has altered.[47]

Intention, above all, constituted the distinction between *exercitium* and other forms of *motus*. In effect, respiratory overload, marked by faster respiration, a speeded-up pulse, and in time sweating, could also take place during work that requires considerable physical effort.

Galenism produced numerous classifications of exercise, based on a number of variables, such as duration, intensity, and velocity, but the most interesting division is that which takes into consideration the effects on health. All authors agreed that physical exercise should be done before meals. According to the *Pantegni,* exercise should perform three precise functions: it should increase the innate heat; ease the expulsion of the superfluous, by expanding the pores in the skin; and harden the body by consolidating its limbs.[48] The increase in innate heat was believed to facilitate the digestive processes that take place in the organism. Its beneficial effects extended not only to the stomach but also to the other parts of the body involved in digestion. The best time for exercise was thus determined by a number of conditions: digestion had to be completed, the body had to be free of a number of superfluities, and the environment had to be temperate, that is, in equilibrium between hot and cold, dry and moist: "it is well to exercise during the more temperate hours of the day. Exercise, then, should be taken in the summer in the early hours of the day and at sundown, in the evening, and in the winter around noon; in the intermediate seasons, one should take exercise in the hours of the afternoon."[49]

The *regimina sanitatis* feature numerous observations concerning the way in which one should exercise, which give us an idea of the importance of exercise in the context of medieval hygiene. The recommended sports were simple and related directly to the contemporary way of life; there were no bookish references to sports practiced in ancient times. The chief sporting activities discussed were walking and running, but other activities were encouraged as well, from simple calisthenics, such as climbing a rope or lifting weights to horseback riding. Bernard de Gordon explained the medical and social benefits of variety in sports:

> It is well that there should be a great variety of exercises, so as to take into account the number and diversity of individuals. Indeed, there are those with foot problems, who cannot take their exercise by walking, while others have hand problems and cannot do exercise that involves the use of the hands; others have sore throats and cannot exercise by singing and playing wind instruments. Lastly, there are the strong and the weak, the rich and the poor, prelates with delicate bodies and those who are not so constituted, and it is therefore appropriate that there should be a great variety of exercises.[50]

Like the ancient Latin physicians, the authors of the *regimina sanitatis* considered walking the simplest and best of exercises. Bernard de Gordon touted walking's benefits, claiming that when the body moves as a whole and in every part it enjoys an optimal state of equilibrium.[51] Maynus de Mayneriis placed walking above all other activities: "It is evident that walking is better exercise than riding on a horse or a cart. While walking, the members of the body work in a more regular and uniform manner than in other sports."[52] The best setting was a clean area, with pure air: "It should be done in a clean place that is exposed to pure air, and you should enjoy the view both nearby and in the distance, as well as the sky, the sea, and the greenery."[53] Angelo dell'Aquila wrote: "In another season, you should leave the house and walk through the greenery or in other pleasant areas, looking at the mountains in the morning and at springs or other pleasant things in the evening."[54]

Horseback riding was reserved for members of the higher social classes. Barnaba da Reggio wrote to an anonymous recipient: "Your regimen should be moderate . . . in accordance with your way of life, riding horses or other forms of exercise in accordance with the requirements of your nobility."[55] And in his *Regimen sanitatis ad regem Aragonum* [Rules of health for the king of Aragon], Arnald of Villanova excluded all sports (playing ball, throwing the javelin, wrestling) except horseback riding, the only form of exercise that could be considered compatible with his patient's royal rank.[56] Bernard de Gordon reserved horseback riding expressly for "the wealthy."[57] These authors also mentioned playing ball; Galen had already devoted a brief work to this subject. It comes up in Arnald of Villanova's *Regimen sanitatis ad regem Aragonum* and *De confortacione visu;* in the regimen written by Maynus de Mayneriis for Antoine de Flisco; in the rules of health written by Saint Benedict of Nursia; and in the *Concordantiae* by Pierre de Saint-Flour, a Parisian physician who practiced around 1360.

Among the physical exercises less frequently mentioned in our sources are wrestling (advised against by both Bernard de Gordon and Arnald of Villanova),[58] sailing (defended by Bernard for those who suffer from cachexia, since it causes nausea and vomiting),[59] throwing rocks, and jumping. Bernard and Maynus both advised riding in a chariot or a carriage. In referring to this exercise Bernard quoted Avicenna as advising one to turn the head toward the back of the cart, to protect oneself from wind and dust.[60]

According to Bernard, each person should try to do exercises that are best suited to his rank. Were there forms of exercise particularly suited to prelates and high ecclesiastical dignitaries? Yes, indeed there were: medieval physicians do offer advice that takes into account the necessity of preserving the dignity of such important people.[61] In this connection, the *Regimen sanitatis* by Bernard de Gordon is a remarkable document. It describes an array of exercises to be practiced by the clergy. What all these exercises had in common was that they could be practiced *in cella*, in a hall that had been converted, temporarily or permanently, into a gymnasium. The foremost exercise was climbing up a rope: "In the room, there should be a stout rope full of knots, hanging from the ceiling: the man should seize the rope with both hands and hold his body straight, without touching the ground, and hang that way for some time."[62]

Baths and massages completed the hygienic practices related to the pair of *motus* and *quies*. Baths, the far more important consideration of the two, were classified in different ways, depending on the regimen in question. Many authors—taking inspiration from the *Pantegni* or the *Ysagoge*—considered baths to be a complementary activity to sports. Others placed baths in the context of the fifth nonnatural thing, believing that the principal action of baths was the elimination of excess substances. By contrast, only passing reference was made to massages, in spite of the importance placed on them by ancient authors.

Food and Drink

Authors of this period saw good nutrition and proper digestion as the most important means to preserving health. Since food becomes part of the body, it was easy to understand that, if lacking the necessary properties, food could alter health. Food also had a number of social and cultural functions, and a physician might take considerable interest in the "art of the table," of which the Middle Ages has left us such testimony. Thus, through cooking, one could treat both the human body and the social body.

The most surprising aspect of these medieval diets concerns the regulation of quantity. All of the authors underscored the importance of frugality. On the one hand, we can link this insistence to Greek and Arabic sources, which contain descriptions of small and infrequent meals. This helps us understand the declaration of Johannes de Toleto, according to whom "modern people are the children of gluttony."[63] On the other hand, the insistence of physicians on this matter suggests that their prescriptions were widely being ignored.

The number of meals and their timing corresponded to this appeal to frugality. Arab authors recommended three meals every two days, distributed as follows: the first day, two meals, in the morning and in the evening; the next day, only a light, quick meal.[64] This schedule was justified by the time needed for digestion, a process that could last from twelve to twenty-four hours. One should therefore try to avoid adding other food to the food that had not yet been digested. Latin physicians, with a few exceptions, adopted this tradition. According to Johannes de Toleto, who made reference to the authority of Galen, one should never take more than one meal a day, because diseases caused by overeating were more numerous than those caused by starvation. The saying "Gluttony killed more than the sword" is his.[65] Maynus de Mayneriis advised eating once or twice a day, with an average of three meals every two days.[66]

Do these statements reflect actual custom? One may well doubt this; for instance, let us look at Jacques Despars's commentary on the recommendations of the "Canon" by Avicenna concerning frequency of meals: "Out of ten thousand, there is not one man who follows this rule."[67] One would tend to think that the custom was to eat more frequently, although our sources provide no confirmation of the system of four meals that is often attributed to the Middle Ages:[68] *ieiunium,* or breakfast, every morning; *prandium,* a meal at nine o'clock; *merenda,* the midday meal; and *cena,* the final meal, at about six in the evening. The *regimina* mention only *prandium* and *cena.* The ongoing debate as to which of the two meals ought to be larger tended to favor the *cena.*

The fact that the suggested foodstuffs were among the most expensive on the market indicates that these regimens were intended for the higher classes of society. White bread was recommended; in this period it was consumed only by the wealthy. Among the meats, great praise was accorded to poultry, considered particularly close to the human complexion. At that time, however, even the bishop of Arles ate poultry only rarely: thirteen times in 1424, seven times in 1429, and nine times in 1430.[69] The same was true of fish. Physicians recommended the most expensive types and criticized the consumption of dried and salted fish, which was the customary method of preparing fish. People of the Middle Ages were great eaters of fish, considering the 150 days of abstinence in the liturgical calendar. This offers some idea of the economic consequences that might ensue from widely respected hygienic prescriptions. The *regimina* roundly condemned the consumption of dried vegetables, one of the fundamental components of the diet of the lower and middle classes of society.

It was with an unheard of competence in the field of cooking that physicians, notably Arnald of Villanova and Maynus de Mayneriis, introduced into their regimens recipes that can be found in ancient culinary texts.[70]

How can we explain this incursion of physicians into the realm of fine cuisine? We may formulate three hypotheses. First, they felt the need to render the food presented to patients as appetizing as possible, thus explaining the presence, in the *regimina,* of chapters devoted to seasonings, *de saporibus.* There might be another reason of a therapeutic sort: a familiarity with the most savory seasonings might allow a physician to care for patients who had problems with either their appetite or their digestion. Third, looking to the social sphere, we see that the *regimina* were a code allowing the physician partly to control the patient's way of life; the realm of nutrition, which formed part of the sphere of private life of each individual, could hardly be left out of this type of regulation. We can thus glimpse, beyond the matter of dietetic norms, the physician's interest in making his patients' behavior suit their social standing.

The Hygiene of Sleep

Aristotle's treatise *De somno et vigilia*, with scholastic commentaries and glosses, constitutes the theoretical framework needed to deal with the fourth of nonnatural things, the pair of sleeping and waking.

According to the *Speculum medicinae* by Arnald of Villanova, sleep is a lulling of the cognitive forces, that is, of the senses, rather than a lulling of the voluntary motor function. It is caused by an ebb of animal spirits present in the brain, which in turn prompts a reduced emission of these same animal spirits by the brain toward sensory and motor organs.[71] Medieval physiology gave the following explanation of sleep: innate heat is summoned back to the internal members, which trigger an ebb in the spirits present in the brain, a drop that leads to an interruption in the functioning of the senses and the motor functions. This interruption has the appearance of a certain quietude, specifically, the somnolence that precedes sleep proper. At the same time, heat increases in the organs of digestion, causing the emanation of vapors toward the brain. Encountering a cold and moist brain, these vapors cause condensation and the obstruction of the passages through which spirits are conveyed toward the sensory and motor organs. When these conduits are wholly blocked, one falls asleep. The reverse mechanism, that of waking up, is explained less clearly. We can try to summarize it as follows: innate heat, no longer required for the use of the digestive organs, spreads throughout the body; when it reaches the brain, it dissolves the humid substances, which evaporate, freeing the conduits and allowing the spirits to flow freely. Awakening occurs when these spirits reach the sensory and motor organs once again.

Sleep plays a threefold role: it warms the innermost parts of the body, through the movement of heat toward the viscera, and especially toward the two digestive organs, the stomach and the liver. It therefore facilitates both the first and the second digestions. It moistens the internal organs through the condensation of vapors emitted by the organs of nutrition. And it permits the repose of the *virtutes animales*—which perform sensory and relational functions—while activating the *virtutes naturales*, especially those of digestion and retention.

The regimens of health insisted on the importance of setting aside the most propitious hours for sleep; they severely deplored the habit of taking afternoon naps. As for how many hours should be devoted to sleep, Maynus de Mayneriis wrote: "taking into account the age and the complexion, I think that the time spent sleeping should range from a maximum of twelve hours to a minimum of eight. It is important to sleep longer after eating heavy and hard-to-digest foods; less, when one has eaten easy-to-digest foods."[72]

The *regimina* recommended a slightly different sort of bed than those we sleep in today. They advised raising slightly the head of the bed, to create a gentle slope toward the feet. Medical texts justified this habit as a way of preventing the regurgitation of food. The position of the body, they urged, should change through the different phases of sleep: at first, one should sleep on the right side, then one should turn onto the left side, and finally one should return to the initial position on the right side. This recommendation, present for the first time in the "Canon,"[73] was over time cited by all of the physicians of the Middle Ages. Other positions were strongly contraindicated, as they could lead to various disorders.

The Hygiene of Waste

The pair of starvation and repletion came fifth in the list of nonnatural things. According to medieval authors, starvation is the state that ensues once an organism has been emptied of everything superfluous or detrimental to the body. Repletion is a plethoric state, produced following the absorption of food or drink. Health requires a balance between these two extremes. Among the substances to be evacuated, it was necessary to distinguish among (1) the waste products from the three physiological digestions; (2) the numerous substances produced by the other organs, such as sperm, developed by the testicles; and (3) the humors, found either in the blood or in their own receptacles. The evacuation of humors required a series of techniques: phlebotomy, the application of suction cups, and the use of leeches for blood; the administration of emetics or of specific purgatives for the three other humors.

The most propitious moment for purging was in the early morning. In general, this was the time for bowel movements, even if physicians stressed the importance of respecting the habitual rhythms of the body. Treatises offered suggestions for treating constipation or diarrhea, among them, starting meals with dried fruit (figs or raisins) or eating bran bread, in the proportion of one-sixth bran to five-sixths flour. The kidneys and the bladder were thought to eliminate superfluous products of the second digestion, and it was therefore necessary to empty the bladder entirely in the morning and again each time one might feel the need.

The third digestion completely assimilated—into the limbs—the nutritious elements borne by the blood. This digestion produced many diverse waste products: hairs, sweat, *sordicies,* tears, nasal mucus, expectoration from the lungs, and the wax secreted by the ears. The purpose of the daily toilet was to rid the body of all these waste products. "In summer, wash with cold water your hands, your face, your mouth, and your head. In winter, contrariwise, use hot water."[74] After washing the face and the hands, it was necessary to rinse the eyes: "Upon rising, you should rinse your eyes with cold water, to eliminate the gummy clots on the eyelashes and all around the eyes." After the manner of Avicenna, the Salernitan regimen advised keeping one's eyes open under water, "as long as possible."[75] Then one was advised to shave and brush one's hair, and even to pluck other parts of the body clean of hair, such as the armpits and the pubis.[76] Dental hygiene also played an important part, and the justifications adduced were often perfectly reasonable: "If a man must wash and rub his teeth, it is because the impurities that are deposited there produce a foul breath. Moreover, dirty teeth emanate spirits that disturb the brain, without considering the fact that the mixture of tartar and food can lead to the corruption of the food in the stomach."[77] The morning toilet could not eliminate all the waste products of the third digestion; it was also necessary to eliminate the superfluous products of the nose, the ears, the chest, and so on. It was also necessary to wash one's hands before and after meals. Bartholomew of Varignana recommended doing so in rose water.[78] Literary sources confirm this practice; failing to do so was scandalous.[79] In the evening, before going to bed was the time to wash one's feet, but only if one had not dined that day. There was a link between the hygiene of one's lower extremities and the good health of sight and hearing; its meaning eludes us. "In the evening, before going to bed, on days when one has not dined, then one should wash and rub one's feet with warm water, to preserve the health of one's hearing, sight, and memory."[80] This operation completed the daily cycle of natural evacuations. After a night of refreshing sleep, another day would dawn, and with it, one would face again all the demands of daily hygiene.

In connection with the pair of starvation and repletion, the regimens of health also offered advice concerning sexual activity. These sources provide a limited image of sexuality, considered solely as a means for the evacuation of a product of the third digestion, the sperm produced by the testicles. There is no mention of pleasure or the emotions involved in sexuality, nothing about fertility or about the moral rules that govern sexual practices. When speaking to patients who had taken a vow of chastity, the *regimina* offered some rules making it easier to maintain those vows.

Emotions

Medieval medicine postulated exceedingly close ties between body and soul; this connection engendered the doctrine of the *accidentes animae* or *passiones*. These were emotions generated in the soul and expressed through movements of the body. Modern psychology identifies passions as propensities that perturb psychic equilibrium. In the Middle Ages, quite to the contrary, the passions were all the emotional impulses of the sensitive soul, and were thus much closer to what we would call "feelings" or "emotions." Passions were psychosomatic movements directly affecting the body, and indirectly affecting the soul. They were a sort of psychophysiological complex: triggered at the level of the spirit or imagination, they had immediate effects on the body, where they produced a series of vital reactions.

Medieval physicians were particularly interested in the somatic modifications caused by passions. They reduced the number of passions from twelve to four or five, but they described in detail the somatic processes that they caused.

The central organ of the process that generates passions was the heart. The emotional dynamic was triggered by the introduction of heat and spirits into the heart or by their outflow from the heart. A modification of the blood ensued, causing in turn all of the different somatic manifestations that are characteristic of the passions (heightened skin color, accelerated heartbeat, hot flushes, chills, and so on). The medical diagram of the passions could be directly superimposed on the philosophical diagram of the passions, with the only difference being that physicians placed greater emphasis on the physiological substrate. The pairs cited by physicians—slow/fast and centripetal/centrifugal—corresponded to the pairs cited by philosophers, peaceable/irascible and withdrawn/vigorous.

In terms of hygiene, there were healthful passions, such as joy, which had no contraindications. To encourage joy, physicians offered bountiful advice, such as eating properly, enjoying life, seeing friends, surrounding oneself with lovely women, and living according to one's rank.[81] There were other, unhealthful passions, chief among them sadness and anxiety, two states of mind contrary to vital dynamism, which tended to chill and dry out the body and the heart.[82] Fear, too, was a pernicious state of mind, for it brought about an entire series of unpleasant somatic alterations: trembling, chills, pallor, and often diarrhea.[83] The fourth unhealthful passion was wrath, characterized by a faster and centripetal movement of heat and spirits. The symptoms were a powerful racing of the heart, a diffuse redness in the face, bulging eyes, and so forth. The attitudes of physicians toward wrath were varied. Some felt that its effects were harmful to health and warned against it; others felt that in certain situations an outburst of wrath might be a good thing. To soothe a state of wrath, physicians recommended music, reading, and especially a sound and restorative sleep.

Hygiene of the Ages of Life

In addition to the *regimina sanitatis* structured according to the six non-natural things, there were other regimens, known as the university *regimina sanitatis*, because they contained scholastic elements, in particular, *quaestiones*. They were assembled in accordance with age or certain specific conditions of life. The scheme of ages or complexions, a legacy of Galen through the medium of Avicenna, can be found in *regimina sanitatis* written during the first half of the fourteenth century by such respected physicians as Bernard de Gordon and Maynus de Mayneriis. What interests us here is their approach to childhood and old age, the ages most often overlooked by the *regimina sanitatis*. One exception, the treatise by Aldobrandino da Siena, was excessively bound up with Arab sources. In certain other cases, it was the age of the recipient of the regimen that prompted remarks concerning the extreme ages of life. Such was the case with the regimen drawn up by Guido da Vigevano for Philip VI of Valois, the *Liber conservacionis sanitatis senis;* such was also the case with the anonymous treatise written for the use of the young princes of the house of Burgundy.

The Regimens of Childhood

In accordance with Galen, medieval physicians strongly recommended that a mother suckle her child. The arguments offered in favor of this practice are exceedingly varied: through mother's milk, it was possible to transmit to the child a number of substances necessary to its development; suckling by a wet nurse might alter the behavior of a newborn, causing it—once it had reached adulthood—not to behave according to its rank.

314

The fact that physicians so emphasized the point is a fair indication, however, that suckling by wet nurses was a fairly widespread practice. In effect, sources mention it frequently. If we take a closer look, we see that the attitudes of physicians were ambivalent. Alongside the many criticisms of wet nurses, we also find arguments in their favor, provided that their age and complexion are appropriate: "Many women are noble, or delicate, or want to avoid the effort, or have no milk. It may also happen that the nipple is too short, or that the woman is ill, and so forth, and that it is therefore not possible to suckle the newborn; in that case, the proper solution is to hire a wet nurse of good repute."[84]

Male children were generally weaned at age three, female children at two and a half. Girls did not have to be as strong as boys, since their activity was limited to caring for home and hearth. Once a child cut his or her first teeth, it was recommended that the milk diet be filled out with soft foods, such as bread soaked in honey water or wine cut with water, meat broth, various forms of boiled wheat, and foods that had previously been masticated, either by the mother or the wet nurse.

The child's day was spent sleeping, eating, and bathing. The morning bath was drawn in lukewarm water and repeated during the day, followed by a short session of massages. The child was to be suckled three or four times a day, at a fixed time, according to some authors, or upon request, according to others. The swaddling clothes were to be changed as needed: "Above all, one should take care that the child's linen is not dirty. Whenever he dirties his linen, it should be changed."[85] "If the swaddling baby cries, one should hasten to undo the swaddling and change it."[86] The daily cycle ended with sleep, induced by a soothing lullaby, *dulcibus cantilenis*.

Once a child had been weaned, it entered the world of adults. At the age of six, a child was ready for school; between the ages of three and six was the time the child learned to walk, became toilet trained, and learned to speak. Children were closely watched, to prevent domestic accidents or malformations produced by bad habits. Children were not forced to learn to walk, lest this result in deformation of the limbs. Children also were not forced to sit in excessively hard or sharp-edged chairs. Care was advised to keep dangerous objects out of children's reach, such as sticks or swords. Play was the child's chief activity during this happy period. Maynus wrote: "Following the nap time, the child should bathe until his skin becomes red. Then, you should allow the child to play for an hour, after which he should eat well. After his meal, he may be allowed to play freely at some length. Later, he should have another bath, and he should eat a second time."[87] Bernard de Gordon added to this scheme a short noonday nap, to allow the child to recover spent energy.

Schooling began at age six. The pedagogy recommended by these physicians was exceedingly latitudinarian: "One should almost always accommodate the wishes of the child, without contradicting it, because to do so might make the child timorous. Anger, according to Galen, leads to rage, and fear leads to the paralysis of the whole being." It was necessary to impart a good education and good habits to a child, for this foundation was fundamental to continued good health and future.

The school years ended at the age of fourteen, when the child's future place in society was selected. Bernard de Gordon described with precision the three choices open to an adolescent of the social classes to which the *regimina sanitatis* were addressed: arms, the mechanical arts of the city, and philosophy, meaning the intellectual life. Each choice required a specific form of training. To prepare for the soldier's life, the young man would have to develop the strength required to defend with courage the banner that he had chosen to follow. He would have to sleep on the ground and ride on horseback, to strengthen his leg muscles; he would have to use a mace with his right hand and his left, to strengthen his arms; he would have to wear a suit of mail to strengthen his shoulders. He would have to be able to withstand heat, chill, and hunger. The adolescent should then be surrounded by strong and intrepid men. He should know how to master fear and panic. He would have to accustom himself to seeing the dead scattered across a field of battle and watch men fight duels lest he quail in the face of the terrible sights of war. All the same, he should never lose his judgment or forget his senses of proportion and justice.

The second path, that of the mechanical arts, included commerce. They actually covered all of the trades and occupations. Bernard de Gordon held them in high consideration, for they were the source of the city's life. One who chose this path should prepare for it by receiving massages only slightly less vigorous than those recommended for knights. Depending on the exact trade chosen, one should do a series of different exercises.

For those who chose the intellectual life, a lighter series of massages and exercises was recommended, for it was thought that soft muscles tended to make a man more reflective.

The Regimen of Old Age

Ever since antiquity, medical literature had established with some precision the parameters of old age. It was thought that old age began around forty-five or fifty-five, which was considered the extreme limit of *pulchri-tudo*. From this point on until the age of seventy-two, one spoke of old men *(senes a senectute)* and very old men *(senes a senio)*.

Old men suffered from declines in warmth and natural moisture. All of the physiological changes they suffered were linked to this preponderance of dryness and cold. With the passage of years, the quantity of heat available to the organism progressively diminished. The cause of this diminution was—aside from the passing years themselves—the accumulation of such other factors as dry air, physical effort, or inappropriate diet. The first thing to be affected was the body's set of digestive functions, at this point incapable of entirely processing the substances ingested. There was an ensuing excess in the production of cold and wet humors, such as natural phlegm and the nonnatural phlegms. A vicious circle thus developed, which proportionately throttled the natural heat; the regimen was meant to break this cycle. It was therefore necessary to ply the organism with warm and wet substances, through nutrition, sleep, and so on. The house should be oriented eastward so that the sun could penetrate into it in the morning. While, during the summer it was necessary to moderate the temperature indoors by sprinkling the house with cold substances, in winter it was necessary to warm the house steadily, with a fire burning night and day.[88] For physical exercise, Bernard de Gordon recommended walking or riding a horse.[89] Other *regimina* called for massages and rubdowns: "One should give them a rubdown every day, both in order to prepare them for exercise and to compensate for the absence of exercise."[90] Baths too could help to humidify and warm the elderly; they were especially helpful if, taken three or four times in each season, aromatic and moistening herbs were added to the water. It was necessary to get out of the bath as soon as wrinkles and roughness began to appear on the skin of the fleshiest parts of the fingers.[91]

As far as diet was concerned, the most important characteristic of the dishes served to the aged was their ease of digestion. Old men should eat less, and only once a day. But it was recommended that exceedingly old men eat several times a day and always in limited quantities. Foods that produce either phlegm or black bile—the two cold humors of the organism—were forbidden, as were dishes described as "viscous," for these could produce obstructions. Bread should have a higher percentage of bran than normal bread. The meat of chicken or waterfowl was recommended, the latter because it lives near lakes and ponds. Lamb, veal, and pork were also accepted, provided they were nice and tender. Fish—an animal with a phlegmatic complexion—was forbidden, especially if dried, salted, or without scales. Eggs were recommended (to be drunk raw)—it was thought that they produced blood. Also recommended were honey and mare's and ass's milk—they were believed to have moistening properties and were to be consumed with a pinch of salt or sweetened with honey.[92] Warm and moist fresh vegetables were also allowed (such as fennel and borage); dried fruit, too, and especially figs, were thought to prevent constipation when eaten just before and just after meals. Wine, a warm and moist food, could be consumed in moderation and was thought to be the best medication for the elderly and the exceedingly old.

Sleep made it possible to recover natural warmth, facilitated digestion, and activated the faculties of the organism; sleep was therefore greatly recommended. In the pair of repletion and starvation, the important thing was to find the golden mean, so as to avoid, on the one hand, a plethoric state or, on the other, a state of malnutrition.[93] It was also necessary to tend to the proper evacuation of the residues of organic digestions, as well as to the rhythms of intestinal activity. The *regimina* offered numerous prescriptions for bowel movements, either through natural methods, such as diet, or artificial means, such as the use of laxatives or enemas. Lastly, as far as the accidents of the soul were concerned, the aged should shun sadness and fear, in favor of joy or wrath; in small doses, wrath increased the natural heat.[94]

As a last consideration, we must distinguish between the *regimina* steeped in Galenism and solid common sense, and another gerontological literature of the Middle Ages: that of the *Regimen senium*, or the *De conservanda iuventute et retardanda senectute*, definitively attributed to Arnald of Villanova. In effect, while the former meant to preserve health at all ages of life, the objective of the latter was merely to delay aging and to prevent the diseases caused by old age.

~ 12 ~

Diseases in Europe: Equilibrium and Breakdown of the Pathocenosis

JEAN-NOËL BIRABEN

We know next to nothing about the health conditions, and even less about the medical ideas, of the earliest humans to populate Europe, over a million years ago.[1] The exceedingly rare evidence offered by paleopathology is in fact wholly inadequate to allow us to form any solid hypotheses concerning this subject. One can safely state that there were a great many accidents, especially hunting accidents.[2] It may be that certain practices of bonesetting date from this period.

Paleopathology of Prehistoric Times

It was, for the most part, not until much later, roughly ten thousand years ago, that the physical, climatic, and biological environment of Europe as we now know it came into being. Roughly 8500 B.C., in fact, the warming of the climate brought about not only a retreat of the glaciers and a major rise in sea level, but also an overall botanical and zoological shakeup throughout Europe. Over the course of a few centuries, forests had replaced the steppe and tundra, while the vast herds of animals vanished.

Two consequences of this, one nutritional in nature, the other medical, are of concern in the context of this book. The harsh climatic shift seems to have been quite unfavorable to the peoples of Europe. The decline in living conditions and in the level of culture coincided with a general famine, and the first millennium of the Mesolithic was marked by a sharp drop in population—save for in northern Europe, where living conditions actually improved—followed by a slow recovery, which began to manifest itself in the next millennium. This appears to have been a fundamental period, for over the course of these two millennia, humans became familiar with the new vegetation surrounding them. In this process of learning, through experiments that were in some cases successful and at other times disastrous, humans accumulated a body of knowledge concerning not only the alimentary qualities of plants, but also their toxic or medicinal virtues.

Very few diseases left traces on bones; paleopathology offers an exceedingly narrow and less than representative sampling of the pathocenosis of these earliest eras.[3]

In the Paleolithic, we note that there were relatively few hereditary or congenital malformations, as well as few cases of infectious osteitis or dental cavities, while it is common to find evidence of trauma (sprains, dislocations, and fractures) and arthropathy (spondylarthrosis and arthrosis, of the hip, in particular).

In the Mesolithic, we find on the whole the same pattern, but abscesses and bone infections seem to have been more common. Tuberculosis of bones and joints is probable, if not absolutely established, while it is quite common to see marks of violent combat (arrowheads embedded in a bone, facial fractures, and so on), especially in male skeletons.

In the Neolithic, hereditary or congenital malformations of the bones, which for the most part affect the spinal column, remained fairly infrequent, while the consequences of trauma (sprains; dislocations, especially of the shoulder; and fractures, especially of the forearm, and broken fingers and toes) are relatively common. The consequences of violence seem to increase greatly. We also see a sharp increase in infections from pyogenic germs: osteitis or osteomyelitis and tuberculosis of the bones or joints. There was also an increase in dental cavities and abscesses, while there seems to have been an almost total absence of bone cancers, though this is probably because, being little calcified, or calcified not at all, they tended not to fossilize. Degenerative conditions were chiefly vertebral, because arthrosis tends to reach the other joints only at a later age.

The considerable volume of vertebral arthrosis, which in some cases can be found in roughly two-thirds of the skeletons of individuals aged forty or over, is a clear reminder of how fragile these spinal columns tended to be. Adaptation in humans to an upright posture was not yet complete, for one thing, and prehistoric peoples may have led far more sedentary lives than we might imagine. Another, less frequent arthrosis is that of the temporomaxillary joint. This condition is almost always associated with heavy dental abrasion, pointing clearly to a diet of material that was exceedingly tough to chew. Dental cavities were less of a phenomenon than they were in the preceding period.

The pathological pattern of the Copper Age and of the subsequent Bronze Age and Iron Age is not notably different from that of the Neolithic, with the exception of the increased frequency of traumas from combat.

The only way we can trace the influence of this pathocenosis (now reduced to nothing more than the traces it left on bones) on a body of medical thought about which we know practically nothing is through observation of the two procedures that left observable marks on the bones. While, in fact, it is impossible to single out the reduced dislocations, we can note a considerable number of dislocations that never were reduced; moreover, although the diaphyseal fractures, almost all of them inflicted to the forearm, remained with fragments piled one upon another, it is at the same time also true that the consolidation, nearly always rectilinear, presupposes the use of splints or some analogous system. The other type of treatment—cranial trepanation—is more surprising. This form of surgery was practiced in the Neolithic, as long ago as 3000 B.C. in western Europe, and quickly fanned out over all the territory of what is now Europe. The operation involves perforating the calvaria without causing lesions to the meninges. Trepanation was more frequent in the Copper Age and in the Bronze Age, becoming rare during the Iron Age. The operation was performed at first with a flint, and later on with a bronze scalpel; it is remarkable that the wound often healed without pyogenic infection, and that fairly frequently the patients survived. It was originally interpreted as a magical ritual (the operation was sometimes performed on cadavers), but the discovery of fractures and preoperative inflammatory lesions on skulls subjected to trepanation leaves little doubt concerning the therapeutic nature of the operation, at least in certain cases. Diaphyseal fractures, on the one hand, and conditions of the cranium, the meninges, and the encephalon, on the other, led the shamans-doctors of the Neolithic to perform new operations, with a degree of success that we are hard put to evaluate with any certainty.

To this drastically limited picture of the pathocenosis offered by the field of paleopathology, we can add the first, tentative hypotheses of the early history of diseases—tentative, but quite probable. The emergence of infectious and parasitic diseases usually occurs in conjunction with a change in the habitat and the ecology of the infected host; more rarely, it occurs in conjunction with a mutation of the germ or the animal or plant parasite. In humans, over the course of the last ten thousand years, cultural changes have played an increasing, and by now practically exclusive, role in the appearance of new diseases. The evolution of diseases follows the laws of biological equilibrium, which tend to lead, over generations, to a reciprocal adaptation between host and parasite. This means that the most recent diseases are the most serious, while the most ancient ones are generally the most benign. Many diseases, moreover, immunize, and given that human populations are split up into groups—farming communities, villages, cities, or nomadic encampments—diseases tend to dwindle away when groups have few contacts and are small in size, or else diseases return only when reintroduced (as is the case on small islands). In order for the disease to persist, there must be, among other things, either frequent contacts among the groups or groups themselves that reach given thresholds (from 30,000 to 300,000 persons, depending on the disease's epidemiology); this explains the importance of the role played by urbanization. Diseases may then disappear along with the conditions that first led them to emerge and encouraged their survival.

The first major cultural transition of European man, which coincided with the Neolithic, almost certainly meant the expansion of the pathocenosis to include numerous afflictions that had not emerged till that time. Increasingly sedentary ways of life led to increasing accumulations of waste—and hence of germs and parasites—around dwellings; monoculture encouraged the development of plant parasites, while the herding and breeding of domestic or commensal animals led to zoonosis and parasitism. Dozens of diseases, some now rare, others still common, were thus introduced into European societies beginning around 6000 B.C., generally spreading from south to north and from east to west. The majority of these diseases have their origins with the earliest domesticated species. For instance, we can list, in declining order of frequency, dogs (scabies, hydatid disease, roundworm), cattle (measles, smallpox, tuberculosis, beef tapeworm), sheep and goats (fluke disease, anthrax, brucellosis), pigs (pork tapeworm, trichinosis), horses (rotz and glanders), water birds (influenza), and rodents (plague, melioidosis).

Clearly, these diseases did not all appear at the same time; rather, they emerged bit by bit and, in some cases, quite late. For many infectious diseases, such as chicken pox, mumps, and diphtheria, we know neither the origin nor the period of first manifestation.[4] We do know, however, that the spread of other diseases, such as typhoid fever and salmonellosis, was facilitated by the use of excrements as fertilizer. Malaria spread two ways: it was borne by travelers and by the surging population of the vector mosquitos, caused by irrigation of fields and the use of man-made fish ponds. Marshy regions and coastal lagoons, areas where malaria was common, were reputed to be areas in which the air was especially unhealthy, hence the name of the disease ("mal-aria," or "bad air").

The division of labor led to the appearance of occupational diseases: silicosis, or grinder's disease, affected miners and stonecutters; saturnism, or lead poisoning, afflicted potters (since lead sulphide was used as a varnish); and hydrargyrism, or mercury poisoning, was found among manufacturers of cinnabar (at Vinca, in Serbia, for instance).

Protohistory and the Archaic Period

We can divide into four categories the causes of death of the Homeric heroes: violent death (in combat or by accident), death as the result of disease, sudden death without any evident cause, and death from grief.[5] Homer principally described wounds. Treatment remained simple and basic: compression in case of hemorrhaging, extraction of foreign bodies, cleaning of wounds, and application of balms and powdered roots. Only rarely did Homer provide descriptions of diseases, such as the "pestilence" of the first book of the *Iliad*, fevers, the madness of Ulysses' men, or the melancholy of Bellerophon.

A certain number of other diseases are described, or in some cases only mentioned, prior to Hippocrates. Cases of madness or epilepsy were inevitably considered to be of divine origin. We also find skin diseases, ulcers, blindness, rheumatic afflictions, dropsy, lumbagos, fevers, and "plagues." This is an exceedingly narrow picture, and it would seem that only diseases indicative of an outside intervention, meaning a divine intervention, were considered worthy of attention.

The Classical Era

Concerning the classical period taken as a whole, we can determine the nature of the pathocenosis by working essentially on medical writings, primarily on the Hippocratic treatises. Any use of the Hippocratic corpus, however, entails numerous difficulties. One of the greatest difficulties unquestionably derives from the conceptual model, that is, the humoral doctrine, which so greatly influenced the way in which clinical observations were recorded. We cannot hope to find correspondences with a precisely defined disease of modern-day nosology for each Hippocratic description. Rather, we should begin with the supposition that one description may cover a number of different diseases, and that a number of different descriptions may cover various forms of a single disease. We thus find, in the Hippocratic corpus, descriptions of sixty or so different afflictions, considered as so many different forms of humoral imbalance. This number agrees, in terms of the general order of magnitude, with the number of diseases generally listed in folk classifications of causes of death, found among peoples the world over. If we further note that this number drops to about fifty when we take as a single disease the various forms of the same disease, then we can clearly see that, in clinical terms, Hippocratic medicine had not really made sufficient progress toward standing alone from traditional folk medicine, at least in terms of diagnostic discrimination.[6]

Fevers are mentioned frequently, but the term "fever" is never defined with any clarity: a physician might find a patient to be warm, but no relation is established with a faster heartbeat or pulse, and there was no means for ascertaining the patient's temperature. The three principal fevers include the *causus* (a continual fever, with a dry tongue and parched throat, intense thirst, nausea, enlarged spleen), the *phrenitis* (another continual fever, but with delirium, a fixed stare, and stupor), and the *lethargus* (according to Galen, intermediate between *causus* and *phrenitis*, with a pseudocontinual fever, somnolence, at times delirium, and abundant, exceedingly fluid, expectorations). These three fevers are probably, for the most part, typhoid and paratyphoid fevers, as well as other salmonellosis, though we also find septicemias, postpartum infections, and the occasional serious jaundice.

We also find, moreover, remittent fevers, with serious outbreaks separated by less feverish intervals, often accompanied by diarrhea or by jaundices, epistaxis (nosebleed), or parotitis. These are chiefly afflictions involving the digestive apparatus, but of fairly diverse varieties.

The intermittent fevers were almost always caused by malaria, which had existed in Greece at least since the Neolithic and had, quite early, emerged in its three forms (caused by *Plasmodium vivax*, *P. malariae*, and *P. falciparum*). The outbreaks of fever were separated by regular intervals of two, three, or four days, hence the names tertian, quartan, and quintan

fever, while the spleen and liver were hypertrophic. The frequency of the
P. falciparum form, the most serious one, can be calculated with some
approximation by noting the relationship between this disease and a genetic defect that leaves marks on the bones—a distinctive cranial porous
hyperostosis—whose frequency in the numerous series of skulls that have
been studied indicates the degree of endemic malaria. We thus find a
frequency of 33 percent in the Mesolithic, 40 percent in the early Neolithic, 19 percent in the later Neolithic, 11 percent in the early Bronze
Age, 17 percent in the middle Bronze Age, 9 percent in the late Bronze
Age, 9 percent in the early Iron Age, 7 percent in the classical period,
14 percent in the Hellenistic period, and 24 percent in Roman times. Of
course, this is an overall evolution, which must have varied from region to
region. It does show that, while malaria in its malignant form may have
been reintroduced at various points, it never entirely disappeared. The
causes of these variations are primarily climatic, but the reclamation of
marshy land probably contributed to some degree, and it is interesting to
note that the periods of greatest prosperity tend to correspond with declines in the frequency of malaria, and vice-versa.[7]

Next we should look at exanthematous typhus. The presence of fleas
is not sufficient to prove its existence. In reality, if we consider that the
so-called plague of Athens of 430 B.C., described by Thucydides, should
be broken down into various diseases, much as Grmek has done for the
"cough of Perinthus," and if we accept that typhus was probably the most
important component, then we are probably faced here with the first
manifestation of this disease in Europe. The description offered by the
historian, detailed though it may be, only deepens our regret that the
authors of the Hippocratic corpus, contemporaries of so noteworthy an
epidemic, should make no mention of it whatsoever. In any case, aside
from the description of the various characteristic clinical signs, the disease's arrival by sea, the particular seriousness of cases linked to under-
nourishment, and the massing of refugees in the besieged city, all the signs
correspond perfectly with what we now know about the disease's epidemiology. Its persistence, however, poses some problems: for reasons that
are unclear, typhus seems to have died out in Europe, only to be reintroduced on various occasions. We should also keep in mind that, for Thucydides as well as for the Athenian physicians who witnessed the epidemic, this was a new disease, never previously encountered.

What the ancients describe as cholera was clearly unrelated to the
Asiatic cholera that appeared at the beginning of the nineteenth century:

this *cholera nostras* is for the most part a food poisoning, not very infectious if infectious at all, that may appear epidemic when it strikes communities or groups that eat together.

J. N. Corvisier has calculated that, for all the cases of fever reported in the Hippocratic corpus, the fatality rate is just over 50 percent. It is possible that such a high fatality rate was produced by selective reporting of the most serious cases, but even if we take this into account, the mortality rate from fevers was assuredly quite high.

Gangrenes are often mentioned in the Hippocratic corpus. Moist gangrene, the most common variety, develops following a sore, an ulcer, a cut in the foot, or an arteritis. In the last-named case, however, infection does not necessarily follow, and the obstruction of the artery can cause a dry gangrene. Two cases are reported of the patient's survival following amputation. Lastly, we should mention dental abscesses, which can provoke necrosis of the lower maxillary.

Afflictions of the respiratory apparatus are quite frequent, beginning with angina. The definition of this condition was fairly vague and involved fever, inflammation of the throat, difficulty in breathing, and pain in swallowing, as well as associated signs that might vary: painful, protruding eyes, a flushed face, an inflamed and swollen neck, hiccoughs, and so forth. It was almost always serious and often was fatal. Membranous angina and stridulous laryngismus were familiar, as was tonsillitis. Also well known were diphtherial pharyngitis and croup. Colds were common (there is a report of an infection that was in all likelihood a sinusitis), but it is hard to be sure whether there were truly outbreaks of influenza. In any case, no serious epidemic of influenza can be identified, and the descriptions report flulike syndromes.

Pneumonia and pleurisy were not clearly separated. Pneumonia was characterized by fourteen to eighteen days of fever and dense expectorations, followed by the formation of a pus sac that could be allowed to break or that could be incised, which causes one to think of a pulmonary abscess or a purulent pleurisy, following a case of pneumonia. The term "pleurisy" is used to indicate pain and inflammation in the side with, in some cases, bloody expectorations, which leads one to think more of rusty sputum than of pneumonia.

Pulmonary tuberculosis was called phthisis, but many other descriptions correspond to cases of tuberculosis: these are slight torpid fevers accompanied by pains in the chest and back, dry cough, and loss of weight. All these symptoms should manifest themselves for at least a year. Other forms can be identified nowadays, such as laryngeal phthisis, a wounded or ulcerated trachea, and others still. A number of ancient authors, not physicians, were persuaded that phthisis was contagious; in effect, considering the living conditions and especially the living quarters of the lower classes of the time, transmission must have been common. Asthma, though not thought of as a disease, is present in the Hippocratic writings, where three alterations of respiration are cited: dyspnea, if breathing was labored and heavy; orthopnea, when breathing was feeble; and asthma, when respiration was light, short, and frequent.

Afflictions of the digestive apparatus were as important as those of the respiratory apparatus, but they are also difficult to interpret, since we know little indeed about the diet of each patient, when we know anything at all. Certainly, afflictions deriving from toxic or spoiled foods, or from infected beverages, must have been common. The recommendation to check for the presence of a leech in the throat, if the throat was filled with blood, shows clearly that drinking water was taken directly from streams or wells, and this in an age when even running streams were often infected upstream by human or animal waste. Diarrhea, vomit, enlarged livers, enlarged spleen, and fever all form part of a frequent pattern that is not sufficiently characteristic. Bloody diarrhea restricts the number of possible diagnoses, but can we really speak of bacillary dysentery when in the presence of a single, isolated case?

Jaundices are often mentioned. They are classified according only to the color of the skin or the season in which they appeared; it is therefore legitimate to suspect that they included, in addition to viral hepatitis, cases of obstructive jaundices or even cases of spirochetosis icterohaemorrhagica, leaving aside alcohol poisoning or other intoxications. We also find reports of hepatic colic. Colics are quite difficult to identify, since abdominal pain can be caused by a number of factors: simple bloat or grave intestinal hemorrhage, mushroom poisoning, mucomembranous colitis, gastroduodenal ulcer, intestinal tumor, intestinal occlusion, peritonitis, or appendicitis that developed in a drastic manner following an inopportune purge.

One cannot sufficiently emphasize the importance of parasites in the digestive tract, the subject of frequent mentions in the Hippocratic texts, though only in passing, as of a common occurrence. Numerous mentions are made of patients expelling intestinal worms from the mouth, an unquestionable sign of an intense ascariasis. Tapeworms, too, are described with precision, although we do not know which species were present.

Nutrition was surely at the origin of serious diseases, in some cases fatal ones. I have mentioned poisonous mushrooms and alcohol poisoning; we should also keep in mind that lead was used in water pipes and in the varnishes of terra-cotta vessels, thus causing a slight lead poisoning, which often resulted in outbreaks of gout. The Hippocratic texts describe podagra. It seems that the diet was fairly well balanced, on the whole. Caloric intake seems to have been adequate; there was also a healthy balance among proteins, sugars, and fats. Certain vitamins may not have been present in adequate dosage; hence the cases of avitaminosis, found especially among the poorer classes. In fact, hunting, fishing, and herding seem always to have been sufficiently bountiful to provide plenty of meat, while in the Neolithic, the progressive replacement of the gathering of a wide variety of plants with a more limited array of cultivated plants led to cases of vitamin deficiencies. Grains, despite their abundance, do not include the full range of indispensable vitamins and amino acids. Especially during the archaic period people seem generally to have consumed insufficient quantities of vitamin A, which protects the eyes, lungs, and skin; vitamin C, which prevents scurvy; and vitamin D, which prevents rickets. Then, with every new contact between Greece and the outside world—the Persian wars (end of the sixth, turn of the fifth centuries B.C.), the Hellenistic period (end of the fourth, turn of the third centuries B.C.), the Roman period (from the second to the third centuries A.D.)—the variety of plants being cultivated increased, trade thrived, and the vitamin intake became better balanced, especially with the advent of carrots (vitamin A), peaches, and apricots (vitamin C) in the third and second centuries B.C. We should note that dental cavities became more common, too.

Concerning the urinary tract, strangury, hematuria, and lithiasis are the only afflictions to be described in the Hippocratic corpus as diseases of renal origin; to these syndromes, which in fact cover various diseases, we should add renal colic, renal infections, and pyelonephritis. We can be sure that Greeks in the classical period suffered from urinary lithiasis, renal colic, various forms of nephritis, albuminuria, serious cases of cystitis, and abscesses of the urethra or the prostate.

Given the state of ignorance concerning the circulation of the blood, the circulatory system was not examined as such, and no one seemed to think that the heart could have or cause diseases. At any rate, we find at least one mention of a case of angina pectoris. I have already spoken of gangrenes from arteritis; it would seem, in effect, that most of the cases of *phlegmasia alba dolens* were infectious phlebitis, while certain cases of dropsy were, quite likely, due to cardiac insufficiency.

Afflictions of bones and joints are the subject of two Hippocratic treatises, which describe in detail nearly all known cases of fractures and dislocations. The most interesting cases involve rheumatism and arthrosis. Arthritis with fever, pain, and inflammation of the joints in a young person leads us to think of acute articular rheumatism. Lumbago, however frequent it may have been (vertebral arthrosis was common in the paleopathology of Greece and all of Europe, in all periods), is not described in the Hippocratic texts, while sciatica is described perfectly. One case, mentioned in an aphorism ("Such as become hump-backed before puberty from asthma or cough, do not recover"),[8] can in all likelihood be linked to a dorsolumbar Pott's disease caused by pulmonary tuberculosis. The great number of the lame provides testimony to the widespread incidence of ankylosis of the hip, as a result of badly reduced fractures or clubfoot. Osteomyelitis was not uncommon.

Diseases of the skin and of the mucous membranes, aside from erysipelas, are generally left undifferentiated and appear under the generic names of ulcer, lichen, aphtha. It is exceedingly difficult to identify them. Mention is also made of "leprosy," sometimes benign, and "itches," which probably corresponds to scabies.

Diseases of the nervous system are mentioned frequently throughout the Hippocratic corpus, often without clearly identifying their nature; generally speaking, they are classified on the basis of the part of the body affected, and many of the descriptions are too vague or too bound up with the concepts of the period to allow a reliable identification. This is the case with "sphacelation of the brain," which presents pains in the head, the spinal column, and the heart, and fainting spells or bouts of swelling, pallor, and fever. "Caries in the bone of the cranium," or else "water in the encephalon," gives rise to pain in the bregma and the temples and pain in the eyes, for which the ultimate remedy is trepanation. This last-named case may have been an instance of tubercular meningitis. We should also note a cerebral hemorrhage with aphasia following excessive consumption of alcoholic beverages, and many other forms of stroke with hemorrhage or cerebral thrombosis, followed by paralysis. At times, paralysis originated from an otitic meningitis, or a diphtheria, or simply a bad fall resulting in lesion of the spinal cord. Brain tumors, though completely misunderstood, are also mentioned. Finally, there appears tetanic infection, with frequent references to a sore or wound, as well as a description of a terrible tetanic crisis. Only one case might suggest the aftermath of poliomyelitis: a man from the mountains, with emaciated thighs, who had experienced difficulty in walking for some time. This isolated description, however, is far too laconic to allow us to use it as the basis for a reliable retrospective diagnosis.

It is important to recognize that epilepsy is presented as a disease of physical—and not divine—origin. The other mental afflictions—neurosis, psychosis, dementia—are treated with extreme discretion.

Diseases of the sensory organs, by contrast, are mentioned quite frequently, especially those of the sight. Like the other Mediterranean countries, Greece is a sunny place, and various ophthalmias (trachoma, blepharitis, cheratitis, leaving aside simple cases of conjunctivitis) were common. Cases of these diseases were exceedingly frequent, and blindness often ensued. Aside from these infections, encouraged by bright sunlight and ultraviolet rays, we also find descriptions of hemeralopia, or day blindness, a clear indication of a deficiency of vitamin A; myopia; glaucoma; and cataracts, which are at least partly genetic in origin.

The endocrine glands—whose function was almost entirely unknown, with the partial exception of the testicles—are rarely mentioned in Hippocratic pathology. We can, all the same, point to one case of mumps orchitis and two probable cases of diabetes.

First Historical Pathocenosis

The absence of certain diseases from the Hippocratic texts, admittedly incomplete, is not particularly significant. Certain missing diseases are mentioned in other texts of the classical period. The Hippocratic treatises report external clinical symptoms, which rarely correspond to a single disease, as they are generally common to more than one disease. Thus, the number of diseases actually observed was far larger than those specifically listed.

I have examined at length the Hippocratic corpus, because it is the earliest source sufficiently rich to form—with the complementary testimony of the era, literary, medical, or paleopathological as it may be—the starting point for the various pathocenoses that have ensued, from antiquity to the Middle Ages. Another factor in this decision is the shadow that this corpus extends over two thousand years of history. So powerful is its influence that it blocks any and all efforts to establish new knowledge, such as that of the Hellenistic school in Alexandria. It even leads to falsification of observations: thus, even such great authors as Galen tried less to discover new diseases than to find those described by Hippocrates, evincing amazement when they encountered differences.

This earliest known pathocenosis in Europe, which will remain our point of reference, was marked by a sharp prevalence of infectious and parasitic diseases. To evaluate the respective importance of the various afflictions, some scholars have compiled statistics on their frequency in a few fundamental books of the Hippocratic corpus, comparing them with other reference sources, such as the votive offerings of Epidaurus. Tables 1 and 2 are derived from those prepared by Corvisier,[9] reclassified by major categories.

Each of these tables has its own significance: the *Epidemiae* are primarily collections of cases; they allow us to establish, with considerable caution, a modern diagnosis. The breakdown of infectious and noninfectious diseases has some indicative value. The *Aphorismi*, by contrast, is a sort of compendium of medical maxims and contains only diseases that were known at the time, which is to say, symptoms or syndromes that can be attributed to a wide variety of etiologies. The subdivision shown in this table, therefore, is less reliable.

The subdivision of diseases and cases need not reflect their actual frequency in the population, but rather indicates their importance to medical concerns. We should note, all the same, that French statistics for causes of death in the middle of the nineteenth century show a frequency of roughly 75 percent for infectious and parasitic diseases, a proportion quite close to what we find in the *Epidemiae* for the whole of all pathology (causes of death and disease, combined).

Other sources, such as the charts of votive offerings from Epidaurus, tend to mention long-term infirmities, such as physical afflictions that had already been suffered over long periods and that were likely to last an entire lifetime. It is worth noting that ocular afflictions, along with cases of sterility, were particularly frequent.

The best source from the classical era—the Hippocratic books known as *Epidemiae*—describes a general pathology quite similar to what remained the situation in Europe up until the middle of the nineteenth century; there were a few major differences, foremost among them the notable absence of several diseases common in the nineteenth century, such as measles, rubella, and a few other viral diseases. Likewise, there is not a trace in Greek literature of venereal infections, such as gonorrhea or

331

Table 1. Frequency of the cases mentioned in *Epidemiae*

Type of case	Number	Percent
With infection:		
Fevers	46	18
Digestive tract	15	6
Respiratory tract	38	15
Traumas, wounds, and injuries	27	11
Postpartum conditions	16	6
Other infections	45	18
Snakebite	1	0.5
Subtotal	188	74.5
Without infection:		
Digestive tract	26	10
Respiratory tract	2	1
Traumas, wounds, and injuries	11	4
Abortions	5	2
Others	23	9
Subtotal	67	26
Total cases	255	100

syphilis. Descriptions of diseases of the genitalia can all be linked either to minor infectious germs or to such sexually transmitted germs as *Trichomonas vaginalis* (a protozoan) or *Candida xx albicans* (a fungus); we find no reference whatever to inguinal tumefaction in connection with ulceration of the penis or urethritis. Yet we must note a detailed description of Behçet's disease and the existence of infections caused by *Chlamydia trachomatis*.

Also absent were such great endemic diseases as smallpox and leprosy, mentioned only once in the Hippocratic corpus with the name "Phoenician disease." Greek physicians during the classical age were not

Table 2. Frequency of the cases mentioned in Aphorismi

Type of case	Number	Percent
With infection:		
Fevers	65	22
Digestive tract	45	15
Respiratory tract	41	14
Nervous system (tetanus)	5	2
Other infections	25	8
Subtotal	181	61
Without infection:		
Digestive tract	11	4
Respiratory tract	5	2
Sprains	2	1
Nervous system	27	9
Others	69	23
Subtotal	114	39
Total cases	295	100

familiar with leprosy, save for the occasional imported case, that is, among patients who had lived in the Middle East.[10] Also missing was polio; rather it was so ubiquitous in its mild form that it could not, "in the demographic and hygienic situation of Greece in the fifth century B.C., provoke numerous cases of paralysis."[11]

The Earliest Historical Epidemics

Equally rare were the "great epidemics": there was no plague, no cholera, no influenza. The only major epidemic was the famous plague of Athens of 428 B.C., which originated in Ethiopia, it is said, first struck in Egypt, and thereafter spread to the Persian empire and into Greece, where it raged in Lemnos and in "other regions," in the Piraeus and at Athens. The Lacedaemonians, or Spartans, who were besieging the city, did not attack but continued to raid and plunder in the surrounding countryside, without being infected by the disease. And while Agnon, with his reinforcements, brought the infection among the Athenian troops surrounding Potidea, in Chalcidica, it does not seem that Greece, on the whole, was affected. Even though we cannot be absolutely certain, we can guess that this was the first appearance of exanthematous typhus in Europe.[12]

For the rest of Europe, we have only indirect testimony. Diodorus Siculus speaks of epidemics that struck the various armies besieging Syracuse. The first such troops were Athenian, in 413 B.C.: the pestilence began in the early days of August, and the fact that he speaks of intermittent fever in this swampy region has led many to conclude it was an outbreak of pernicious malaria. Then, in 396 B.C., it was the turn of the Carthaginians: for these soldiers, the disease began with catarrh and a swelling of the neck, followed later by fever and osphyalgia and a heaviness in the legs, dysentery, and the eruption of pustules all over the body. A number of the sick broke into delirium and ran through the camp. Death frequently occurred on the fifth or sixth day, amid atrocious suffering. This mysterious epidemic, which forced the Carthaginians to lift their siege, has been interpreted variously. Haeser has called it petechial typhus, Krause instead believes it was smallpox. Whether it was one or the other, or a third disease entirely, this remained a localized epidemic.[13]

The same can be said of epidemics reported in Rome by chroniclers, epidemics that rarely extended beyond the surrounding towns.[14] The first of these, which occurred in 738 B.C., according to Dionysius of Halicarnassus and Plutarch, was too deformed through the lens of legend to be reliably identified.

We know nothing about the nature of the epidemics that raged in 707 B.C., in Rome and in Italy at large; in 645 B.C. under the rule of Tullus Hostilius on the Alban Hills; in 508 B.C. under Tarquinius Superbus in Rome, when an epidemic caused the deaths of many pregnant women, young maidens, and children; and in 490 B.C., when a famine was joined by a serious epidemic that spread among the Volsci, striking with particular ferocity the town of Velletri. Two years later, a number of women seized by divine fury announced an impending epidemic. It did occur, striking almost the entire population, though with a low rate of mortality. At the feast of Capitoline Jove, so many of the dancers were ill that the sacred dances were performed in an unsatisfactory manner. Some commentators have claimed that this account, by Dionysius of Halicarnassus, describes the first epidemic of influenza in Europe; still, nothing in this clearly anecdotal account seems to provide solid evidence.

In 471 B.C., following sinister omens, the women of Rome were stricken with a contagious disease; those who were pregnant gave premature birth, their infants dying with them. Once this epidemic ended, another one followed. This second epidemic presented such severe conditions of catarrh that no human succor could in any way alleviate it. Fortunately, the disease did not last long. Some have identified this epidemic, too, as influenza, whereas others conclude it was pneumonia. The mention of epidemic catarrh leads us to think of an acute contagious pneumonopathy, a flu syndrome.

Ten years later, in 461 B.C., another epidemic broke out. This one was far more deadly, and it affected people of both sexes, all ages, and every rank of power and wealth in the same way: it killed both consuls, all the tribunes, and a quarter of the senators. According to Dionysius of Halicarnassus and Livy, the epidemic raged in Rome for a year, but it also struck neighboring peoples, such as the Equii and the Volsci. Town and country were equally afflicted, and according to Paulus Orosius, the epidemic continued for three years in Italy. What we do know is that it seemed to be transmitted both through direct contagion and through infected air, which is not sufficient to allow us to establish a retrospective diagnosis.

In 411 (or 408) B.C., according to Livy, a highly "pernicious" epidemic devastated Rome and Latium, causing few deaths but so debilitating the population that work was abandoned in the fields, resulting in a famine the following year. Here, too, Schnurrer and Haeser speak of influenza, but nothing in the text allows us to advance such a hypothesis.[15]

The epidemic of 329 B.C., linked, according to Livy and Paulus Orosius, to bad weather, was attributed to corruption of the air, a likely indicator of the degree of penetration of the ideas of Greek medicine.

In 295 B.C., during the war against the Samnites, the Romans were struck by a pestilence. With varying intensity, the epidemic continued the following year. The Sibylline Books were then consulted; their advice was to send emissaries to Epidaurus, there to obtain a statue of Aesculapius and bring it back to Rome. The epidemic was not a terribly virulent one, and the pressing needs of war caused the consuls to delay sending the emissaries to Epidaurus. After the disease had raged for three years, the emissaries returned, the cult of Aesculapius was established in Rome, and the epidemic ceased.

In addition to these texts concerning Sicily, Rome, and Latium, we can find some scattered information regarding Iberian or Carthaginian Spain: in 476 B.C., in response to the epidemics that had hit the Mediterranean coast of Spain, the Carthaginians sacrificed a number of animals and humans to the gods. In 404 B.C., a pestilence decimated the Carthaginian army in Sicily, and Himilco, forced to sign a peace treaty, sent home—where they had apparently contracted the disease—his Balearic and Iberian mercenaries. In 383 B.C., once again, the Iberian mercenaries who were fighting in Sicily were sent back home, as the epidemic raged through the Carthaginian army. Perhaps, we should connect this mass return to the serious epidemic that struck the fortified city of Sagunto (383 B.C.). Most of the city's notables and leaders died.

Epidemics of the Hellenistic and Roman Periods

Every period in the history of Europe is marked by a particular pathogenic complex, differentiated regionally, formed of a fairly stable set of current diseases; some of these are hereditary and can be linked to the population's gene pool, while others, such as accidental injuries, commonplace infectious diseases, poisonings, and certain degenerative conditions, are instead a product of everyday family or occupational living. Dwellings, dress, diet, work, play, and so forth, are all subject to seasonal variations.

The establishment of a Neolithic culture in Europe, marked by farming, herding, an increasingly sedentary way of life, and rapid population growth, was certainly the factor that triggered a rupture in the pathocenosis between 6000 and 3000 B.C. During classical antiquity, the pathological equilibrium was upset once again by a major cultural transition, specifically, by urbanization, which led to the appearance of the great epidemics.

And so, aside from the more commonplace afflictions, found in every era, which we encountered in the Hippocratic corpus, every period in European history has been characterized by a specific pathocenosis, featuring other diseases, which either form part of the set of common diseases or else contribute to the array of major epidemics. Other diseases still, which may have been limited geographically until that point, extend their range, while others retreat or even disappear.

In Europe, from the end of the classical age onward, there was a succession of ten or so pathocenoses; the ones related to this context are the first six, all prior to the year 1500, the start of the great era of exploration. In the first of these pathocenoses, which covers the Hellenistic age and the establishment of the Roman empire (roughly the first three centuries B.C. and the first half of the first century A.D.), the major epidemics were relatively limited and few in number. For two years, from 278 to 276 B.C., a serious pestilence ravaged the city of Rome and its surrounding region: the Romans were losing all hope when the extremely cold winter of 277–276 halted the epidemic; so harsh was that winter that the Forum was covered with snow for forty days. In 212 B.C., during the Roman siege of Syracuse, the Roman army was stricken with a serious epidemic, though Livy offers no symptoms in his description. Much later, during the reign of Nero, Silius Italicus wrote a poem concerning this siege, and in it he described the symptoms of a malignant pneumonia.

We know nothing concerning the nature of the epidemics which laid low the Carthaginian army during its siege of Sagunto, on the Iberian peninsula, in 218 B.C.; raged in Rome and in surrounding areas in 208 B.C.; ravaged both the Carthaginian and the Roman armies in Calabria in 205 B.C.; and struck the galley slaves of the Roman fleet in Lycia in 190 B.C. So serious was this last epidemic that the fleet was obliged to weigh anchor and sail away from the infected harbor. All of these epidemics, at any rate, remained local. Only one, brought back by the troops in Iberia in 214 B.C., spread throughout the country, but we know little about its nature.

The epidemic that devastated Italy for three years, from 182 to 180 B.C., would seem to have been more serious, since the high number of those who fell ill with it prevented the departure of an entire army. Livy states that, once the prayers that had been offered to the deities proved useless, the public accused evil men of spreading the disease (later, they would be called "plague spreaders").

In 175 B.C., a particularly virulent epidemic struck the entire peninsula, sowing death among free men and slaves. So high was the death count that, in many cities, the dead were left unburied. Its symptoms varied and were contradictory, in some cases reminiscent of the symptoms of a tertian fever or those of a quartan fever, in other cases similar to symptoms of a rheumatic fever or even those of cutaneous scabies. A. Corradi believes that it was an intermittent malarial fever, a hypothesis that strikes me as decidedly audacious.

In 142 B.C., a new epidemic struck the city of Rome. According to Livy, "even in the most secluded parts of the body, and under the tongue, there were red and hard pustules with a black and livid head." It would be tempting to consider these pustules, which were the most distinctive feature of the clinical picture, as the first appearance of smallpox in Europe; this would hardly seem remarkable in a period in which the Romans built a network of roads to the Middle East, after conquering Corinth and Anatolia.

This disease did not take root, as it were; another disease, however, brought back from Syria by the troops of Pompeii in 60 B.C., began silently and slowly to spread throughout the Italian and Iberian peninsulas: leprosy, at the time known as "elephantiasis." In 43 and in 23 B.C., two unidentified epidemics ravaged Italy, while from A.D. 14 until 37, an affliction of the skin slowly spread throughout the land; some scholars believe it was a form of leprosy, others think it was a common dermatitis.

It is natural, then, to wonder what influence the diseases and epidemics, either common or new, just briefly sketched, had on the medical thought of the period. In the Greek world, clinical observation hardly ended with Hippocrates, and new information enriched both the body of knowledge and the perceptions of certain physiological and pathological phenomena. Alexandria, at any rate, was the true center of progress. Ever since the foundation of the museum—to limit ourselves narrowly to the direct influence of the observation of diseases—Herophilus of Chalcedon had drawn a link between fever and rapid pulse rate. In 280 B.C., Erasistratus proclaimed himself, by experience, opposed to harsh diets and bloodletting, while in 50 B.C. Heraclides of Tarentum introduced opium—which had long been used by the peasants of the Mideast—as a therapeutic drug. Gentius, an Illyrian king, revealed to Greek physicians the fever-relieving virtues of this herb, which thus took the name of gentian. As late as the eighteenth century, it was considered to be the best febrifuge, after cinchona.

Around the first century of the Christian era, a new pathocenosis began that was to last for four centuries. This period, when the West was united under the Roman empire, was marked by a number of pandemics, some of which outdid—in terms of extent and virulence—anything that had been seen before. The first, and the weakest, appeared in A.D. 46, carried from Asia to Italy by a Roman knight. This new disease, called *lichen* by the Greeks and *mentagra* by the Romans, appeared as a skin disease that generally began from the chin, then extended to the face, following the outline of the eyes, and ran down toward the neck, the chest, and the hands. Even though Pliny the Elder, a witness of the disease, fails to describe it in detail, it would seem to have been different from the sycosis known to Greek physicians and to Celsus. Celsus presents two forms of it: tubercular sycosis, which is based on the face, and moist sycosis, which tends to affect the scalp most of all. Some scholars believe that it was a form of leprosy, and others speak of syphilis or herpes. Nowadays most scholars feel that it was pityriasis and sycosis, which is to say, a parasitic form. But, as contagious as it may have been, it is difficult to believe that it could have constituted a full-fledged epidemic, extending over all of Italy, Illyria, Gaul, and the Iberian peninsula, thereafter returning to a sporadic form.[16]

A few years later, in A.D. 65, Rome was hit by a serious epidemic that, according to Tacitus, spared no one, striking all age groups, both genders, and all social classes. Tacitus tells us that it killed 30,000, including nobles and senators, in the city in the three months of autumn. He offers no specific information on the nature of the epidemic but speaks of the frequent epidemics that four years later, in A.D. 69, spread all over Europe, especially in Gaul and in Germany.

The so-called Antonine plague struck like lightning out of a blue sky.[17] In 167, the victorious troops of the emperor Lucius Verus returned to Rome from the East, where they had conquered Mesopotamia and defeated the Parthians. These soldiers, however, brought with them a terrible disease. Legend has it that the disease originated in the temple of Apollo at Seleucia, which Roman soldiers sacked in 166. Ammianus Marcellinus, however, in the fourth century, stated that this was the interpretation of the Chaldean priests of the sun (assimilated with Apollo), who wanted people to believe that this was a divine punishment, thus demonstrating the power of their god. It is true, however—he added—that "in Babylonia the naphtha wells emit vapors that are harmful to man and beast," and that these vapors can corrupt the air. The epidemic spread, between A.D. 167 and 172, over much of western Europe, especially through Gaul and Germany, reaching beyond the natural boundary of the Rhine at certain points. No social category escaped it: even one of the sons of Marcus Aurelius died of it.

This time, there is an abundance of medical descriptions of the epidemic, perhaps even too many, as the picture that emerges is rather murky. Galen fled Rome to escape the disease, offering descriptions of the disease in seven different passages of his work. He called it *megas loimos*, or "great pestilence." He declared that it was similar to the plague of Athens described by Thucydides, but in reality only the social context was comparable, while the symptoms presented differed sharply. Galen noted a flushed or livid face, fever, vomit, and ventral flux at the onset and, after nine days, exanthems that evolved into pustules. This pattern has led many authors to lean strongly toward identifying the Antonine plague as smallpox. Further evidence in favor of this interpretation comes from Galen's description of the disease as recurring more or less seasonally for fourteen or fifteen years, or perhaps for even longer, and returning, more than once, in the same location. Some authors have suggested measles, others have spoken of contagious erysipelas or even dengue. When all is said and done, smallpox remains the most plausible hypothesis. What remains to be understood is why the disease disappeared, only to return, apparently, on two separate occasions.

In A.D. 189, a new pandemic ravaged the West. Italy, one of the most heavily populated regions of the empire, and Rome, the empire's largest city, were particularly hard-hit. According to Dio Cassius, there were as many as two thousand deaths a day in Rome, as a famine coincided with the pandemic. The emperor Commodus, on the advice of his physicians, retired to Laurentum, where the odor of the laurels, it was believed, made the air healthier.

Galen speaks about the epidemic at the beginning of his book *De probis pravisque alimentorum sucis* (= *De bonis malisque sucis*), which he wrote in Rome in his old age, during the last years of the second century. He explains that the epidemic began after several months of famine and appeared to have struck various regions of the empire. The essential symptom was an exanthem. In certain patients this symptom was reminiscent of an erysipelas, while in others it resembled an acute abscess. In still others it looked like a herpes cluster or a patch of psoriasis or even leprosy and, in the most serious cases, it resembled a gangrenous carbuncle. It was accompanied by fever and by a fetid ventral flux, which evolved into dysentery with tenesmus. A number of authors have claimed that this clinical pattern marked a return of smallpox, while others are torn between scarlet fever and measles. A first appearance of measles would explain both the symptoms and the overall pattern of this epidemic. The disease remained endemic thereafter, since the population level required for its maintenance is sharply lower than that required, for example, for smallpox.

As serious as its political effects may have been, the epidemic of "mortal fevers" that in 232 decimated in Dalmatia the army sent to fight the Persians, and even infected the emperor Alexander Severus, seems to have been a local epidemic, though we know little about it. The same may be said of the disease that in 238 ravaged the army of Maximinus near Aquileia, preventing the emperor from punishing the rebellious Romans.

A few years later, in 252, another terrible epidemic shook the empire to its foundations for fifteen years. It took the name "plague of Saint Cyprian" since it was that saint, then bishop of Carthage, who left us the most complete picture of the disease, in the absence of any medical description. The disease, he wrote, came from Ethiopia, and it spread throughout the West, sparing not a single city. It began in the autumn of 251 and ended in July of 266. The clinical picture is not equally clear: the disease began with a ventral flux and proceeded with an ulcerous angina, vomit, and bloodshot eyes. In some of those afflicted, it culminated in gangrene of the foot, while others experienced a languor of the legs or, still worse, were left deaf or blind.

In 302 a new epidemic began to spread. A number of authors have theorized that the "malignant pustules" spreading over the entire body, even reaching the eyes, were signs of a malignant smallpox, whereas others have suggested these were carbuncles. There is no decisive evidence to allow us to settle on a precise diagnosis; the fact remains that the intervals between the epidemics allow us to suppose that the population must have been severely decimated. The epidemic of the pustules broke out again in 312. In 359, a serious pestilence struck in Armida (modern Diyarbakir, on the Tigris), during a war between Rome and Persia. The historian Ammianus Marcellinus set down an exceedingly detailed description.[18] In 376, in the Balkans, a "plague" began, quite virulent at times, following the arrival of the barbarians south of the Danube. The same can be said of the epidemics that accompanied the vast turmoil of the period, breaking out locally; one prime example is the plague that ravaged a famine-stricken Rome under siege by the Visigoths between 408 and 410.

Although Roman medicine continued to seek its inspiration in Greek thought, it began to produce some original ideas, at times very accurate ones, such as that found in this passage by Marcus Terentius Varro from his book *De re rustica:* "Precautions must also be taken in the neighbourhood of swamps, both for the reasons given, and because there are bred certain minute creatures which cannot be seen by the eyes, which float in the air and enter the body through the mouth and nose and there cause serious diseases."[19]

The Diseases of the High Middle Ages

Toward the middle of the fifth century, a new period began in the history of health in Europe. Trade declined but invading peoples moved frequently from place to place, at times en masse, exacerbating the chances of the spread of certain diseases. Moreover, the documentation concerning this period was no longer limited to the Mediterranean regions but slowly extended to include first the west, and then the center and the north, finally covering eastern Europe as well.

In 444, the Britons of what is now Great Britain were, tradition recounts, ravaged by an epidemic and had to call on the Saxons to ward off the attacks of the Picts. If there is a historical foundation to this story, then we may gather that the epidemic in question had enormous repercussions on world history.

Evagrius, known as Scholasticus, reports that, in 455, in the wake of a drought and a famine, a major epidemic originating in Asia Minor spread to the Balkan peninsula, continuing along the course of the Danube as far as Vienna. This disease, against which the efforts of physicians proved fruitless, could kill in three days, following the appearance of coughing and an intumescence, accompanied by inflammation of the entire body. In these signs, Schnurrer believes one can recognize measles.

Up until the sixth century, chroniclers make no mention of any significant epidemic; nonetheless, the texts of legislation and regulations, both civil and religious, show a growing concern about certain endemic diseases, especially leprosy.[20] Quite rare in the first century, according to Celsus, leprosy gradually took on an importance that it had never previously had, marking the beginning of a new period. Shunned by the population at large because of the reputation of the disease, which was considered contagious and incurable, lepers were often forced to lead a marginal and grim existence. The church, which assumed responsibility for their care, decided to open leprosariums. The first of these, a modest dwelling, was established in A.D. 460, not far from the abbey of Saint-Oyan (now Saint-Claude, in the Jura). This type of institution was to proliferate throughout Italy and Gaul, on the Iberian peninsula, and, finally, in the British Isles and in Germany.

During the course of the sixth century, many different ecclesiastical councils (in particular, the council of Orléans, in 549) made it obligatory for bishops to see to the care of lepers. Lepers were forbidden to continue to live among their families or to circulate freely among the population at large. It may be that the effects of these early measures of segregation were less drastic than has long been thought. In any case, the progress of the disease, which till that point had been quite rapid, seems to have slowed sharply over the course of the seventh century. Other phenomena about which we know little or nothing may have accentuated this development, but the fact remains that this slight remission of the disease was not lasting. Beginning in the eighth century, the authorities became aware of a new and more serious outbreak of the disease. Between the ninth and eleventh centuries, leprosy once again seems to have regressed.

Another major epidemic, smallpox, which seemed to have vanished, made its return in the sixth century, with unprecedented virulence. Beginning in 541, the disease raged through France, Germany, Belgium, and the British Isles, especially Ireland, where J. F. D. Shrewsbury has identified its appearance in 543, and again in 548, 550, and 555.[21] In France, Gregory of Tours described it in Touraine in 581, where it struck adults in particular, as if this had been its first appearance. Among the disease's victims were Gregory himself, his cleric, and the seventy-year-old bishop of Nantes, who died in 582. Apparently, it did not become endemic, as the population in general and the urban agglomerations in particular seem to have been below the necessary threshold in many regions. In the British Isles, it seems to have vanished for a century, only to return, as virulent as its first appearance, in 664, finally establishing itself as endemic from 675 onward. A number of episodes indicate the disease's path: in 709, Saint Bertin healed a man suffering from smallpox at Saint-Omer; in 711, the disease reached or perhaps reappeared in Spain, in the wake of the troops of Tariq; and lastly, in 996, Hugh Capet, king of France, died of smallpox.

In the East, in 622, a physician-priest of Alexandria named Aaron set down the first medical description of smallpox. This description remained unknown in the West, where it was not until the eleventh century that we find a medical manuscript, written in the area around Orléans, offering a first, summary description (eighteen lines long) of the disease and its treatment. Three other medical manuscripts cite smallpox: one from the beginning of the ninth century, from the region of Dijon, and two others from the eleventh century, one from Vendôme, the other from Rouen. Later on, smallpox seems once again to have vanished, at least in northern Europe.

After leprosy and smallpox, the third great scourge to sweep across Europe, making its very first appearance, was the bubonic plague. The first wave was known as the "plague of Justinian."[22] It arrived from the Red Sea, at the Egyptian port of Pelusium; in 542 it was then transported to Constantinople by ship. From this city it spread, the same year, to Thrace, Macedonia, Dalmatia, and Spain. In 543 it reached Rome and Italy and spread to Marseilles and Provence, traveling along the Rhône valley as far as Treves, or Trier. This initial outbreak caused untold damage, and indeed the consequences were so devastating that they can be blamed for the ultimate failure of Justinian's policy of reconquest. Nevertheless, only Europe's Mediterranean coasts were hit, possibly because they were the only areas heavily enough populated to allow the disease to thrive. And so the plague returned regularly, in successive waves with intervals that ranged from nine to thirteen years. Of the twenty or so waves of plague between 541 and 767, at least eleven affected Mediterranean Europe, penetrating only slightly toward the north. Then, for reasons that still escape us, the plague vanished, both from Europe and from Africa and Asia.

Following the year 800, a new pathocenosis made its appearance and was to last three centuries: leprosy retreated, epidemics of smallpox became less frequent, the plague disappeared, and two new epidemics made their appearance.

The most remarkable of these epidemics, and the most serious in this period, was the so-called holy fire (or Saint Anthony's fire). In 857, along the shores of the Rhine, a disease appeared that had already been familiar to the Romans and that had been described in Germany in the second century. Most had forgotten this local affliction, however, and when it reappeared in the form of an epidemic, it sowed terror with its devastating mortality, spreading panic as it advanced. In reality, it was not an infection at all but food poisoning from rye ergot, the fungus *Claviceps purpurea*. Originating in central Asia, this parasitic fungus spread in waves when the annual climate was favorable. Mixed with flour, it produced two different forms of illness, depending on whether the poisoning was serious or mild. In the acute or convulsive form, spasms with violent contractions tormented the patient, developing toward delirium and death. In the weak or gangrenous form, the patient's sleep was disturbed by nightmares, enormous subcutaneous blisters full of serous fluid developed, and the limbs were tormented by shooting pains. Then the limbs blackened, dried out, and finally broke at the joints. It was this blackening that led people to think of a mysterious internal fire that charred the limbs from within, hence the name of holy fire.

Having begun on a small scale in 857 on the left bank of the Rhine, near Xanten, the epidemic reached the Parisian region about a half-century later, finding in France an ideal climate. The first two appearances in a terrifying series occurred in the Île-de-France in 912, and in the Île-de-France and the Champagne region in 945. Beginning in 993, ergotism struck one or more province of France every year, causing tens of thousands of atrocious deaths and leaving in its wake as many cripples. This torment visited the inhabitants of the Île-de-France, Artois, Champagne, Lorraine, Limousine, Aquitania, León in Spain, Wallonia, Flanders, Dauphiné, and Marseilles, and then Germany in 1105 and England in 1109. Ergotism reached its acme in western Europe.[23]

The other great epidemic was influenza. This viral infection made its first brutal appearance in the winter of 876–877. It was far more serious than the flu syndromes and the coryzas of antiquity. Certain authors wrote of measles and pneumonia, but according to the studies done by A. Proust,[24] a diagnosis of influenza is inescapable. Striking several countries in the course of just a few months, influenza returned often, causing unprecedented and widespread mass deaths once or twice a century, especially in 927 and 1105.

It is thought that in this period, another serious but endemic disease, malaria, which till this point had been confined to the eastern shores of the Mediterranean, was transported to the Atlantic coasts and all the way to the shores of the North Sea by Vikings on their way back from raids in the Mediterranean and on Africa. In this way, *Plasmodium vivax* was established on the Danish, German, Dutch, Belgian, and French coasts, whence it spread, along the rivers, into the marshy areas further inland, such as the Sologne and the Brenne in France, Hannover, the western area of the mouth of the Elbe, and the Westphalian lowlands in Germany.

The existence of a census of the Latin medical manuscripts from the high Middle Ages preserved in French libraries, compiled by Ernest Wickersheimer,[25] has made it possible to prepare an overall chart of the pathocenosis of that period (Table 3). The 118 texts listed, which date from the seventh to the eleventh centuries, come largely from the libraries of French monasteries, though a few are from England, Belgium, Luxembourg, Germany, Switzerland, and Italy; among those classified as being of unknown origin, two take their inspiration from Spain, though they may not come directly from there. The fact that the manuscripts appear to copy one from another leads us to believe that these constitute, if not a proper statistic of the diseases of the era, at least a reflection of the health concerns of western European society at a time when medicine was practiced

Table 3. Diseases mentioned in the manuscripts from the high Middle Ages in western Europe

Type of case	Number	Percent
With infection (or parasitosis):		
Fevers	60	5.5
Digestive tract	46	4
Respiratory tract	69	6
Traumas, wounds, and injuries	18	2
Postpartum conditions	1	0.1
Other infections (or parasites)	138	13
Snakebite	8	1
Nervous system (tetanus)	4	0.4
Subtotal	344	32
Without infection:		
Digestive tract	129	12
Respiratory tract	43	4
Traumas, sprains, wounds	9	1
Nervous system	133	12
Abortions	7	1
Others	426	38
Subtotal	747	68
Total cases	1,091	100

in the monasteries. For greater ease of reading, I have counted mentions of a disease or prescriptions to counter the disease (many diseases, in fact, are mentioned solely in this case), grouping them just as I grouped the diseases mentioned in the Hippocratic corpus. I have not taken into account thirty prescriptions for minor conditions.

A detailed examination is certain to be of interest: out of 60 mentions of fevers, 13 concern intermittent fevers, 5 concern other fevers, and 42 concern various febrifuges. The 175 mentions of the digestive tract are far more varied: 18 concern the mouth (gums, tongue, teeth, throat), 35 concern afflictions of the stomach, 24 concern the intestine and belly, without counting the 27 cases of diarrhea, the 7 cases involving the anus, and the 10 having to do with laxatives or enemas. Another 22 involve liver problems, 7 concern vomit and nausea, 5 concern loss of appetite, and 4 have to do with hernias. Of the 112 mentions of the respiratory tract, 11 have to do with angina, another 11 concern dyspnea, 30 involve coughs and catarrh, 5 involve colds and rhinitis, 15 have to do with the chest and lungs, 3 concern the bronchi, 14 have to do with pleurisy, 16 involve phthisis, and 2 concern empyema. And of the 137 mentions of the nervous system, 29 have to do with migraines and their treatment, 22 involve paralysis and apoplexy, 15 concern epilepsy, 13 are prescriptions for pain, 2 are for sciatica, 12 are for problems with sleeping, plus there are 2 preparations for surgical anesthesia, 5 for vertigo, 17 for psychosis, and 4 for spasms and tremors.

The major epidemic diseases are mentioned quite rarely: smallpox 4 times, carbuncles 7 times (*carbunculus, anthrax,* and *pustula maligna,* though the description does not allow us to identify these terms), leprosy only once, holy fire 12 times, and rabies 6 times.

The other diseases, which are troublesome in any comparison with the diseases of antiquity, are those affecting women, mentioned 58 times; among them are 18 preparations meant to restore interrupted menstruation, 5 against sterility, 1 contraceptive, 5 concerning the breasts, 10 concerning lactation, 9 for the uterus, 8 for childbirth, and 3 concerning stillbirth of the child; the single mention of gonorrhea shows just how limited the presence of the disease still was.

There are 27 mentions of traumas and wounds, uniformly subdivided among fractures and wounds; there are few dislocations. Blood is mentioned 23 times, chiefly due to hemorrhages; the heart is mentioned 22 times, the spleen 13 times, and the urinary tract 55 times, 29 of which concern calcules, 14 the kidneys, and 7 urine. We should note the significance of gout, which receives no fewer than 57 mentions and which chiefly afflicted the upper classes. In A.D. 599 Pope Gregory I the Great noted that he was writing in bed, following a bout of gout that had lain him low for the previous fourteen months. The varnishing of terra-cotta and the bottling of wine were regularly done with lead-based products, leading to an alimentary lead poisoning that helped cause widespread gout. Arthrosis, with 14 mentions, was significant, as it had been in every other period. Skin diseases—with 43 mentions—were one of the major health concerns of the time; they were described in an imprecise manner, however, and the term "scabies" covers every sort of dermatosis. Hydropsy, with only 9 mentions, occupied a less important ranking. Parasites, however, were mentioned 49 times: for the most part, intestinal worms (tapeworms, with 23 mentions, and roundworms) or fleas were involved.

Greater pride of place is given to the sensory organs, especially the eyes (80 mentions), in an era when dwellings, without fireplaces and badly lit by tiny windows, were regularly filled with smoke from the braziers used for heating or the oil lamps used for illumination. This was a period, moreover, when eyeglasses were simply not manufactured. After the eyes come the ears, with 18 mentions, and the nose, with 9.

The humors, difficult as they were to identify, occupied a major role in the nosology of the period, with 56 mentions: we find 8 mentions of cancer. There were also antidotes against poisoning (8 mentions), which were normally quite specific, incantations against evil spirits, and some thirty-odd prescriptions against the minor miseries of everyday life (phlyctenae, blisters, scars, warts, and so on).

This summary presentation in no way is meant as a depiction of the distribution of diseases in the high Middle Ages. Rather, it reflects the everyday health concerns of western Europe, leaving aside major sweeping epidemics.

The Diseases of the Low Middle Ages

From the twelfth century onward, the foundation of the pathocenosis established in Europe following the Crusaders' return home at the turn of the century remained substantially unchanged, with respect to the various diseases discussed in the previous section. Nevertheless, certain endemic diseases did change owing to the new and frequent contacts with the Middle East.

In the first place, smallpox—which seems to have disappeared in

Europe during the eleventh century—reappeared toward the end of the twelfth century, but only in the Mediterranean region. Here, from the thirteenth century onward, we begin to find descriptions of the disease in the writings of the physicians of the southern regions.

By contrast, leprosy, which had retreated from the ninth century onward, became invasive starting in the twelfth century. This sudden expansion throughout Europe may have been a result of the previously mentioned contacts with the Middle East, where it was quite common. Shortly after the fall of Jerusalem, the Hospitaler Order of Saint Lazarus was founded in Palestine; this order was consecrated to the care of lepers. From the twelfth to the thirteenth century, there was a sharp increase in the foundation of leprosariums by the church, by the Hospitaler Order of Saint Lazarus, by kings, by lords, and by cities. At the end of the thirteenth century, it is estimated that there were some nineteen thousand of them throughout Europe. If we accept an average of fifteen or sixteen lepers per leprosarium (according to the lists dating from this period, they ranged from two or three lepers to more than a hundred, in the larger cities), and suppose that—as modern epidemiology informs us—half of all cases are practically undetectable, then in Europe, around the year 1300, there must have been some six hundred thousand lepers, out of a population of 75 or 80 million, if we include Russia. This amounts to 0.82 percent. For reasons that are entirely unknown, leprosy began to retreat beginning in the first half of the fourteenth century.[26]

The holy fire, still widespread and quite common around the year 1100, began a rapid retreat around the beginning of the period that we are now examining. To combat this scourge, an order of Hospitalers was founded in Saint-Antoine-de-Viennois in 1095. This order provided appropriate care to the needs of those suffering from the holy fire, which thus came to be known as Saint Anthony's fire. Good wheat bread, on which the ill were fed, certainly helped in their recovery, but the retreat of the disease may also be partly explained by the custom of no longer sowing rye alone and mixing it with wheat instead. Another factor may have been the shift in the climate, which was unfavorable to *Claviceps purpurea*. At the start of the thirteenth century, the disease spread once again in Spain, where the Antonine Hospitalers opened a hospital in every place where it was reported. The retreat of the disease became increasingly marked, however, and by the beginning of the fourteenth century it had almost entirely disappeared, causing only rare and weak epidemic outbreaks in limited areas.

Another noninfectious scourge, scurvy, acquired major importance at this juncture. This avitaminosis, which strikes only populations that have long subsisted solely on sausages and salted foods, probably made an early, minor appearance in the major cities, where winters are long. Armies fell victim to it, especially armies bound on distant expeditions, such as the crusade led by King Louis IX of France to Damietta, in 1248.

Tuberculosis continued to reap its harvest of victims, but if phthisis seemed far more worrisome (15 mentions) in the high Middle Ages than did scrofula (2 mentions), it was the latter form that became—if not more common—at least more visible in the twelfth century. Underlying this European outbreak of tuberculous adenitis was the large-scale export of bovines from Lombardy to the rest of western Europe. It seems that these animals, often tuberculotic, then propagated bovine strains of the Koch bacillus, encouraging the ganglionic form of the disease. What we do know is that in the twelfth century, throughout England and France spread the belief that the royal touch could cure scrofula, or king's evil, as it was called. In England, tradition has it that this power was first exhibited by Edward III, the Confessor; in France, it was by Clovis. In fact, the royal touch was always accompanied by a sizable almsgiving by the king, and these gold pieces improved the living conditions of the poor people, thus reinforcing the efficacy of the treatment.

As for other epidemics, leaving aside influenza, which may have come from Venice by sea in 1172, and which then ran wild through Italy, France, Saxony, and England, we essentially see only local ones.

The Black Death

The return of the plague in 1347 brought a devastating end to this centuries-long equilibrium. For the next one hundred and fifty years, the plague caused the establishment of a new pathocenosis.[27] Having reached Europe from the east through trade with the East and Central Asia, first it raged through the southern plains of the Volga and Don, striking the tribes of the Golden Horde. The khan Gani Bek, or Djanibeg, who was laying siege to Caffa, which was Genoa's trading outpost in the Crimea, saw to it that the disease was spread to the encircled city by catapulting cadavers of plague victims over the city walls. From Caffa, Genoese galleys brought the plague to Pera, another Genoese trading outpost in the harbor of Constantinople; that city was struck by the plague in July of 1347. It then spread to Messina in September of 1347, and to Marseilles on November

1, after the city of Genoa had refused to allow its own galleys to dock. Other ports along the coastal routes were hit: Venice, Split, Leghorn, Barcelona, Valencia, Almeria, and all the islands of the Mediterranean. At the beginning of 1348, during the winter, the plague spread inland and took a pneumonic form. Passing directly from person to person by coughing, the pneumonic plague sowed terror through the populace, killing in two or three days with a fatality rate of 100 percent. It was all the more terrifying since, having vanished for roughly five centuries, no memory of it remained, and it was viewed as a completely mysterious scourge.

In the spring, having resumed its bubonic form, the plague slowly continued to spread through the trade routes, following the rivers upstream, and then descending downstream at a far more rapid pace. It hit Toulouse in April, Bordeaux at the end of June, and then arrived by ship in southern England, in Ireland, and in Rouen. On August 20, it arrived in Paris via the Seine; on September 29, it was brought overland to London, and then it hit Calais. Winter came and the plague seemed to diminish in fury. In the spring of 1349, however, it continued its progress in an uneven fashion: in Burgundy it seems to have lost its force, while Norway, Denmark, and Germany were infected from London through the coastline of the North Sea. The Netherlands, which had broken off all trade with England for the previous two years, remained undamaged. The central Rhine was devastated in 1349, as were Portugal, Austria, and Hungary.

From Lübeck, infected overland in the summer of 1350, the plague spread to Sweden and to the Baltic port cities, at the same time spreading to central Germany and northern Poland; in 1351, it reached Courland (a region of modern-day Latvia) and Byelorussia. In 1352, the Russian principality of Novgorod was decimated in turn, as the epidemic spread into the forests and across the tundra. In five years, the plague had killed a fourth or a fifth of the inhabitants of Europe, and only a few regions— such as Galicia in Spain, the Netherlands, Iceland, Bohemia, Finland, Polish Galicia, and the Romanian principalities—escaped this catastrophe.

The turmoil swept all before it, and it was all the more devastating because, in 1360, the plague reappeared in Franconia, raging through Europe once again and reappearing periodically every ten or twelve years or so. Two sorts of attempts were made to flee the plague; one was physical flight, which only served to spread the disease; the other was moral flight, to patron saints and miracle workers. Another sort of reaction was violent; in 1348, in Toulon, there began a movement to persecute the Jews, falsely accused of spreading the disease. This movement later expanded to much of the rest of Europe. In August of 1348, in Venice, flagellants first appeared, turning the aggressive drives against themselves, making pilgrimages to Austria, Hungary, Moravia, southern Poland, and Germany, ranging from east to west, and finally arriving in Flanders. Condemned by the pope and by civil authorities, the two movements died out in December 1349 and early 1350.

The disappearance of much of the regular clergy, which had done so much to assure the intellectual formation of society, caused a sharp decline in knowledge throughout Europe and the resurgence of superstition and witchcraft, which in turn contributed greatly to a sense of disorientation. This may ultimately have been the cause of the appearance of a new epidemic entirely specific to this period, Saint Vitus's dance. On numerous occasions, various authors have described scenes of dancing mania among the Germanic peoples: the chronicle of Erfurt mentions it in 1237 in connection with the children of the town. The chronicle of Maastricht cites it in 1278, when the dancers caused the collapse of the bridge over the Moselle; many of the dancers were drowned. Finally, in Lusitze, a small village along the Bohemian border, as the Black Death approached in 1349, girls and women danced for days at a time before a painting of the Madonna. Then, on July 15, 1374, in many different cities of the central Rhine, groups of boys and girls appeared, apparently out of nowhere, and danced in their hundreds in the town squares, singing at the top of their lungs. The movement spread throughout the region. Everywhere, spectators, infected with the spirit, joined the dance and followed the group in its wanderings. The prohibitions ordered by town governments and foul weather put an end to the movement in late November, but every summer, from 1375 until 1381, the dancing began again. In 1381, the clergy decided to lead the young people in pilgrimage to the church of Saint John the Baptist of Kilburg, where calm was restored. In 1414, however, the epidemic broke out again in Strasbourg and spread through Baden-Württemberg and Bavaria. This time, it was through the good offices of Saint Vitus—hence the name of the phenomenon—that the clergy managed to end it, and it was now to Saint Vitus that all appeals were directed when the strange epidemic resumed (for example, in 1463 at Metz and in 1518 at Strasbourg).

Most of the epidemics, far from retreating, spread extensively. Suffice it to consider influenza, which was described at Montpellier in 1387 by Valescus of Taranto, in Paris in 1403 and 1413, throughout Europe and especially in Italy in 1438, and in France in 1482. Smallpox seems to have reappeared in central and northern Europe over the course of the fifteenth century; dysentery was increasingly common, and it often forced armies to retreat, with enormous losses. Such was the case with victorious armies, as well, such as that of the Black Prince, the prince of Wales, in Spain. The only epidemics that clearly retreated were Saint Anthony's fire and leprosy.

The plague of the fourteenth century, the Black Death, played a major part in upsetting all certainty in medical thinking. This tremendous epidemic disease, found in the writings of neither Hippocrates nor Galen, appeared exceedingly contagious in popular experience, contradicting the traditional ideas of physicians. In 1377, the Republic of Dubrovnik ordered the first quarantine.[28] Measures to isolate the sick were considered effective. Bit by bit, the dogma of transmission through corrupted air (miasmatic dogma) began to wear thin. In the fifteenth century, municipal regulations of public hygiene, isolation, and disinfection, organized in an exemplary manner by the government of Venice, spread throughout Europe. People's minds were ready for the idea of contagion, which Girolamo Fracastoro expressed clearly in the sixteenth century. It did not fully catch on, however, until the nineteenth century.

Notes

1. Introduction

1. *De prisca medicina*, ed. Jouanna, 3–5; see also Herter (1963a), 464–483. For the earliest period of historiography of the medical art, see in particular Smith (1989) and Pigeaud (1992).

2. Pap. Lit. Lond. 165, British Museum, London; ed. and trans. Jones, 1947.

3. Celsus, *De medicina*, preface, 1–11. See Mudry (1982), 15–17.

4. Ibn Abi Usaybi'a, [sources of information concerning the categories of physicians]. For an overall perspective on the historiography of medicine in ancient authors writing in Arabic, see Ullmann (1970), 228–233, and Hau (1983).

5. This text remained a manuscript until it was published, and also translated into Italian, by Schullian and Belloni, 1954.

6. *Histoire de la médecine, où, l'on voit l'origine et le progrès de cet art*, partial ed., 1696; complete ed., 1702; rev. ed., 1723; Eng. trans., 1699.

7. *The History of Physick, from the Time of Galen to the Beginning of the Sixteenth century*, 2 vols., 1725–1726; Lat. trans., 1734.

8. See Heischkel, in Artelt (1949), 208–237.

9. *Versuch einer pragmatischen Geschichte der Arzneykunde*, 4 vols., 1792–1799; rev. ed., 5 vols., completed 1803.

10. *Geschichte der Heilkunde nach den Quellen bearbeitet*, 2 vols., 1822–1829.

11. *Lehrbuch der Geschichte der Medizin und der Volkskrankheiten*, 1845.

12. *Storia della medicina italiana*, 5 vols., 1845–1848. This general history of medicine is set in the context of a national history.

13. *Storia della medicina*, 3 vols., 1850–1866.

14. *Geschichte der Medizin*, 1859. For the debate between Wunderlich and Haeser, see Temkin and Temkin (1958).

15. *Grundriss der Geschichte der Medizin und des heilenden Standes*, 1876; Eng. trans., 1889.

16. See, for example, Littré (1872).

17. *Oeuvres complètes d'Hippocrate* (= *Opera omnia*), 10 vols., 1839–1861.

18. *Histoire des sciences médicales, comprenant l'anatomie, la physiologie, la médecine, la chirurgie et les doctrines de pathologie générale*, 2 vols., 1870.

19. Starobinski (1953).

20. Numerous volumes of his *Cabinet secret de l'histoire* appeared from 1895 until 1912.

21. *Kurzes Handbuch der Geschichte der Medizin,* 1922.

22. *Geschichte der Medizin,* 2 vols., 1906–1911.

23. *An Introduction to the History of Medicine,* 1913; see the 4th ed., 1929. Garrison was a pioneer in the field of modern bibliographical documentation in the area of medicine at large, and in the history of medicine in particular. He made use of and developed the catalogs by Johann Ludwig Choulant (1828 and 1841) and Alphonse Pauly (1874). See Brodman (1954) and Garrison and Morton (1983).

24. *Storia della medicina,* 1927; 3d rev. ed., 2 vols., 1948.

25. *Geschichte der Medizin,* 3 vols., 1949–1955.

26. I should also mention, primarily because of their educational value, the manuals by Adalberto Pazzini (1947 and 1974), Erwin Ackerknecht (1955 and 1982), Maurice Bariéty and Charles Coury (1963). The manual by Charles Lichtenthaeler (1975), which was intended to introduce the physiological method of Magendie into the history of medicine, fails to keep the promises made in the preface. For an overall view of medical historiograpy, see Clarke (1971) and Webster, in Corsi and Weindling (1983), 29–43.

27. *A Short History of Medicine;* the first edition dates from 1928; the new edition, revised by E. Ashworth Underwood (1962), has been completed with information of a more strictly medical nature.

28. *Handbuch der Geschichte der Medizin,* 3 vols., 1901–1905.

29. Laignel-Lavastine and Guégan (1936–1949); completely redone under the direction of Poulet, Martiny, and Sournia (1977–1980); Laín Entralgo (1972–1975).

30. Sarton did not achieve this goal until late, and in an incomplete fashion. The *Introduction to the History of Science* (1927–1948), a vast and precious collection of biobibliographical information, does not progress past the Middle Ages, while his more synthetic work stops at the dawn of the Christian era (*A History of Science,* 1952–1959).

31. Sarton (1918); see Grmek (1965).

32. See especially Taton (1957–1964); Geymonat (1970–1976); Rossi (1988).

33. See, for example, Nordenskiöld (1928) and Montalenti, in Abbagnano (1962). See also Jacob (1970), Judson (1979), and Mayr (1982) as models of different types of histories of certain branches of biology.

34. Sigerist (1935) and Sarton (1935). For this debate, see Grmek (1965).

35. See Sigerist (1960).

36. See, for example, Léonard (1981) for France, Cosmacini (1988) for Italy, and Rosenberg (1992) for the United States.

37. *A History of Medicine,* 2 vols., 1951–1961.

38. *The Development of Modern Medicine: An Interpretation of the Social and Scientific Factors Involved,* 1936.

39. See the proceedings of the symposium published by Crombie (1963). For a number of aspects of this disagreement, especially in the United States, see Reingold (1981), and for criticism of externalism, Koyré (1966).

40. For a well-balanced summary of the situation, see Fruton (1992).

41. See Hall (1983).

42. *The Structure of Scientific Revolutions* (1962).

43. In the history of medicine, constructivism can be traced back to a Polish hematologist, Ludvik Fleck (1935), but it did not really begin to develop until the work done by Americans in the 1980s. For Fleck and the Polish school of medical philosophy, see Löwy (1990).

44. This expression is taken from Leonard Wilson (1980), who roundly criticized the abuses of the sociological approach in American medical historiography. See also Rothschuh (1980).

45. See Grmek (1979).

46. *History of the Peloponnesian War*, 1.22.

2. The Birth of Western Medical Art

1. Concerning the whole of this chapter, see Jouanna (1992).

2. "Suda," under the name of Hippocrates I.

3. *De diaeta acutorum*, 1.

4. Xenophon, *Memorabilia*, 4.2.

5. *De articulis*, 33.

6. *De prisca medicina*, 1.

7. *De diaeta acutorum*, 1.

8. A. J. Festugière, in the commentary on his edition of the treatise *De prisca medicina* (Paris, 1948), 32.

9. Plato, *Sophist*, 232d–e.

10. *De arte*, 1.

11. Plato, *Protagoras*, 311d–c.

12. Plato, *Phaedrus*, 270c.

13. Aristotle, *Politics*, 4.4.1326a15.

14. Pinault (1992).

15. Galen, *Methodus medendi*, 1.1.

16. Compare the Presbeutikos and the inscriptions of Delphi: Inv. 2255 and Inv. 6687 A and B + 8131.

17. *Prorrheticon*, 1.72.

18. Ibid., 1.34.

19. The Presbeutikos is thought to have been delivered before the Assembly of the Athenians by Thessalos, the son of Hippocrates, in a plea in favor of Kos.

20. Herodotus, 3.131. It is quite surprising that Herodotus fails to mention, among the renowned centers of that period, the physicians of Kos or those of Cnidus.

Was it that they were too close to Halicarnassus, the birthplace of Herodotus? Local rivalries might well explain the silence of the historian.

21. The listing of the various different Hippocrates can be found in the "Suda"; the inscription was published by Benedum (1977), 272–274.

22. Galen, *Administrationes anatomicae*, 2.1.

23. Lichtenthaeler (1984).

24. The various testimonies on this text have been collected by Rosenthal (1956), 52–87.

25. Plato, *Protagoras*, 311b–c.

26. See Galen, *In Hippocratis de natura hominis commentarii* (preamble), and *Quod optimus medicus sit quoque philosophus*, 3.

27. He was born in Cyprus according to Aristotle (*Historia animalium*, 511b23ff.). In the *Life of Brussels*, he is mentioned as one of the disciples born in Kos. The statement by Aristotle, being much older, is more trustworthy.

28. Oribasius, *Collectiones medicae*, 8.8.

29. Andreas, *Genealogy of the Physicians*, in the *Life of Hippocrates* by Soranos.

30. Commentarius in *Hippocratem de articulis*, 4.40.

31. See Galen, *Methodus medendi*, 1.1. Galen makes a comparison between this healthy rivalry among the ancients to the ill-natured rivalries among the moderns, in particular the methodic physician Thessalos in his critique of Hippocrates.

32. See his *Commentary upon "De diaeta acutorum" of Hippocrates*, 1.1.

33. Inv. 6687 A and B + 8131. First published by J. Bousquet (1956), this inscription became well known in the milieu of specialists in Hippocrates especially beginning with the report by Kudlien (1977b).

34. Sherwin-White (1978), 257.

35. Littré (1839–1861).

36. Aristotle, *Historia animalium*, 3.3.512b12–513a7.

37. *De natura hominis*, 11. This description can also be found in *De natura ossium*, 9.

38. Aristotle, *Historia animalium*, 3.3.511b23–50.

39. *De natura ossium*, 8.

40. Herodotus, 2.84.

41. The bibliography on the matter of Hippocrates is exceedingly vast. A few recent works include Joly (1961a), Lloyd (1975b), Smith (1979), Langholf (1986).

42. Erotian, *Vocum Hippocraticarum collectio*, ed. Nachmanson, 9.1ff.

43. *Anonymus Londinensis*, 5.35–7.3.

44. Galen, *Commentarius in Hippocratem de articulis*, 4.40.

45. Galen, *In Hippocratis epidemiarum librum I commentarii*, 3.2 (= Diocles, frag. 97 Wellmann).

46. Celius Aurelianus, *Tardae passiones*, 4.8.113 (= Herophilus, frag. 261 Von Staden); cf. Galen, *In Hippocratis prognosticum commentarii*, 3.1.4 (= Herophilus, frag. 33 Von Staden).

47. The study by Deichgräber (1933) is a classic in this connection.

48. Whereas Jouanna (1974) and Grensemann (1975), in two independent efforts concerning the Cnidean treatises in the *Corpus Hippocraticum*, were particularly careful to work out the criteria of membership in the Cnidean school and the relationships among the treatises, especially through a study of the parallel constructions (supposing a common model of the *Cnidean Maxims*), Smith (1973) has questioned the validity of a distinction between the Cnidean treatises and the Koan treatises while reexamining the testimony of Galen concerning Cnidus and Kos. Smith's article was of great historical importance in Hippocratic studies, for it threw the problem of medical schools into a state of crisis. There are numerous studies on this matter: Kudlien (1977b); Kollesch (1977); Di Benedetto (1980); Lonie (1978); Thivel (1981); Joly (1983); *De morbis II,* ed. Jouanna; Grensemann (1987); Kollesch (1989); Langholf (1990).

49. For a detailed presentation of each of the treatises that make up the *Corpus Hippocraticum* with a bibliograpy of the editions, see Jouanna (1992), 527–563.

50. *Epidemiae I* and *III:* around the years 410–400; *Epidemiae II, IV,* and *VI:* around the years 400–390; *Epidemiae V* and *VII:* around the years 350–340.

51. Aside from *De humoribus,* see *Prorrheticon I, Prorrheticon II, Praenotiones Coacae, Aphorismi, De diaeta acutorum,* and Appendix to *De diaeta acutorum.*

52. This is the title of the treatise in Erotian and also in an ancient manuscript (Parisinus gr. 2253).

53. For these testimonies, see Grensemann (1975), 1ff., and *De morbis II,* 29ff.

54. See especially *De morbis II,* 2, 66, 68, 70, and 73; *De affectionibus interioribus,* 3, 6, 13, 16, and 48.

55. *De affectionibus interioribus,* 10 (three cases of consumption, or phthisis); 14 (four cases of kidney disease); 35 (four cases of icterus); 52 (three cases of tetanus). The Cnidean subdivision of diseases is set forth by Galen in his *Commentary upon "De diaeta acutorum" by Hippocrates,* 1.7: seven cases of imbalance of bile; twelve cases of bladder disease; four cases of kidney disease; four cases of strangury; three cases of tetanus; four cases of icterus; three cases of consumption, or phthisis.

56. For an analysis of this complex array of factors, see Grensemann (1975 and 1987).

57. Jouanna (1974).

58. Bourgey (1953).

59. This treatise, almost entirely lost in Greek, has been preserved in an ancient Latin translation, discovered by Littré. It has not been possible to establish with certainty whether it was glossed by Erotian.

60. *De prisca medicina,* 22–85.

61. Manuli and Vegetti (1977).

62. *Praeceptiones,* 6. Concerning these treatises, see Gourevitch (1984).

63. Lanata (1967); Nörenberg (1968); Thivel (1975); Kudlien (1977a); Lloyd (1979); Jouanna (1989).

64. *De aere, aquis, locis,* 22.
65. *De diaeta* [*Regimen*], 89, 90.
66. *Prognosticon,* 1; see *De natura muliebri,* 1.
67. *Plutus,* v. 411.
68. Herzog (1931).
69. Strabo, *Geographia,* 14.2.19.
70. *De morbo sacro,* 1, 2.
71. *De aere, aquis, locis,* 22.
72. *De morbo sacro,* 18.
73. *De natura hominis,* 4–7.
74. Schöner (1964).
75. Sarton (1952), 368.
76. *De aere, aquis, locis,* 6, 11.
77. Ibid., 16, 23.
78. Ibid., 13.
79. Aeschylus, *Prometheus Bound,* vv. 442ff.; Sophocles, *Antigone,* vv. 332ff.; Euripides, *Suppliants,* vv. 201ff.; Thucydides, 1.2ff.; see Romilly (1966).
80. Aeschylus, *Prometheus Bound,* vv. 482ff.; Sophocles, *Antigone,* vv. 362ff.
81. Herter (1963a).
82. *De prisca medicina,* 3.
83. Ibid., 5.
84. Ibid., 12.
85. *De locis in homine,* 46; *De arte,* 8.
86. Stückelberger (1984); *De prisca medicina,* 45–49.
87. Heinimann (1961); Lloyd (1979).
88. *De arte,* ed. Jouanna, 167–190.
89. *De arte,* 2.
90. Euripides, *Alcestis,* vv. 785ff. (See also Agathon, frag. 6 and 8 Snell.)
91. Joos (1957).
92. *De prisca medicina,* 1.
93. Ibid., 12.
94. *De arte,* 4.
95. Ibid., 5.
96. *De prisca medicina,* 9.
97. *Iliad,* 11.514.
98. Plato, *Protagoras,* 322c–d.
99. *De arte,* 6.
100. Diels and Kranz (1951), 67 B 2.
101. Aristotle, *Metaphysics,* 1.1.981a28–30: "Men of experience know well that a thing exists, but they do not know why, while men of the art know the reason why [*dia ti*] and the cause."
102. *De arte,* 11.

103. *De flatibus*, 1.

104. *De prisca medicina*, 20.

105. See in particular the use of "prophasis" both in the sense of "apparent or triggering cause" of the disease, in opposition to *aition* (see *De aere, aquis, locis*, 4), and as a synonym of *aition* in the sense of cause (see *De natura hominis*, 13). There have been many studies of this idea. See most recently Rechenauer (1991), 38–109.

106. Lloyd (1979), 147ff. Concerning the level of experimentation among the Hippocratic physicians, see Grmek (1990), 17–43.

107. Jones (1946); Kühn (1956); Longrigg (1963); Lloyd (1975b).

108. *De diaeta* [*Regimen*], 2.

109. *De flatibus*, 2ff.

110. Joly (1960).

111. *De diaeta* [*Regimen*], 10.

112. *De carnibus*, 2.

113. Plato, *Phaedo*, 96a–c.

114. *De hebdomadibus* [*De septimanis*], 10. Mansfeld (1971).

115. *De arte*, 25–29.

116. Longrigg (1963 and 1983).

117. *De prisca medicina*, 1.

118. *De natura hominis*, 1.

119. Ibid., 2–3.

120. *De prisca medicina*, 20.

121. *De natura hominis*, 1.

122. Bourgey (1953); Joly (1966); Kudlien (1967); Lloyd (1979); Grmek (1983b).

123. *Epidemiae VI*, 6, 17. See also *De officina medici*, 1, and *Epidemiae IV*, 43.

124. *De capitis vulneribus*, 10.

125. *Prognosticon*, 2.

126. Coury (1968).

127. See in particular *De morbis II*, 59 ("sound of leather"), 61 ("sound of vinegar"); 47 and 61 ("auscultation by shaking"); *De morbis II*, 51–57.

128. *De officina medici*, 1; *Epidemiae IV*, 43; *Epidemiae VI*, 8, 129.

129. *Prognosticon*, 15, 25.

130. Galen, *De diebus criticis*, 2.4. In this book, as we know it, there are many more; many cases are repeated however in *Epidemiae VII*.

131. Kudlien (1969).

132. Ioannidi (1983).

133. The failure to distinguish is evident in the older treatises. Certain treatises, however, do distinguish arteries from veins. On the one hand, we find this distinction as early as the surgical treatises (see, for example, *De articulis*, 45) and in *Epidemiae V*, 46; all the same, we do not know what constituted the distinction in these two passages; the author of *Articulations* says at 45 that he will discuss communications

between veins and arteries in another work, which unfortunately has not survived. On the other hand, in the post-Hippocratic treatise *De alimento,* 31, the distinction is clearly between the veins, which transport blood, and the arteries, which transport air; Harris (1973).

134. And in the plural these arteries correspond to what we call the bronchi.

135. The pulse first appears in the treatise *De alimento,* 31; but this work dates from after the Hippocratic age (influenced especially by Stoicism).

136. For one of numerous examples, see *Praenotiones Coacae,* 125.

137. Duminil (1983).

138. Principal descriptions appear in *Epidemiae II,* 4.1 (= *De natura ossium,* 10); *De natura hominis,* 11 (= *De natura ossium,* 9); *De morbo sacro,* 6; *De carnibus,* 5.

139. *De locis in homine,* 47: "Diseases that are designated as feminines. The uterus is the cause of all such diseases."

140. *De natura muliebri,* 3 (liver), 8 (hips), 14 (loins), 38 (ribs), 48 (head), 49 (legs and feet), 63 (heart).

141. *De mulierum affectibus* [= *De morbis mulierum*], 2.7.

142. Ibid., 2.145.

143. *De articulis,* 45; cf. *Mochlikon,* 1.

144. *De articulis,* 46.

145. See *Prognosticon,* 5.

146. *De morbo sacro,* 7.

147. See, for example, *De prisca medicina,* 11.

148. Of considerable importance is the treatise *De carnibus,* which explains the original formation of man. The author devotes special attention to each of the main organs: brain (4), heart (5), lung (7), liver (8), spleen and kidney (9). Similar attention is not devoted to the stomach, which is simply mentioned in passing.

149. These three explicatory models are found in *De prisca medicina,* 11.

150. Aristotle, *Meteorologica,* 4.3.381b7.

151. *De prisca medicina,* 18.

152. *De locis in homine,* 1; *De glandulis,* 11.

153. See, among others, *De affectionibus,* 1, and *De morbis I,* 2.

154. *De natura hominis,* 4.

155. *De prisca medicina,* 22.

156. Diels and Kranz (1951), 59 B 21 a; see Diller (1932).

157. Diels and Kranz (1951), 31 B 100.

158. He is also the author of the strate C (Grensemann) of the gynecological treatises.

159. See *De flatibus,* 8.

160. *De morbis IV,* 51, 52.

161. *De arte,* 12.

162. Ibid.

163. F. Bacon, *De dignitate et augmentis scientiarum,* 2.2.

164. *Epidemiae I,* 5.

165. *De fracturis,* 36. Concerning the theoretical foundation, see *De arte,* 8.

166. See, for example, *De fracturis,* 1.

167. See, for example, *Epidemiae V,* 27; see Plutarch, *De profectibus in virtute,* 82d.

168. *Epidemiae I,* 2, 5. Trans. Jones (1923), 165.

169. *De flatibus,* 1.

170. *Epidemiae VI,* 2, 24.

171. Ibid., 4, 7.

172. *Iusiurandum,* trans. Jones (1923), 2–3; see Lichtenthaeler (1984).

173. Especially *De flatibus* and *De arte;* see ed. Jouanna (1988), 10–24, 167–174.

174. Pigeaud (1981); Jouanna (1987).

175. *De flatibus,* 1.

176. *Poetics,* 1149b.

177. *De natura hominis,* 9.

178. Clement of Alexandria, *Stromates VI* (frag. 917 Nauck).

179. *De flatibus,* 1.

180. Brandenburg (1976); Rechenauer (1991).

181. Herodotus, 2.77.

182. *Aphorismi,* 3.1.

183. Thucydides, 7.87.

184. Ibid., 2.47–54.

185. Ibid., 2.47, 4.

186. Ibid., 2.51, 4.

187. Ibid., 1.23, 6.

188. Romilly (1990), 121–124.

189. See in particular the references to medicine in the dispute between Nicias and Alcibiades in 4.14 and 18, with the studies by Romilly (1976) and Jouanna (1980).

190. Diels and Kranz (1951), 82 B 11 (14).

191. Schuhl (1960); Joly (1961b); Herter (1963b); Vegetti (1966–1969); Joly (1974), 233–246; Manuli and Vegetti (1977); Jouanna (1978).

192. Plato, *Gorgias,* 522a.

193. Plato, *Phaedrus,* 261a.

194. Ibid., 271c; see Joly (1961a); Herter (1976); Jouanna (1977); Mansfeld (1980); Joly (1983); *De prisca medicina,* 77–81.

195. *Lois,* 4.659, 6–660a2.

196. Ibid., 4.720ff., 9.857c–d.

197. Olerud (1951); Jouanna (1966); *De diaeta* [*Regimen*], ed. Joly and Byl, 46; Joubaud (1991).

198. Plato, *Republic,* 3.405c–408b.

199. Plato, *Timaeus,* 89a–d. Concerning the *pharmakon* in Plato, see Derrida (1968).

200. Celsus, *De medicina,* preface.

201. See Galen, *Quod optimus medicus sit quoque philosophus; De placitis Hippocratis et Platonis.*

3. Hellenistic Medicine

1. For the chronology of Praxagoras, see *Fragmenta,* ed. Steckerl, 1958; see also Capriglione (1985). For Herophilus, see Von Staden (1989)—a fundamental work for an understanding of Herophilus and of all Hellenistic medicine. For Erasistratus, see Von Staden (1989) and *Fragmenta,* ed. Garofalo, 1988—indispensable for the edition of the fragments. Fraser (1969) denies the presence of Erasistratus in Alexandria; the arguments offered by Lloyd (1975a) in favor of the opposite opinion appear quite persuasive to me; see also Von Staden (1989), 141–142.

2. For the epistemological level of Hippocratic medicine, see Joly (1966); also Vegetti (1983), 41ff., and Jouanna (1992).

3. Frag. 42 Von Staden.

4. Frag. 32 Garofalo.

5. Polybius, *Historiae,* 12, 25d2–6; Herophilus, frag. 56 Von Staden.

6. *De prisca medicina,* 20. The words of the author of *De prisca medicina* do not (as one might suppose) go beyond the "clinical" limits of Hippocratism.

7. The Aristotelian doctrine of the makeup of living beings was to become canonical in medicine (except for schools following the atomist beliefs). There is a first level formed of the fundamental qualities *(dynameis)* of matter (hot/cold, solid/fluid); these are in turn surrounded by the primary elements (fire, air, earth, water, known as the *stoicheia*). At the second level, the aggregation of qualities results in the creation of the "homeomeric parts" or homogeneous parts, which correspond to the various tissues (flesh, bones, blood, etc.). At the third level, there is the aggregation of homogeneous parts, which gives rise to organs with specific functions (hand, eye, etc.). A proper mixture, or temperament *(krasis),* of elements or qualities in the constitution of the body would necessarily ensure the good health of that body; therapeutic action consists of restoring a defective *krasis* to a proper condition.

8. *De sensu et sensibilibus I,* trans. and comm. Mugnier (1953) 22, and Lanza and Vegetti (1971).

9. See Vegetti (1986), 15ff.

10. For this interpretation, see Vegetti (1971), 503ff.

11. For the thermic paradigm and for the cardiocentrism of Aristotle, see Manuli and Vegetti (1977), 113ff.

12. The lack of vital heat in the female made her unable to transform excess blood into semen; the blood therefore was evacuated through the menstrual flow. At the moment of impregnation, this excess of female blood served as the material on

which the male semen acted, transforming it into an embryo, through a further process of coction. For the relationship between the Aristotelian theory of reproduction and ancient gynecology, see the essays by Manuli and Sissa, in Campese, Manuli, and Sissa (1983).

13. *De motu animalium,* ed. Nussbaum, 163. In relation to the pneuma in Aristotle, see (following Jaeger 1913) in particular Peck (1963), and Lanza (1971), 788ff.

14. *De generatione animalium,* 2.6.744a2.

15. *De motu animalium,* 10.

16. *De generatione animalium,* 2.3.736b34.

17. See Solmsen (1968), 563, 605ff.

18. The expression is taken from Hahm (1977).

19. Harris (1973), 106ff.

20. One of the direct links between Aristotelianism and medicine is the compilation of the *Problemata medica,* which constitutes the first book of the pseudo-Aristotelian *Problemata.* The assembly of this compilation began in a Peripatetic milieu, probably at the turn of the third century B.C., and also included material taken from Aristotle and Theophrastus. In the form that has come down to us, this compilation dates back only to the second century A.D. Concerning the *Problemata,* see the commentaries by Marenghi, 1965, and Louis, in the edition of 1991.

21. For the "high" dating of Diocles, see Kudlien (1971a), 192–201 (in opposition to Jaeger, 1938).

22. Frag. 112 Wellmann.

23. We would be obliged to consider as roughly contemporary Diocles and the treatise *De corde* of the *Corpus Hippocraticum* (trans. and comm. Manuli and Vegetti 1977, 101ff.), if we accept the early date, toward the middle of the fourth century B.C. That would be our opinion, but most scholars now prefer a sharply later date.

24. Frag. 30, 62, 72 Steckerl.

25. Frag. 85, 9 Steckerl.

26. See Harris (1973), 108. The "error" of Praxagoras fits into the context of a debate concerning the energy principle *(dynamis, rhome, ischus),* which offered an equally satisfactory explanation of voluntary and involuntary movements. This debate was in time to involve all of the great physiologists, from Praxagoras himself (see frag. 29) all the way up to Herophilus and Erasistratus (see frag. 111 Garofalo). According to the latter, pneuma belonging to the system of the heart and the arteries necessarily played a central role.

27. Frag. 32, 32A Steckerl.

28. Frag. 19, 31 Steckerl.

29. Frag. 18, 21, 22, 46 Steckerl.

30. Frag. 109, 115, 117 Steckerl.

31. See Pliny in Erasistratus, frag. 8 Garofalo (for phlebotomy, frag. 62A, B Garofalo).

32. Frag. 6, 7, 8 Garofalo.

33. In opposition to the remarks of Diels (1893) (= 1969, 239ff.), see the well-founded comments of Repici (1988), 1ff., 32ff., 85ff.

34. In this connection, see Fraser (1972) (for the medicine, see 338ff.).

35. See in this connection Von Staden (1989), 28ff.

36. See frag. 63A Von Staden. In connection with Alexandrian anatomy, one fundamental source remains Edelstein (1967), 254ff.; for the chronological boundaries (first half of the third century B.C.), see Kudlien (1968a and 1969). See also Von Staden (1989), 138ff.

37. *De partibus animalium,* 1.1.640b35.

38. Galen, *Administrationes anatomicae,* 1.2 (Kühn, 2:220–222).

39. See Von Staden (1989), 3ff., 149ff.

40. See in this connection Kudlien (1979), 64, 119. We know that the king Antiochos made a major gift (one hundred talents) to Erasistratus.

41. The writings of Herophilus include essays on anatomy, the pulse, therapy, regimens, and obstetrics. He may also have written a critical commentary on the Hippocratic *Prognosticon;* the title of another work, *Against Common Opinions,* suggests that he had in any case engaged in a critical revision—doxographic in nature—of common medical knowledge.

42. Frag. 42 Von Staden.

43. Concerning the development of the technological models of antiquity, see Ferrari (1985), 163ff., and (1984), 225ff.

44. Frag. 50B Von Staden.

45. Frag. 233 Von Staden.

46. Frag. 59A Von Staden.

47. Kudlien (1979), 280ff. For the relations between skepticism and medicine, see Viano (1981).

48. Frag. 50A, 54, and 232 Von Staden.

49. See in this connection Viano (1984), 346ff.

50. See also Viano (1984), 347ff.

51. See, for example, frag. 114 Von Staden.

52. Celsus, *De medicina,* preface, 23–26. See also frag. 63A Von Staden.

53. Among those who criticized this practice, see Tertullian (*De anima,* 10, 4). According to him, Herophilus had carried out 600 vivisections, "thus using a hatred of man to understand man," becoming at the same time a "physician and a butcher." His cruelty, for that matter, was perfectly useless, for dying in horrible pain supposedly altered the structures that the vivisectionist wished to observe. Concerning the "cruel zeal" of the anatomists, see also St. Augustine, *De civitate Dei,* 22, 24, 145. See Scarborough (1976).

54. There are, all the same, exceptions concerning the use of human dissection. The *rete mirabile* of vessels at the base of the brain, described by Herophilus (frag. 121 Von Staden), exists solely in cows and pigs. It is an irony of fate that Galen should

have considered this nonhuman structure to be the site of the development of psychic pneuma.

55. Frag. 81 Von Staden.

56. Frag. 141 Von Staden.

57. See Galen, *De placitis Hippocratis et Platonis,* 7.4 (trans. De Lacy, 448).

58. Frag. 85, 86, and 140A Von Staden.

59. See in this connection Von Staden (1988).

60. Frag. 146 Von Staden.

61. Frag. 145A Von Staden.

62. Frag. 143B Von Staden.

63. Frag. 182 Von Staden; see in this connection West (1973) and Grmek (1990), 33–36.

64. Frag. 173 Von Staden.

65. Fraser (1972), 354; see also Von Staden (1989), 246ff., who speaks of a "striking instance of the persistence of tradition within an innovative scientific community."

66. Frag. 64A Von Staden.

67. Frag. 130, 131, 205A and B Von Staden.

68. Frag. 248B and C Von Staden. See Pigeaud (1982).

69. Frag. 1 Von Staden.

70. See Fraser (1972), 86ff.

71. See in this connection Von Staden (1982), 76ff.

72. Garofalo (1988), 22, speaks of an Erasistratus "scientifically posterior" to Herophilus. The principal works by Erasistratus are the *General Discourses* (anatomo-physiology), *Fevers* (anatomy and pathology of the heart and blood vessels), *Paralyses* (anatomy and pathology of the nervous system), and *Regimen.*

73. Frag. 32 Garofalo.

74. Frag. 80 Garofalo.

75. Frag. 81 and 82 Garofalo.

76. Frag. 149 Garofalo.

77. Frag. 289. Still, we must not forget the polemic by Aristotle against the thesis put forth by Anaxagoras, who stated that man was the most intelligent animal because of his hands. Aristotle replied that man had hands because he was the most intelligent (*De partibus animalium,* 4.10).

78. Frag. 86 Garofalo. In connection with this language, see Von Staden (1975), 187.

79. Frag. 87, 88. The idea of *logoi theoreton* (the invisible emanations of matter from a body through the pores) also appears in Herophilus, though with no particular epistemological emphasis (frag. 142 Von Staden). It arises, quite naturally from the language of Epicurus (see *Letter to Herodotus,* 47, 62, in which it is linked to the timing of the movement of atoms). Sedley (1989) translated the expression as "viewed by reason," with reference to the process of forming concepts by analogy. The adop-

tion of this idea in the key passage of Erasistratus's anatomophysiology offers a fine epitome of that author's thinking. For an interesting attempt by Erasistratus to demonstrate experimentally a phenomenon through the *logoi theoreton,* see Von Staden (1975), 180 and Grmek (1990), 37–38. Erasistratus had caught a bird and caged it for some time without feeding it. In the end, he weighed the bird with its droppings and found that the overall weight was now less than the initial weight.

80. Frag. 78 Garofalo. The concept of "government" *(dioikesis)* plays a central role in the thought of the Stoics, who believed that providence, destiny, and pneuma were responsible for ruling the entire universe (see, for example, *Stoicorum veterum fragmenta,* 2, 945).

81. Frag. 86 Garofalo.

82. Frag. 86–89 Garofalo.

83. Frag. 88, 89, and 103 Garofalo.

84. Frag. 90 Garofalo.

85. Frag. 86 Garofalo.

86. Frag. 147 Garofalo.

87. In connection with Hellenistic artillery, see Marsden (1968), 17, 58ff., 106ff. For research on ballistics in Alexandria in the middle of the third century, see Fraser (1972), 429. For the chronology of Ctesibius, more or less a contemporary of Erasistratus, see Fraser (1972), 2:662. Concerning the relationship between medicine and mechanics (as well as the problem model or metaphor), see Vegetti (1990) (esp. n. 11). For a more general summary, see Schürmann (1991).

88. The expression is taken from Harris (1973), 204.

89. Frag. 93 Garofalo.

90. See Furley and Wilkie (1984), 32ff.; Repici (1988), 32ff.

91. Frag. 136 Garofalo.

92. Frag. 138 Garofalo.

93. Frag. 101 Garofalo.

94. The subject was the effort to build an *aerotonos,* a catapult that had been invented by Ctesibius, in which the compressed air in the cylinders was meant to replace the driving energy of the springs. Concerning this effort to create a hybrid of mechanics and pneumatics, see Marsden (1968), 128; Ferrari (1984), 258. For the biological analogies with this machine, see Vegetti (1990), 18ff. Concerning pneumatics in general, see Drachmann (1948).

95. Frag. 42A and 47 Garofalo.

96. Frag. 101 Garofalo.

97. Frag. 111B and 203 Garofalo.

98. Frag. 119 and 144 Garofalo.

99. Frag. 201 Garofalo. Concerning Erasistratus's ideas regarding the heart, see Harris (1973), 196ff.; Furley and Wilkie (1984), 26ff.; Garofalo (1988), 24ff. For a number of similar devices in Alexandrian technology, see Lonie (1973). For the

revision of the theory in a sense closer to that of Aristotle, developed by the disciples of Erasistratus during the period of Galen, see Lonie (1964).

100. Frag. 54 and 105 Garofalo.

101. Frag. 112 Garofalo.

102. Frag. 39 Garofalo.

103. Frag. 240 Garofalo.

104. See in this sense Viano (1984), 340.

105. See Harris (1973), 221.

106. Frag. 198 Garofalo. Harris (1973), 196, speaks of "invention rather than the discovery" of capillaries by Erasistratus; see Wilson (1959).

107. Frag. 44 Garofalo.

108. Frag. 158 and 161–162 Garofalo.

109. Frag. 198; "a sole cause," frag. 169 Garofalo.

110. Frag. 198 and 200 Garofalo.

111. Frag. 240 Garofalo.

112. Frag. 212 Garofalo.

113. In reference to this therapeutic tradition Smith (1982) attempted to reduce the originality of Erasistratus, putting him within the larger current of Hippocratism. Smith (p. 409) did recognize, all the same, that the "pneumatics and hydraulics" of Erasistratus had directed him in his use of dietetic medicine.

114. Frag. 62A Garofalo.

115. Frag. 184B Garofalo.

116. For the relationships and differences beween Erasistratus and the Stoics concerning the theory of pneuma, see Verbeke (1945), 177ff. Concerning pneumatic medicine, see Kudlien (1962 and 1968b).

117. See the discussion between Galen and Chrysippus in *On the Doctrines of Hippocrates and Plato*, 4.5–6, ed. and trans. P. De Lacy (Berlin, 1984), 258–260. In this connection, see Vegetti (1990).

118. See *Stoicorum veterum fragmenta*, 2.897; Solmsen (1968), 578ff.; Isnardi Parente (1989), 61.

119. Concerning the links between Erasistratus and Asclepiades, see Vallance (1990), 130ff.

120. For these problems, see Vegetti (1981).

4. Medicine in the Roman World

1. See Fraser (1972), Von Staden (1989), and Gourevitch (1992).

2. See Herophilus's *Fragmenta*, ed. Von Staden, 1989 (the second part lists all the members of the sect, from 250 B.C. to A.D. 50).

3. According to Caelius Aurelianus, *De morbis acutis*, 2.6, 32.

4. See Temkin (1935a) and Von Staden (1982).

5. For the text in general, see Mudry (1982); for this matter, Temkin (1935a) is still pertinent.

6. For the first of these three texts, see ed. Atzpodien; for the other two, see ed. Walzer and Frede, 1984.

7. This work, certainly, is nothing more than pseudo-Galenic (see Kollesch [1973]) and probably just slightly prior to the prime of Galen, even though it never contradicts the thought of Galen.

8. *Definitiones medicae,* 15, 16, 17 (Kühn, 19:353).

9. *Introductio,* 4 (Kühn, 14:683).

10. *Inscriptiones Graecae,* 14.1759. See Benedum (1977).

11. *De medicina,* preface, 18.

12. See, for example, Scarborough (1976) and Ferngren (1982).

13. *De pulsuum differentiis,* 4.2 (Kühn, 8:715).

14. Brain (1986).

15. Deichgräber (1930).

16. *Introductio,* 4 (Kühn, 14:683).

17. See, for example, Hankinson (1987).

18. Celsus, *De medicina,* preface, 27.

19. Pliny, *Historia naturalis,* 29.5.

20. Celsus, *De medicina,* preface, 38.

21. Ibid., 52.

22. One can always benefit from reading Allbutt (1921). See also Albert (1894), Scarborough (1969), and Gourevitch (1984).

23. We think that he died later, in 91. See Rawson (1982) and Gourevitch (1984).

24. Vallance (1990).

25. See, concerning methodism and Soranos, Gourevitch (1988 and 1991).

26. *De medicina,* preface, 56.

27. *De morbis acutis,* 2.6, 26.

28. *De morbis diuturnis,* 1.4.

29. This, at least, is the point of view defended by E. Dezeimeris in an article in *Journal complémentaire du Dictionnaire des sciences médicales,* 1824, 3–17 and 80–88 ("Des principes du méthodisme, considérés comme source de la doctrine physiologique").

30. *Definitiones medicae,* 14 (Kühn, 19:353).

31. Anonymous of Bamberg, L. III, 8.

32. See, for example, Galen, *De pulsuum differentiis,* 1.7 (Kühn, 8:295). Caelius Aurelianus, *De morbis acutis,* 2.6, and CIG 6292.

33. Galen, *De pulsuum differentiis,* 3 (Kühn, 8:646).

34. Ibid., 4.2 (Kühn, 8:719).

35. Garofalo (1992), 91–106.

36. Grmek and Gourevitch (1988 and 1994).
37. *De tremore,* 7 (Kühn, 7:635–636).
38. See Temkin (1973).
39. See Kudlien (1964b).
40. The edition of Hude (1958) is worth rereading, as Kudlien himself points out (preceding note).
41. See Boulle, Grmek, et al. (1982), 88.
42. Celsus, *De medicina,* preface, 4. Soranos, *Gynaecia,* 1.2–3; see Gourevitch (1988b).
43. *Rufus von Ephesos Krankenjournale,* 1978.
44. Pliny, *Historia naturalis,* 29.17.
45. Concerning his biography, properly speaking, the most recent book is by Moraux (1985); for a special aspect of that biography, see Grmek and Gourevitch (1986). For Galen in general, see Sarton (1954) and García Ballester (1972); and above all, for the state of the Galenic question, see Nutton (1981) and Scarborough (1981).
46. Unpublished letter to Ernest Renan dated July 29, 1868, Bibliothèque Nationale, Nouvelles Acquisitions Françaises, 11459, 58.
47. Same collection, 14188, 364–369.
48. *La Médecine: Histoire et doctrines,* 2d ed., 1866, esp. folio 368, page 95.
49. For this period, see especially Nutton (1973).
50. See Meyerhof (1929).
51. See Gourevitch (1987b).
52. *De formatione foetuum* (Kühn, 4:701–702).
53. See especially Frede (1987), chap. 15, "On Galen's Epistemology."
54. See *De placitis Hippocratis et Platonis,* ed. and trans. De Lacy.
55. See Moraux (1984), pt. 5, "Medizin und Philosophie: Galen von Pergamon," 687–808.
56. *Ars medica,* 4 (Kühn, 1.314–315).
57. *De bono habitu* (Kühn, 4:750).
58. *Definitiones medicae,* 131 (Kühn, 19:384).
59. *De bono habitu* (Kühn, 4:752).
60. Kühn, 5:833.
61. *De usu partium corporis humani,* 13.1 (Kühn, 4:142).
62. Ibid., 11.14 (Kühn, 3:899ff.).
63. Ibid. (Kühn, 3:906).
64. In this connection, Souques (1936) remains excellent.
65. See Siegel (1968).
66. See Smith (1979), chap. 2.
67. See Amacher (1964) and A. Debru, "Expérimentation chez Galien," in Haase (1993–94), 1719–1756.

371

68. *In Hippocratis de humoribus commentarii III,* 7 (Kühn, 16:80–81).

69. We now have a series of editions: ed. Simon, 1906; ed. Duckworth, Lyons, and Towers, 1962; ed. Garofalo, 1991.

70. See Harris (1973).

71. See *De causis respirationis* [On respiration and arteries], ed. Furley and Wilkie.

72. See Temkin (1935b).

73. *De compositione medicamentorum per genera,* 3.7 (Kühn, 13:634).

74. *De simplicium medicamentorum temperamentis et facultatibus,* 9.1, 2 (Kühn, 12:171).

75. *Liber simplicis medicinae,* 1.21 (Kühn, 11:418–419). See Grmek and Gourevitch (1985).

76. *Historia naturalis,* 23.56.

77. See Gourevitch (1988a).

78. *De praenotione* (Kühn, 14:625).

79. Kühn, 9:218–219.

80. See *Methodus medendi* and the proceedings of the symposium devoted to it in 1982, Kudlien and Durling (1991).

81. See Nutton (1984).

82. *Greek Anthology,* 16, 270.

83. *Inferno,* 4.143–144.

84. Temkin (1935b).

85. See ed. Pritchet, 1982.

5. Medicine in the Byzantine and Arab World

1. *Memoirs of an Arab-Syrian Gentleman,* ed. P. K. Hitti (Beirut, 1964), 162ff.

2. Galen, *De simplicium medicamentorum temperamentis et facultatibus,* 8, s.v. *napy* and *skorodon* (Kühn, 12:85, 126).

3. *Memoirs,* 162ff.

4. Ullmann (1970), 182–184; Savage-Smith (1987), 3–28.

5. Jagailloux (1986), esp. 19–25; Michalla (1989).

6. Bibliography in Strohmaier (1989b), 12ff.

7. Baader (1984), 251–259.

8. German trans. G. Strohmaier, *Über die Verschiedenheit der homoiomeren Körperteile,* 1970.

9. Hunayn ibn Ishaq, *Über die syrischen und arabischen Galen-Übersetzungen,* [On the Syriac and Arabic translations of Galen], ed. and trans. Bergsträsser, work cited at n. 124; *Compendium Timaei Platonis aliorumque dialogorum synopsis,* ed. P. Kraus and R. Walzer, 1951.

10. Johannes Philoponus, *De aeternitate mundi contra Proclum,* 17.5, ed. H. Raabe (Leipzig, 1899; 1st ed., Hildesheim, 1963), 599.

11. Penella (1990), 1–9.

12. Oribasius, *Collectiones medicae; Synopsis ad Eustathium; Libri ad Eunapium.*

13. Penella (1990), 115–117; Nutton (1984), 3ff.

14. Lieber (1981), 171–180; Strohmaier, "Der syrische und der arabische Galen," in Haase (1993–94).

15. Hunayn ibn Ishaq, *Galen-Übersetzungen,* n. 20.

16. Strohmaier (1991), 28ff.

17. Pfaff (1931).

18. Strohmaier (1974), 321; Degen (1986, 276ff., and 1989).

19. Concerning the identity of the author, see Wolska-Conus (1989).

20. Ullmann (1970), 82; Sezgin (1970), 3:161.

21. Strohmaier, "Der syrische und der arabische Galen," chaps. 2, 6.

22. Strohmaier (1987).

23. Strohmaier, "Der syrische und der arabische Galen," chap. 3.

24. Ibid., chap. 2.

25. Sachau (1870) (anthology), 101–124; Baumstark (1922), 168ff.; see Galen, *De diebus decretoriis,* 3 (Kühn, 9:900–941, esp. 913).

26. Strohmaier (1980).

27. Yuhanna ibn Masawayh, *Le Livres des axiomes médicaux,* ed. and trans. Jacquart and Troupeau, 222.

28. Strohmaier (1969), 77–85; Spies and Müller-Bütow (1971), 49–55.

29. Müller (1891).

30. Ibn Abi Usaybi'a, [Sources of information concerning the categories of physicians], ed. Müller, 1:185, 4.

31. See al-Biruni, [Selected works], ed. Strohmaier.

32. Zimmermann (1976), 407ff.

33. Strohmaier (1989a), 169.

34. Al-Biruni, [Book of stones], ed. Krenkow, 204–206.

35. Dietrich (1988), 40.

36. Anna Comnena, *Alexiad XV,* vol. 3, ed. B. Leib (Paris, 1945), 229–242.

37. Hohlweg (1988), 39–49.

38. Leven (1990).

39. *Arabian Nights,* 449th–454th nights.

40. Temkin (1960); Oesterle (1980).

41. Avicenna, *Poème de la médecine* (Poem on medicine), trans. H. Jahier and A. Noureddine (Paris, 1956), n. 1257.

42. See the glosses (not part of the text of Galen) in *Sieben Bücher der Anatomie des Galen,* ed. M. Simon (Leipzig, 1906), 1:58 (Arabic); 2:42 (German).

43. Barhebraeus, *The Laughable Stories,* ed. E. A. Wallis Budge (London, 1897), n. 356.

44. See, for example, 'Ali ibn al-'Abbas, [Complete exposition of the medical art], Bulaq, 1:254–281.

45. Baader (1984), 254ff.
46. See the edition by Grand'Henry, 1984, 29–31, 60–62.
47. *Axiomes médicaux*, n. 43.
48. Sudhoff (1916).
49. Baader (1984), 256ff.; Kuhne (1989), 3–20, 291–327.
50. Ed. Kuhne, 1987, 343–366.
51. 'Ali ibn Rabban Tabari, [Paradise of wisdom], ed. M. Z. Siddiqi (Berlin, 1928), 280; other material in Ullmann (1978), 108.
52. See especially Ullmann (1977).
53. Ullmann (1970) discusses the *Sefer Hanisyonot*, a Jewish medical text linked to Arab magical medicine.
54. See *De elementis secundum Hippocratem*, 2.5.
55. *De simplicium medicamentorum temperamentis et facultatibus*, 11.1, 48 (Kühn, 12:365); see *De locis affectis*, 6.5 (Kühn, 8:421ff.); Ibn Sina [Avicenna], [Canon of medicine], 2, 2, 2, 20; see Dols (1988), 263ff.
56. *Fi tahqiq ma li-l-Hind*, ed. E. Sachau (London, 1887), 95.
57. For the exact form of the name, see Iskandar (1984), 6ff.
58. Ibn Butlan, *Das Aerztebankett* [Banquet of physicians], Germ. trans. F. Klein-Franke (Stuttgart, 1984), 187.
59. *Therapeutica*, ed. Puschmann, 1:571–573.
60. Al-Gazzali, [Restoration of the religious sciences] (Beirut, n.d.), 4:300–310.
61. See the bibliography in *Arabische Volksmärchen*, ed. S. al-Azharia Jahn (Berlin, 1970), 474.
62. Migne, *Patrologia Graeca*, 87:3, cols. 3513–3520; see Nutton (1984), 6, and Duffy (1985), 23ff.
63. *In Hippocratis aphorismos*, 2:53, 256.
64. Ibn Hindu, [Key of medicine], ed. Mohaghegh and Daneshpajuh, 16; see in this connection Rosenthal (1969), 524.
65. Ullmann (1970), 185–189.
66. Al-Gazzali, [Restoration of the religious sciences], 303.
67. For greater documentation, and a partly different interpretation, see Klein-Franke (1982), 118–132.
68. See Hunger (1978), 2:285–316; Nutton (1984), 1–4.
69. Al-Biruni, [Book of stones], 213–215.
70. Al-Mas'udi, *Kitab murug ad-dahab wa ma'adin al-gawhar*, ed. M. M. Qamixa (Beirut, 1986), 4:90–96.
71. Ibn Hindu, [Key of medicine], 48–52.
72. See al-Biruni, [Book of stones].
73. *De venaesectione adversus Erasistrateos Romae degentes*, 23 (Kühn, 11:314ff.); see *De sectis ad eos qui introducuntur*, 1.

74. Ibn Abi Usaybi'a, [Sources of information concerning the categories of physicians], 1:10; see Dols and Gamal (1984), 66.

75. Ibn Butlan, *Das Aerztebankett*, 44.

76. Ibn Hindu, [Key of medicine], 13.

77. *Al-Biruni's Book on Pharmacy and Materia Medica*, ed. H. M. Said (Karachi, 1973), 10.

78. Ibn Ridwan, *Über den Weg zur Glückseligkeit durch den ärztlichen Beruf* [The way to happiness through the medical art], ed. Dietrich, 24–27; see Ibn Gumay', *Treatise to Salah ad-Din on the Revival of the Art of Medicine*, ed. Fähndrich, sections 71–74.

79. Ibid., section 14.

80. Rosenthal (1968), 93–95.

81. Al-Qifti, *Ta'rih al-hukama'*, ed. J. Lippert (Leipzig, 1903), 1.

82. Rosenthal (1956).

83. Meyerhof (1944), 119–134.

84. See the appreciations by Jacquart and Micheau (1990), 57–80; in any case, one should not overestimate the influence of his criticisms on Galen; cf. Weisser (1991), 141–145.

85. Al-Biruni, [Book of stones].

86. Meyerhof (1935b).

87. Hau (1975).

88. [Book of smallpox and measles], ed. Opitz, 1911.

89. Rosenthal (1971), 73ff., 109, 114.

90. Avicenna, [Canon of medicine], 2, s.v. "almas."

91. Al-Biruni, [Book of stones].

92. Schacht (1936), 536ff.

93. [Treatise on diabetes], ed. Thies.

94. Jacquart and Micheau (1990), 188ff.

95. Sezgin (1970), 36, 123.

96. *Rasa'il ihwan as-safa'*, Beirut, 1957, 1:175; Ibn Haldun, *Muqaddima*, 4th ed., 1978, s. l., 82.

97. Al-Farabi, *Kitab as-siyasat al-madaniyya*, ed. Nayyar, 1964, 87.

98. Fück (1952), 74.

99. Ullmann (1970), 86–96.

100. See Nutton (1984), 8.

101. Al-Gazzali, [Restoration of the religious sciences], 308.

102. Ullmann (1970), 92–95.

103. *Abhandlung über die Ansteckung von Qusta ibn Luqa* [Book on infection], ed. Fähndrich, 1987.

104. Ibid., sections 43ff.

105. See Leven (1987).

106. Ibn Abi Usaybi'a, [Sources of information concerning the categories of physicians], 1:242; see Brecher and Lieber (1978).

107. Bulgakov (1972), 298.

108. See his commentary on *De aere, aquis, locis*, ms. in Cairo, Tal 'at Tibb, 550, f. 73v.

109. Baumstark (1922), 168ff.; Galen, *De diebus criticis*, 3 (Kühn, 9:900–941, esp. 913).

110. See, for example, Avicenna, *Poème*, nn. 646–658.

111. *De aere, aquis, locis*, ed. Diller, 26, 19f.

112. Al-Biruni, *Chronology of Ancient Peoples*, 269ff.

113. Klein-Franke (1984); see on this matter Ullmann (1978), 111–114.

114. See, for example, Ritter and Plessner (1962), 164–166.

115. See *In Hippocratis epidemiarum librum VI commentaria I–VI*, ed. Wenkenbach and Pfaff (1956), 483–487; see also Iskandar (1978), 241ff.

116. *Quod animi mores corporis temperamenta sequantur* (Arabic text), ed. H. H. Biesterfeldt (1973); see García Ballester (1972), 132–136, 247–249.

117. Ishaq ibn 'Imran, *Maqala fi l-malihuliya* (= *Constantini Africani libri duo de melancholia*), ed. Garbers, f. 94a–95a; see also Ullmann (1978), 72–77.

118. Avicenna, *Poème*, n. 212.

119. Yuhanna ibn Masawayh, *Axiomes médicaux*, n. 39.

120. Bürgel (1973); Maziar Zafari (1990).

121. Avicenna, [Canon of medicine], 3, 1, 4.

122. Galen, *Prognosticon*, 6, ed. V. Nutton (Berlin, 1979), 100–105; see the commentary by Nutton on this passage.

123. Abu Sa'id ibn Bahtishu', *Ueber die Heilung der Krankheiten der Seele und des Körpers* [Concerning the treatment of diseases of the body and the soul], ed. Klein-Franke, 45–54.

124. Translations in Leclerc (1876), 1:383–388, in Ullmann (1970), 141–144, and in Jacquart and Micheau (1990), 69–73.

125. Ibn Gumay', *Treatise*, section 83.

126. *Administrationes anatomicae*; the part that survives in Arabic was published by Simon in 1906; Duckworth, Lyons and Towers in 1962; and Garofalo in 1986.

127. Ibn Abi Usaybi'a, [Sources of information concerning the categories of physicians], 1:178, 30, 180, 29ff.

128. Ed. Hirschberg and Lippert, 1902, 11–17.

129. 'Abd al-Latif, *The Eastern Key*, ed. Zand and Videan, 274.

130. Meyerhof (1935a), 100–120; Iskandar (1974), 602–606; see Siegel (1968), 48–56, 65ff.

131. Catahier (1989), 74–77.

132. Meyerhof and Schacht (1968).

133. Yuhanna ibn Masawayh, *Axiomes médicaux*, n. 8.

134. See esp. *De placitis Hippocratis et Platonis*, ed. and trans. De Lacy.

135. *Commentaria in Hippocratis prognosticon,* 124–127.

136. Zimmermann (1976), 401–414.

137. [Philosophical works], ed. Badawi, 41ff., 53ff.

138. Al-Farabi, [Catalog of the Sciences], ed. Gonzales Palencia (Madrid, 1932).

139. Abu Sa'id ibn Bahtishu', [Concerning the treatment of diseases of the body and the soul]; see the critical remarks by Dols and Gamal (1984), 22ff.

140. Iskandar (1976), 242.

141. Al-Biruni and Ibn Sina, [Questions and answers], ed. Nasr and Mohaghegh, 13.

142. Gohlmann (1974), 24ff.

143. Avicenna, [Canon of medicine], 3, 11, 1; likewise Aristotle, *Historia animalium,* 1.17.496a4.19ff.; see the contrary opinion of Galen in *Administrationes anatomicae,* ed. Simon, 1.53 (Arabic); 2.39 (German).

144. Avicenna, [Canon of medicine], 1, 1, 5, 1; see the summary in Jacquart and Micheau (1990), 178ff.

145. Karimov (1980), 125ff.

146. Avicenna, [Canon of medicine], 3, 20, 1, 1.

147. An analysis of this exceedingly complex reasoning can be found in Weisser (1983); see esp. 117–140; concerning the opinions of Galen, see also Nickel (1989), 29–60.

148. Nickel (1989), 71–83.

149. Avicenna, [Canon of medicine], 7, 31, 3, 21, 1, 2.

150. Weisser (1983), 244–249.

151. Ibn Tufayl, *Hayy ibn Yaqzan,* 5th ed. (Damascus, Saliba, and 'Ayyad, 1962), 24ff.

152. Bürgel (1968), 263–340.

153. Jacquart and Micheau (1990), 185–188.

6. Charity and Aid in Medieval Christian Civilization

1. See Isidore of Seville, *Etymologiae,* 7.2, 6.

2. See Geremek (1980), 1069–1070.

3. The most significant passages of the Gospels in this connection are Luke 6:36, and Matthew 5:18, and especially Matthew 25:31–34; in the Epistles, James, more than John and Paul, was the apostle of the active practice of charity, expressed through specific works of charity.

4. The distinction is made by Mollat, in Collectif (1978), 65. Thomas Aquinas, in *Summa Theologiae,* 2a2ae, q. 30, a. 4, ad 3, established a distinction between charity (which unites us with God by the *affectum*) and mercy or assistance (which makes us similar to Him in the *effectum*).

5. See Imbert (1947), 13, and Geremek (1987).

6. Baudry de Bourgueil, *De visitatione infirmorum;* see Agrimi and Crisciani (1980), 89.

7. See Agrimi and Crisciani (1978a), 8–9, 20, 76; Agrimi and Crisciani (1980).

8. See Amundsen and Ferngren (1982), 16.

9. For examples of these oppositions, see Fulbert de Chartres, *Himnus seu prosa de sancto Pantaleone,* in Migne, *Patrologia Latina,* 141, cols. 339–341; Pierre Comestor, *Sermo XLII Synodicus,* in Migne, *Patrologia Latina,* 198, cols. 1822–23.

10. See Crisciani (1983b), esp. 40–41.

11. See *De institutione divinarum litterarum,* in Migne, *Patrologia Latina,* 70 (esp. col. 1147) and *Variarum libri,* 12, 6, 19.

12. See Crisciani (1983b), 43–49.

13. The observation is by Humbert de Romans. In a more general context, see Murray (1974).

14. Beginning at the end of the twelfth century and above all in the thirteenth century, scholasticism dealt with charity in theological and pastoral texts. We should point out that, in this case, the theory was ahead of the actual organizational structures for the practice of assistance, which did not come into existence until the end of the fourteenth and the fifteenth centuries.

15. See G. D. Mansi, *Sacrorum conciliorum nova et amplissima collectio* (Venice, 1776), 21.438–439, 459, 528, 1160–61, 1179; 22.373, 670, 831.

16. *Die Chirurgie des Heinrich von Mondeville,* ed. J. L. Pagel (Berlin, 1982), 134–135.

17. *De instructione medici,* in De Renzi (1852–1859), 2:74–75, 5:333–334, 339, 348–349.

18. See Agrimi and Crisciani (1988) (esp. chap. 4) and Amundsen and Ferngren (1982), 17–27.

19. Oratio 43, *In laudem Basilii Magni,* in Migne, *Patrologia Graeca,* 36, cols. 377–380.

20. See Gai (1977), 91.

21. Foucault (1972), 14.

22. See Flint (1989); Sigal (1969); and Agrimi and Crisciani (1978b and 1980).

23. See Cattaneo (1984), 13–29.

24. Cited by Mollat, in Imbert (1982), 2:1.

25. Saint Benedict, *Regula,* ed. G. Penco (Florence, 1958), 115–117, 145–147.

26. See Schipperges (1964b).

27. See Jetter (1978), 313–337.

28. Grmek (1982), 34–36.

29. See Mollat (1982).

30. See Rando (1983).

31. Provided with qualified physicians and nurses, it was divided into five special sectors. See Miller (1985), 12–19.

32. For this and other special statutes cited hereinafter, see Le Grand (1901) and Agrimi and Crisciani (1980), chap. 2.

33. Jacques de Vitry; see Agrimi and Crisciani (1980), 123–126.

34. See the statutes of the Hôtel-Dieu of Angers (thirteenth century), Saint-Julien de Cambrai (1220), and the Hôtel-Dieu-le-Comte de Troyes (1263).

35. The order of Saint-Antoine-du-Viennois took care of the "ardents," literally, "burning ones," who were afflicted with ergotism. In Bordeaux and at Comines, in Flanders, hospices were built for paralytics. Following the example set in Paris, where Saint Louis (King Louis IX) had founded in 1260 the Hôpital des Quinze-Vingts, a number of institutions meant solely for the blind were founded in Chartres, Angers, and Meaux. See Imbert (1947) and Mollat, in Imbert (1982), 2:3.

36. *De laudibus civitatis Ticinensis* (Pavia, 1984), 49.

37. *De magnalibus Mediolani* (Milan, 1974), 54–56.

38. For the differences between the Islamic hospital and the Western hospital, see Jacquart and Micheau (1990), 243–251.

39. See Agrimi and Crisciani (1988), 194.

40. See Guglielmo de Saliceto, *Cirurgia* (Venice, 1490).

41. See P. Amargier, "La Situation hospitalière à Marseille," in Collectif (1978).

42. A *medicus pauperum* was paid in Milan to "medicare gratis infirmos hospitalium civitatis . . . et suburbium Mediolani et carcerum." In connection with municipal physicians, see Grmek (1982), 43–46, 54–56; Naso (1982), 25, 32–33.

43. For this testimony and for others concerning the activity of surgeons and physicians in the hospitals, see Imbert (1947), 139; Jacquart (1981), 127–131; Mollat (1978).

44. See Imbert (1947), 138; Mollat, in Imbert (1982); Saunier (1986), 235–246.

45. See Foucault (1961).

46. Concerning this particular link, see Moore (1990), 45–59.

47. The code of Rotari (643) called for the banishment of lepers from civil society.

48. See, for example, for Bologna, Agrimi, and Crisciani (1980), 137.

49. See Jacquart and Thomasset (1985) and Bériac (1988).

50. Agrimi and Crisciani (1980), 296.

51. Ibid., 78–79.

52. Biraben (1976), 2:99ff.

53. Carpentier (1962), 112.

54. Pietro da Tossignano, *Tractato de la pestilentia,* cited in Agrimi and Crisciani (1980), 299.

55. See, for example, Guy de Chauliac, in Agrimi and Crisciani (1980), 297–298. For the treatises on the plague, see Biraben (1975–76).

56. Pope Clement VI established in 1348 special rites for masses during an outbreak of the plague.

57. In Milan, at the end of the fourteenth century, there was an attempt to regulate the devotional efforts of the Whites (see Albini [1982], 23). For Venice, see Brusatin (1981), 15–17.

58. See Tuchman (1978), 118.

59. See Ariès (1975); Cosmacini (1988), 16; and Albini (1982), 22.

7. Medical Scholasticism

1. Libera (1991), 59.

2. Meyerhof (1930). Concerning the view of Alexandrian teaching offered by Arab authors, see the points made by Iskandar (1976).

3. This was Hippocrates, *De aere, aquis, locis,* 2.

4. *Etymologiae,* 4.13; ed. of the Latin text Lindsay, 1911; Eng. trans. W. D. Sharpe, in *Isidore of Seville: The Medical Writings,* special issue of the *Transactions of the American Philosophical Society* 54–2 (1964).

5. For a summary of these texts, see Sigerist (1958); Baader (1984); Sabbah, Fischer, and Corsetti (1988).

6. Concerning the translations and commentaries from Ravenna, see Beccaria (1959, 1961, 1971) and Palmieri, in his edition of the Latin translation of *De sectis* (1992).

7. Ravenna, *Commentaria in librum de sectis Galeni,* ed. and trans. Westerink.

8. Palmieri (1981).

9. A number of fragments of this commentary on the Hippocratic *Aphorismi* are published in Beccaria (1961). For the text of a version of the pseudo-Soranic *Ysagoge,* see V. Rose, *Anecdota Graeca et Graecolatina,* vol. 2 (Paris, 1870), 163–173, 243–274.

10. Concerning the possibly Hellenistic origin of this division, see Englert (1929), 23. Concerning its application to Alexandria in the later era, see Cunningham (1982).

11. Temkin (1973 and 1935b).

12. For the most recent overviews, see V. von Falkenhausen, in *Dizionario Biografico degli Italiani,* vol. 30, 1984, 321–324; Bloch (1986), 1:93–110, 127–134; Montero-Cartelle (1990).

13. Archivio della Badia, Cod. V, 97, described in Beccaria (1956), 297–303.

14. See Maurach (1978), 148–174 for an edition of the version that has been attributed to Constantine of Africa. For a comparison with the Arabic original, see Jacquart (1986), Weisser (1986), and Newton (1994).

15. Concerning the origin of this concept in medicine and its development in the Middle Ages, see Bono (1984).

16. Stephen of Pisa, treasurer of Antioch, translated the writings of al-'Abbas a second time, probably in 1127, and this time faithfully; his *Regalis dispositio* nonetheless was not as widely distributed; for the date of this translation (1127 or 1154), see Hunt (1950). The *Pantegni* was transcribed in a number of manuscripts; it was published twice during the Renaissance: in Lyons in 1515, and Basel in 1539. For the Latin text and Italian trans. of the first book of the theoretical part, see ed. M. T. Malato and U. De Martini (Rome, 1961). Concerning a comparison between the Arabic and the Latin versions, as well as the general question of the distribution of the *Pantegni*, see Burnett and Jacquart (1994).

17. These principal points were, originally, the preliminary questions that Alexandrian commentators of Aristotle would set for any text they analyzed (its intention, its utility, its author, its title, the part of philosophy to which it belonged, etc.). Diverse sorts of *accessus ad auctores* were used by physicians in the twelfth century. In the *Pantegni*, Constantine of Africa reduced the number of entries to six. Concerning the technique of *accessus ad auctores* in the Middle Ages, see Quain (1945), 215–265.

18. Constantine of Africa probably relied on an Arabic manuscript of the summaries known as the *Summaria Alexandrinorum;* for a description of a manuscript of this type, see Dietrich (1966), 33.

19. The anatomical elements are contained in the treatise entitled *Gynaecia.* The various editions and translations of this text are listed in Sabbah, Corsetti, and Fischer (1988), 155–157.

20. De Koning (1896), 355.

21. *Pantegni,* Lyons, 1515 ("Theorica," 3.25).

22. See Jacquart and Micheau (1990), 120–122.

23. Following Galen, the *Pantegni* distinguished among the *membra similia* (similar parts, such as the bones, muscles, etc.) and the *membra officialia* (instrumental or organic parts, such as the heart, the liver, etc.).

24. As is the case with Constantine of Africa, the bibliography concerning the school of Salerno is abundant and uneven in reliability. Fundamental research can be found in a series of articles listed in Kristeller (1986). There is a detailed bibliography of previous work in Baader (1978). See also Oldoni (1987); this article is reliable only in its references to the activities of the school of Salerno in the tenth century.

25. A Parisian influence on the school of Salerno was recently posited by Morpurgo (1990). This hypothesis is largely based on faulty arguments.

26. Some are published in De Renzi (1852–1859).

27. Concerning the steps that led to the formation of the corpus and to its commentary, see Kristeller (1986) and Jordan (1987 and 1990).

28. This work presented the Galenic principles in a Christian context. See Burkhard, *Nemesii episcopi Premnon physicon,* Leipzig, 1917 (ed. of the version of

Alphanus); and Verbeke and Moncho, *Nemesius of Emesa, De natura hominis,* Leiden, 1975 (ed. of the version of Burgundio da Pisa, twelfth century).

29. Concerning the place of medicine in the heart of the classifications of knowledge, see Amundsen (1979) and Eastwood (1982).

30. See Weisheipl (1965).

31. This is the case with the commentary by Agnellus of Ravenna on the Galenic treatise *Des sectes.*

32. See Jordan (1987) and Jacquart (1992).

33. See Hugonnard-Roche (1984).

34. Boethius, *De Trinitate,* ed. H. F. Stewart and E. K. Rand (Cambridge, 1946), 8. Concerning the semantic field of *physica,* which tends in one of its accepted meanings to qualify rational medicine, see Bylebyl (1990).

35. The Salernitan commentators were among the earliest users of the twelfth-century Greco-Latin versions of these texts; see Birkenmajer (1970), 73–87; Jacquart (1988).

36. Aside from the edition cited in the Bibliography, one will find a summary of the doctrine of Ursus in Stürner (1975).

37. Creutz (1936).

38. See Bazàn, Wippel, Fransen, and Jacquart (1985).

39. See Lawn, *I Quesiti Salernitani,* 1969, and *The Prose Salernitan Questions,* 1979.

40. Concerning the methods of scholastic teaching, see Weijers (1987) and the classical work by Grabmann (1909–1911). The term *punctum* seems to have emerged from the teaching of the law. It was used in medicine in Bologna and Montpellier. In the latter university, the chancellor Jacques Angeli assembled, in the fifteenth century, a great series of scholastic questions, which he entitled the *Puncta medicine.* See Delmas (1966), 23–28.

41. The best general presentation of medical teaching is still the work by Bullough (1966). See also Siraisi (1990), 48–77.

42. This opposition was pointed out especially by Siraisi (1981).

43. See Jacquart (1981), 97–107, 199–217.

44. The *Conciliator* was completed between 1303 and 1310. Peter of Abano had studied at Padua; he spent some time in Paris between 1299 and 1303. Concerning the personality of this scholar, physician, philosopher, astrologer, and translator from the Greek, see Paschetto (1984).

45. Eduard Seidler distinguished in Parisian medicine a *via intellectualis,* a *via scolaris,* and a *via pragmatica;* the first of these three was basically represented by passing foreigners and scholars whose interest in medicine was only occasional. See Seidler (1967). Concerning Jean de Saint-Amand and Pierre de Saint-Flour, see Wickersheimer (1979) (reprint of the ed. of 1936), 476–478 and 634, and Jacquart, supplement, 1979, 179–180. Regarding the plague, see Rebouis (1888). Concerning Guillaume Boucher, see Wickersheimer (1979), 229. Concerning the pragmatic aspect of Parisian medicine, see Jacquart (1994).

46. See Kibre (1978), 213–227.

47. See *Cartulaire de l'Université de Montpellier*, published under the auspices of the Conseil Général des Facultés de Montpellier, Montpellier, 1890, 1:180–183.

48. A list of these questions is published in Siraisi (1981), 305–310.

49. This classification, a product of Galenism, was universally adopted in the Middle Ages in accordance with the scheme outlined in Hunayn ibn Ishaq's *Ysagoge*.

50. [Canon of medicine], I, 2, 2, 1, 15.

51. Siraisi (1981), 16, includes analysis of the treatment of these matters.

52. Taddeo Alderotti is well known for having set forth the Averroist heterodox theory of the uniqueness of the intellectual; all the same, he approached this question with prudence; see Nardi (1949) and Siraisi (1981), 168–174.

53. Question preserved in the Vatican manuscript, Bibl. Apost., Vat. lat., 2418, fol. 165va–166va. There is a recent study of Alberto de Zanchariis by Grmek (1990c).

54. See Siraisi (1981), 265–267.

55. *Quodlibet* preserved in the Escurial manuscript, f. I 14, fol. 9va–10vb; see Beaujouan (1972), 161–221. Concerning Giacomo da Piacenza, physician of the king of Hungary and bishop of Zagreb, see Grmek (1990c).

56. See Kühn, 1:309. For analysis of the Bolognese interpretations, see Ottosson (1982), 178–194. I should point out that Giacomo da Piacenza devoted another question to the degrees of health and disease, a problem bound up with the philosophical notion of the "latitude of the forms" (ms. Escurial, f. I 14, f. 14rb–14vb).

57. Jacquart (1990a), 251–271. For a detailed account of these Hippocratic and Galenic translations, see Kibre (1985) and Durling (1961).

58. This matter of the slow introduction of the new texts is dealt with in McVaugh (1974).

59. Credit for this expression, taken up by modern historians of medieval medicine, is due to García Ballester (1982), 97–158. Concerning the introduction of the "Canon" by Avicenna and its popularity in the Middle Ages, see Siraisi (1987a), 19–76.

60. A great many analyses have been set forth on the controversies linked to the last two problems mentioned; see Preus (1977); Kollesch (1987), 2:17–26; Hewson (1975); Jacquart and Thomasset (1985).

61. This opinion of Aristotle is found especially in *De partibus animalium*, 3.4.666a–666b and 3.5.667b.

62. Concerning the position of Taddeo Alderotti and his disciples, Mondino de' Liuzzi and Pietro Torrigiano, see Siraisi (1981), 186–195.

63. Mondino, Comm. Tegni, ms. Vatican, Bibl. Apost., Vat. lat., 4466, fol. 68v, cited by Siraisi (1981), 193.

64. Concerning the biography and the writings of Arnald of Villanova, see Paniagua (1969 and 1994) and McVaugh (1970). Concerning his place of birth, much debated, see Benton (1982). Beginning in 1975, an international team regularly published the medical writings of Arnald of Villanova in the *Arnaldi de Villanova*

opera medica omnia, in Barcelona. The *Breviarium practice,* which long supported a false interpretation of his medicine, was not written by him at all.

65. One will find an analysis of his treatment of the question in McVaugh (1990).

66. Avicenna, [Canon of medicine] (ed. Venice, 1527), I, 1, 6, 1, cited by McVaugh (1970), 79.

67. Ibid., I, 1, 5, 1.

68. This distinction became a topos in the fourteenth century; see, for example, Demaitre (1980), 79.

69. See McVaugh (1990), 79–80.

70. Peter of Abano, *Conciliator,* fol. 59rb–6orb.

71. See Lonie (1981b), 19–44; Arnald of Villanova, *Opera medica omnia,* 10:95–117; García Ballester and Gil Sotres (1986).

72. *Nicomachean Ethics,* 1140a–1140b; *Metaphysics,* 7.7.1032b.

73. See, concerning this oft-debated question, Agrimi and Crisciani (1988), 21–47.

74. *Physics,* 2.2.195a15–16; Avicenna, [Canon of medicine], I, 1, 1, 2. Concerning Western medieval authors, esp. Pietro Torrigiano, see Ottosson (1982), 247–251, and Siraisi (1981), 186–195.

75. At the beginning of the *Ars medica* (Kühn, 1:305), Galen points out the possibility of three forms of teaching: the first form considers the final purpose as the point of departure and proceeds by analysis or breakdown; the second form consists of the recomposition of that which has been found through analysis; the third form consists of a breakdown of the definition. In the *Analytica posteriora* (2.189b20–25), Aristotle enumerates four forms of pursuit: the fact, the reason why, whether a thing exists, and what it is.

76. Averroës, *Commentum in Physica* (Venice, 1562–1574), fol. 4.

77. One will find a summary of these modern controversies and an analysis of the medieval commentaries in question in Ottosson (1992), 98–126. See also Schmitt (1981), 80–138.

78. A. G. Little and E. Withington, eds., *Opera hactenus inedita Rogeri Baconi,* vol. 9 (Oxford, 1928), 150–179. Concerning the life and work of Roger Bacon, see Crombie and North (1970) and Lindberg (1983).

79. Peter of Spain was the author of both philosophical commentaries and a *Thesaurus pauperum,* a work of medical practice that was quite successful. See the summary of his work in Schipperges (1973), 679–691.

80. At Montpellier, in the second half of the thirteenth century, a rejection of Hippocratic-Galenic medicine and a return to an empirical approach were recommended by the Dominican Nicholas of Poland; see Eamon and Keil (1987).

81. This subject is treated in a great number of modern works concerning medieval medicine, among them two particularly in-depth studies: Schipperges (1982), 25–36; Agrimi and Crisciani (1990).

82. See the commentaries by the Italian masters Taddeo Alderotti, Jacopo da

Forli, and Ugo Benzi, published in Venice, respectively, in 1527, 1547, and 1517. See also Kibre and Siraisi (1975).

83. *Metaphysica,* A, 980b; *Analytica posteriora,* 2.19.100a.

84. Kühn, 17(B):345–887, 18(A):1–195.

85. [Canon of medicine], II, 1, 2. See Crombie (1961), 79–81.

86. Gentile da Foligno, *Comm. Canon* (Venice, 1492), introduction to book 1.

87. A Bolognese author of the fourteenth century (Dino del Garbo or Mondino de' Liuzzi) sums up these difficulties in a brief work on weights and measures: see Siraisi (1981), 291.

88. *Ad Glauconem de medendi methodo,* 1.9 (Kühn, 11:31); see Grmek (1990b), 42–43.

89. See McVaugh, in Arnald of Villanova, *Opera medica omnia,* vol. 2, and Dureau-Lapeyssonie (1966).

90. Gentile da Foligno, *Comm. Canon,* I, 1, 1, 1.

91. For example, this aspect is set forth excessively in Pouchelle (1983).

92. Concerning this problem in general, see Alston (1944).

93. See Grmek (1990c).

94. For analysis of this decree, see Brown (1981); Santi (1987), 861–878; Paravicini-Bagliani (1989).

95. Note that human dissection was practiced in Byzantium. See Bliquez and Kazhdan (1984) and Browning (1985).

96. See O'Neill (1970) and Saffron (1975), 80–83.

97. Experimentation on human beings is attributed to the emperor Frederick II, though it belonged to the realm of legend; see Artelt (1940), 5.

98. Concerning the practice of dissection in Bologna, see Siraisi (1981), 110–114.

99. Concerning the demonstration of Henri de Mondeville, see MacKinney (1962), 233–239. Concerning the insistence of Arnald of Villanova in his summary of *De interioribus* by Galen, see McVaugh (1990), 76–77.

100. See Wickersheimer (1910), 159–169; German trans. in G. Baader and G. Keil, eds., *Medizin im mittelalterlichen Abendland* (Darmstadt, 1982), 60–72.

101. Henri de Mondeville, *Chirurgie,* 32. Jacques Despars, *Expositio supra librum Canonis Avicenne,* I, 1, 5, 1, 2. See Jacquart (1985), 48–52.

102. Concerning the examinations demanded by Innocent III, see O'Neill (1976). Concerning the postmortem examinations in Bologna and Provence, see Münster (1955), 257–271; Ortalli (1965–1968); Shatzmiller (1989).

103. For the Bolognese statutes of 1405, see Malagola (1888), 274–276. Averroës, *Colliget* (Venice, 1497), 1.1.

104. The *Anathomia* by Mondino de' Liuzzi was published repeatedly throughout the Renaissance; a facsimile of the edition of Pavia, 1478, is contained in E. Wickersheimer, *Anatomies de Mondino de' Liuzzi et de Guido da Vigevano* (Paris, 1926); ed. and Italian trans. P. Giorgi and G. F. Pasini (Bologna, 1992).

105. See French (1979), 461–468.

106. Concerning this question, see Jacquart and Thomasset (1985).

107. *Anathomia,* ed. Wickersheimer, 25.

108. Gentile da Foligno, *Comm. Canon,* III, 21, 1, 1.

109. Avicenna, [Canon of medicine], I, 1, 1, 1. Pietro Torrigiano, *Plusquam commentum* (Venice, 1557), fol. 10. For an analysis of the relations between theory and practice, see Agrimi and Crisciani (1988), 20–47.

110. Averroës, [Commentary on the Cantica of Avicenna], in *Aristotelis opera,* vol. 10 (Venice, 1562, repr., Frankfurt, 1962), fol. 221rv. Concerning the position of Arnald of Villanova, see McVaugh (1990).

111. Averroës, *Colliget,* 1.1. Pierre Chauchat, "Comm. De crisibus de Galen," ms. Reims, Bibl. Mun., 1014, fol. 73r. Concerning this master, see Wickersheimer (1979) (reprint of the ed. of 1936), 625–626. Concerning practical teaching in Paris, see Denifle and Chatelain (1891), 2:454.

112. Regarding the problem of an eventual adaptation of the theory as a function of the observations of practice, see McVaugh (1987).

113. Concerning the influence of the thought of William of Ockham and his followers on Tommaso del Garbo, see Park (1985), 202–209.

114. See Jacquart (1990c). On the *scientia ingeniorum,* see Beaujouan (1975), 440–443.

115. Concerning the juridical *Consilia,* see Ascheri (1982) and Herberger (1981). For a summary of the medical *Consilia,* see Agrimi and Crisciani (1994). See also Taddeo Alderotti, *Consilia,* ed. Nardi, and Lockwood (1951). A list of the *Consilia* of Antonio Cermisone appears in Pesenti (1984), 72–89.

116. See McVaugh (1971).

117. See Demaitre (1975), 102–123; Demaitre (1976), 81–95; Riddle (1974); Pesenti (1982).

118. Michele Savonarola, *Practica maior,* prologue; Antonio Guaineri, *De pleuresi,* 10; Ugolino da Montecatini, *De balneis,* 98. See Jacquart (1990b), 140–160, and Park (1985), 214.

119. See, concerning this break, Grmek (1990b), 301–316.

120. See Siraisi (1987b).

121. There is an illuminating analysis of the links between the acceptance of the philosophy of Aristotle and the interest in astrology in Lemay (1962).

122. See ed. V. Tavone (Rome, 1958). A good analysis of the foundations of the application of astrology to medicine can be found in Dell'Anna (1990).

123. Roger Bacon, *De erroribus medicorum,* 1928, 154.

124. Peter of Abano, *Conciliator differentiarum,* 10, 104; see Federici-Vescovini (1987), 19–39.

125. Kühn, 9:900–941.

126. [Canon of medicine], IV, 1, 4, 1, and IV, 2, 2, 2. Also see Mehren (1884), 383–403.

127. Concerning the criticism offered by Nicole Oresme, who attacked Galen

tactfully, see Caroti (1976) and Coopland (1952). Concerning the opinion of Jacques Despars, as expressed in his commentary on Avicenna's "Canon," see Jacquart (1990b). For other criticisms of astrology, see Trinkhaus (1989), 46–68.

128. Pietro da Tossignano, *Consilium pro peste evitanda,* in Johann von Ketham, *Fasciculus medicine* (Venice, 1493).

129. Concerning the links between astrology and magic at the end of the Middle Ages, see Federici-Vescovini (1983), 171–193.

130. See White (1975). The *Astrarium* by Giovanni Dondi has been the subject of a facsimile reproduction and of a critical edition by Emmanuel Poulle (Padua and Paris, 1987–88).

131. Concerning the new idea of nature in the twelfth century, see Gregory (1975); on the chronology of the translations, see Alverny (1982).

132. *Breviarium dictum viaticum,* prologue.

133. Summary of the medical knowledge of William of Conches in Elford (1988), 308–327.

134. See ed. M. Lemoine (Paris, 1988).

135. See S. Van Riet and G. Verbeke, *Avicenna Latinus, Liber de anima* (1968). Summary of the doctrine of Avicenna in Libera (1989), 103–105. We should note that there are a few nuances between the theories set forth respectively in the "Canon" and in *De anima.*

136. See Crombie (1961); McEvoy (1982); Southern (1986).

137. The bibliography on these subjects is abundant; see Hewson (1975); Demaitre and Travill (1980); Siraisi (1980); Jacquart and Thomasset (1981); Anderson (1953).

138. Dante, *Banquet,* or *Convivio,* 4; see the interpretation offered by Libera (1991), 277–286.

139. See Murdoch (1975).

140. See Thomasset (1982) and Michaud-Quantin (1966), 584–588.

141. Concerning Baudry de Bourgueil and André le Chapelain, see respectively Laurie (1991), 11–71, and Jacquart and Thomasset (1985). For an edition of the treatise of Constantine of Africa, see E. Montero-Cartelle, *Constantini Liber de coitu* (Santiago de Compostela, 1983).

142. Concerning the whole set of problems with heroic love and its sources, see Wack (1990).

143. See Klibansky, Panofsky, and Saxl (1964). See also Heger (1967) and Jacquart (1983), 43–53.

8. The Concept of Disease

1. For the array of depictions of disease in accordance with cultural and social classes, see Gourevitch (1964), 437–477; Herzlich (1969); Engelhardt (1975), 125–141; Murdock (1980); Bean (1981); Laplantine (1986).

2. See Buck (1949), under the entries "Sick, Sickness" and "Well, Health."

3. See esp. Engelhardt (1975), Kräupl Taylor (1979), and Currer and Stacey (1986). For the historical roots of this distinction, see in particular Temkin (1961), 629–647.

4. Rothschuh (1975).

5. For the concept of the norm, see Canguilhem (1972) and Susser (1981). The distinction between disease and diseases has been nicely analyzed by Sadegh-Zadeh (1977).

6. See Grmek (1983b), 12–13.

7. For an overall view of the development of these concepts, see Sigerist (1931); Berghoff (1947); Riese (1953); King (1954); Rather (1959); Lush et al. (1961); Grmek (1967); Kudlien (1967); Diepgen, Gruber, and Schadewaldt (1969); Rothschuh (1975); Caplan, Engelhardt, and McCartney (1981); Nordenfelt and Lindahl (1984); Reznek (1987); Pérez Tamayo (1988).

8. The identification of disease as an intruding object is quite widespread in the ancient folklore of all peoples. See Clements (1932) and Sigerist (1951), 1:128–130. For archaic notions of medicine, see also Coury (1967).

9. For the historical precedents of the notion of "disease-intoxication," see in particular Diepgen (1940). It should be noted that the term "toxic" comes from the Greek word for arrow.

10. See Grmek (1984a).

11. See Dodds (1959); Smith (1965); Lanata (1967).

12. See several examples in Jouanna (1988a).

13. See Grmek (1983b), 43–62. The idea of the divine etiology of certain diseases survived throughout antiquity (see in particular Dodds 1959 and Byl 1990) and surfaced again in the Middle Ages with the triumph of Christianity and Islam.

14. Odyssey, 9:410–412.

15. Hesiod, *Works and Days*, 100–104.

16. Kudlien (1967), 51; Grmek (1983b), 66.

17. See Grmek (1983b), 68–69. For an overall view of primitive theories and efforts to classify them, see Murdock (1980) and Pérez Tamayo (1988), vol. 1.

18. Aetius, *Placita*, 5.30.1; according to Stobaeus, *Eclogae*, 4.36.

19. Diels and Kranz (1951), 1:215–216. This version was established by H. Diels in the anthology *Doxographi Graeci*, 1879.

20. Hippocrates, *Epidemiae*, 1.2, 5 (Littré, 2:637). For this "Hippocratic triangle," see in particular Gourevitch (1984).

21. See Cambiano (1982) and Rechenauer (1991), in particular 312.

22. For the general terms designating disease, see Preiser (1976).

23. Galen, *De sanitate tuenda*, 1.4. This definition is given literally by the Stoic philosopher Chrysippus, quoted by Galen in *De placitis Hippocratis et Platonis*, 5.2.

24. Aristotle, *Problemata*, 1.1 (ed. P. Louis, Paris, 1991, 10).

25. Plato's explications were complex and could hardly be limited to pertur-

bances of the elements. Though he clearly showed the influence of earlier medical doctrines and the doctrines of his time, Plato got caught up in the meanderings of philosophical speculation concerning the geometric makeup of the human body and its supposed subordination to the soul. See in this connection Riese (1953), Miller (1962), and the introduction by Luc Brisson to his edition of *Timaeus*, 1992, 55–57.

26. Hippocrates, *De diaeta* [*Regimen*], 1.3, 1 (ed. Joly and Byl, 126–127).

27. Hippocrates, *De prisca medicina*, 14.4 (ed. Jouanna, 136).

28. For the ideas of Empedocles, see in particular O'Brien (1981). For the role played by the four primary qualities in ancient philosophy and medicine, see Lloyd (1964b).

29. See Schöner (1964) and Grmek (1991b).

30. Hippocrates, *De natura hominis*, 4 (ed. Jouanna, 172–175). See Jouanna (1992), 457.

31. Manuli (1985), 38–240, and Grmek (1991b).

32. Jouanna (1988a) and Byl (1990).

33. See Van Brock (1961), Kornexl (1970), and particularly Kudlien (1973).

34. Aristotle, *Problemata*, 7.4 (ed. Louis, 124).

35. Littré, in *Oeuvres complètes d'Hippocrate* (Paris, 1839), 1:453.

36. See Vintró (1972) and Grmek (1983b), 420–423.

37. For this problem as a whole, see Bourgey (1953) and Jouanna (1992); for the school of Kos, see Temkin (1928) and Deichgräber (1933); for the school of Cnidus, see Ilberg (1925), Boncompagni (1972), Grensemann (1975), Wittern (1978), and Kollesch (1989).

38. Daremberg (1870), 1:121.

39. The distinction between the doctrine of Kos and that of Cnidus has been criticized, especially by Smith (1973), Lonie (1978), and Thivel (1981).

40. Erasistratus, *Fragmenta*, ed. Garofalo (1988).

41. See Deichgräber (1930) and Temkin (1961), 249.

42. Galen, *De temperamentis*, 6, and commentaries on the Hippocratic treatises.

43. From this point of view, the most instructive is the Galenic treatise *De locis affectis*.

44. See in particular Riese (1953), Siegel (1968), and Temkin (1973).

45. Skoda (1988); Byl (1992), 77–94; and Jouanna (1992).

46. Laín Entralgo (1961); Vintró (1972), 107–144; Grmek (1983b), 409–437.

47. For the Hippocratic art of diagnosis, see Siegel (1964); Preiser (1978); Wittern (1978); Di Benedetto (1986). For the Hippocratic conceptualization of certain diseases or groups of diseases, see Clarke (1963); Grmek and Wittern (1977); Grmek (1983b); Byl (1988); Potter, Maloney, and Desautels (1990).

48. Temkin (1928); Vust-Mussard (1970); Robert (1975).

49. Stephen of Alexandria, *Commentaria in Galeni librum therapeuticum ad Glauconem*, 1:267; see Temkin (1961), 249–250.

50. Pindar, *Pythian Odes,* 3.47–50. See Benveniste (1945).

51. For the classification of diseases in the writings of the *Corpus Hip-pocraticum,* see Jouanna (1992), 207–220.

52. See Bertier (1972), 13–23, 161–165.

53. Isidore of Seville, *Etymologiae,* 4.5.

54. See, for example, De Renzi (1852–1859), 2:411–412.

55. Especially *Physics,* 7.3 (246b).

56. See Ottosson (1982), 130–135, 194. Although this author is certainly right about medieval Galenism, his line of reasoning is less persuasive where the pathological doctrine of Galen himself is concerned.

57. Baader and Keil (1978), 121–144.

58. See Grmek (1984a).

59. Siebenthal (1950); Diepgen (1958), 5–9; Laín Entralgo (1961).

60. See Pigeaud (1981).

61. See Noye (1977) and Agrimi and Crisciani (1978a).

9. Drugs

1. Concerning this form of therapy, see Lorenz (1990).

2. See Girard (1988 and 1990).

3. See Watson (1966).

4. For the history of medications in general, see Delaveau (1982), 67–117; Kölbing (1985), 12–38; Dousset (1985), 38–55; Bonuzzi (1987), 52–59; Bernabeo (1987), 65–100. For an inventory of ancient sources, see Büchi (1982), 32–90; of Greek antiquity up to the time of Galen, Scarborough (1985), 213–215; of Byzantium, Kritikos and Papadaki (1969). Pigeaud (1982) first examined the theories of medications in antiquity.

5. *Republic,* 405d.

6. Lorenz (1990), 18–22.

7. See, for example, *Odyssey,* 4.230.

8. Concerning the term *pharmakon,* see Artelt (1937).

9. In Greek this would be *anairon* (that which kills), *deleterios* (destroyer), *diaphthartikos* (that which destroys entirely), *thanasimos* (mortal), *phthoroipos* (agent of destruction).

10. See, for example, *De antidotis,* 1.1.5: *thanasima pharmaka.*

11. For an inventory of the *materia medica* of the *Corpus Hippocraticum,* see Dierbach (1824) and Moisan (1990a). On continuity with preceding periods, see Scarborough (1983), 307–308; the case of narcotics is covered in Moisan (1990b).

12. See, for example, *De natura hominis,* 9. This principle does exclude that of a certain "homeopathy" (as in *De locis in homine,* 42).

13. Stannard (1961); Harig (1980).

14. Scarborough (1983).

15. Jouanna (1992), 224–228.

16. Pigeaud (1982), 60.

17. We should carefully consider *De plantis*. Yet before we do that, we should clear up the matter of the various contributions to the work that now survives, which is a translation into the Arabic of a now lost Syriac text, which in turn had been the translation of a new version of the original work by Aristotle, done by Nicolaus of Damascus (around 64 B.C.–A.D. 14). Concerning this question, see Moraux (1973), 487–514.

18. *Problemata*, ed. Louis, xxiii–xxx.

19. Ibid., 1.57.

20. Ibid., 1.42, 47.

21. In Greek: *ta empodia* (literally, "the obstacles"). See *Problemata*, 1.42.864a33.

22. Ibid., 1.40.864a2, and 1.42, 47.

23. Ibid., 1.40.863b32–33 and 864a1–2; 48.865a21.

24. Ibid., 1.41.864a15.

25. Ibid., 1.40.864a9–10, and 1.48.865a23, with the verb *syntheko* (literally, "to fuse into one mass") and its derived adjective *syntektikos* designating, quite precisely, dissolution.

26. The dating of Diocles has given rise to extensive debate, summarized by Kudlien (1963) and reexamined recently by Von Staden (1989), 44–46, who considers Diocles to have been a contemporary of Aristotle.

27. For *dynamis* in the *Corpus Hippocraticum*, see Plamböck (1964). For a potential relationship between the *Corpus Hippocraticum* and Aristotle, see Vizgin (1980).

28. Problemata, 1.30.863a6, and 1.33.863a13.

29. Pseudo-Dioscorides, *De venenatis animalibus*, preface.

30. Garofalo (1988), 71–72 (frag. 35). This fragment appears in the treatise *De causis* (Touwaide 1992a, as opposed to Garofalo 1988, 29).

31. Scarborough and Nutton (1982), 200, translate *dynamis* in Dioscorides as "powers, faculties, or what drugs 'do,'" and no more.

32. Von Staden (1989), 516.

33. The last editor, S. Amigues (Paris, 1988, xxxiv–xxxv), seems to admit the authenticity of this book. For the text, see ed. Hort.

34. Scarborough (1978) is the first study of pharmacology.

35. See, for example, 9.16.8, where Thrasyas and Alexias are mentioned as experts in the field of poisons.

36. Bretzl (1903).

37. Von Staden (1989), 416–417 (frag. 248a–c).

38. Pigeaud (1982), 53; Lloyd (1979); Scarborough (1983), 1, n. 1.

39. Von Staden (1989), 418–419 (frag. 249).

40. Brain (1982).

41. Mudry (1982), 70–71. Concerning the empirical school, see Wellmann (1905); Deichgräber (1930); Edelstein (1933); Galen, *Subfiguratio empirica,* ed. Atzpodien; Pentzopoulou-Valalas (1990).

42. See, for example, Galen, *De sectis,* 8.

43. *De materia medica,* preface, 5 (2.3.13–16, ed. M. Wellmann, Berlin, 1906–1914): *peirasmos* (literally, "essay").

44. Vallance (1990).

45. See *De materia medica,* preface, 2 (2.1.18–20, ed. Wellmann), with Gourevitch (1991), 60–61. For the pharmacology of Asclepiades, see Scarborough (1975).

46. Scarborough (1991).

47. Concerning Dioscorides, see Riddle (1985).

48. See *De materia medica,* preface, 6 (1.3.18, ed. Wellmann).

49. For example, *thermantikos* (heating), *styptikos* (astringent), *psyktikos* (cooling).

50. See, for example, a *dynamis* that "has the property of being active against the pains of the bladder" (*De materia medica,* 3.142).

51. Mantegazza (1989), 33.

52. For this point of view, see Touwaide (1990)—contradicting Riddle (1985), who suggested a system of classification by drug affinity.

53. For an overall view, see Touwaide (1988).

54. Concerning Cratevas, see Wellmann (1897) and Orofino (1992).

55. Von Staden (1989), 400–401, 515–518.

56. Galen, *De antidotis,* 1.1 (ed. L. Winkler [Marburg, 1980], 142–146).

57. For a pharmacological analysis, see Scarborough (1977–1979) and for a historical analysis, Touwaide (1991b).

58. This theory dates from the 1856 edition by O. Schneider (Leipzig), 181–201, and was perpetuated as late as Scarborough (1977), 4. It has been reexamined by Knoefel (1991), who attempted to show its inaccuracy.

59. Touwaide (1991a), 278.

60. Galen, *De antidotis,* 1.1.

61. Galen, ibid., is explicit on this point.

62. The latter is the view of Watson (1966), 76–78, who bases his work on a Galenic treatise of questionable authenticity, *De theriaca ad Pisonem,* 10 (concerning the authenticity, see ed. E. Coturri [Florence, 1959], 16; ed. L. Richter-Bernburg [Göttingen, 1969], 7, 42, n. 1; Nutton [1983], 6, n. 21).

63. *Problemata,* 1.45.864b33–35.

64. *Historia plantarum,* 9.17.1.

65. For the *pharmaka* used in Egypt, from the third century B.C. until as late as the fourth century A.D., see Gazza (1955–56).

66. Concerning this expedition, see Shelag (1968).

67. For trade in exotic products in Rome, see Miller (1969) and Raschke (1978).

68. An inventory of the pharmacology of Celsus is found in the work of Caturegli (1966).

69. For Scribonius Largus, see *Compositiones,* ed. Sconocchia, 5–9.

70. Books 20–32. Concerning Pliny, see Reynolds (1986) and Scarborough (1986).

71. For an analysis of their authenticity and their origin, see Touwaide (1984 and 1992a).

72. For example, see Scribonius Largus, *Compositiones,* 170, 173, 176.

73. Galen, *De antidotis,* 1; *De theriaca ad Pisonem* (of doubtful authenticity); see Watson (1966).

74. See Scarborough (1985), 216–221.

75. *De simplicium medicamentorum temperamentis et facultatibus,* 1–11.

76. *De compositione medicamentorum per genera,* 1–7.

77. *De compositione medicamentorum secundum locos,* 1–10.

78. *De antidotis,* 1–2.

79. *De locis affectis,* 3.

80. See, for example, *De simplicium medicamentorum temperamentis et facultatibus:* Kühn, 11:421, mandrake and hemlock; 11:820, aconite; 12:55, hemlock; 12:79–80, mushrooms; 12:127, yew; 12:212, arsenic; 12:235, sandarac; for theriac, see *De antidotis,* 1.1.

81. For example, *De simplicium medicamentorum temperamentis et facultatibus* (Kühn, 12:235): "participates in the caustic dynamis." Concerning the Platonism of the era, see Donini (1984), 359.

82. For the system of Galenic pharmacology, see Riddle (1985), 169–176; Scarborough (1989). The theory of degrees is set forth by Harig (1974).

83. *De locis affectis* (Kühn, 8:194–197).

84. For an overall presentation of Byzantine *materia medica,* see Stannard (1985) and Scarborough (1985).

85. For Byzantine medical teachings, see Duffy (1985).

86. Lemerle (1971), 109–307; Wilson (1983a), 63–147.

87. Vatican, Biblioteca Apostolica, Cod. Graecus 284 (Touwaide 1985).

88. Concerning Theophanes Chrysobalantes, also known as Theophanes Nonnos, see Sonderkamp (1985 and 1987).

89. For Greek southern Italy, which perpetuates ancient traditions, see Ieraci Bio (1989).

90. A general account is to be found in Baader (1984). For Dioscorides, see Riddle (1980), 4–8, 20–27. For Galen, see Baader (1981). An inventory of the treatises of pharmacology may be found in Opsomer (1989), x–xlix, and of *materia medica,* on pp. 19–89 of the same work.

91. Concerning the school of Ravenna, see Mazzini and Palmieri (1991).

92. For the influence of this treatise in the West, see Mazzini and Palmieri (1991), 294–309 (on Ravenna); Agnellus of Ravenna, *Commentaria in librum de sectis*

Galeni, ed. Westerlink; John of Alexandria, *Commentaria in librum de sectis Galeni,* ed. Pritchet; Wilson (1983b) (on Greek manuscripts copied in the West); Alverny (1985), 21–22 (on Burgundio da Pisa).

10. Surgery

1. Grmek (1989), chap. 2.
2. LeVay (1990), 20–42.
3. Michler (1968a).
4. Michler (1968b).
5. Gurlt (1898), 354–394, is still valuable.
6. Jackson (1990).
7. See Mani (1991).
8. Michler (1969).
9. *Epitomae medicae,* ed. Adams, 2:247–511; Gurlt (1898), 562–590.
10. Siraisi (1990), chap. 6.
11. Constantine of Africa, *Liber de chirurgia,* ed. Malato and Loria, 12–19.
12. Text in Sudhoff (1914–1918), 103–147; see Corner (1937a).
13. Text in Sudhoff (1914–1918), 148–236.
14. Corner (1937b).
15. In Guy de Chauliac, *Ars chirurgica,* 1546, f. 200v.
16. Ibid., ff. 189r–v, 197r–v.
17. Ibid., f. 197.
18. Keil and Loechel (1975); Keil (1983–84).
19. *On Surgery and Instruments,* ed. Spink and Lewis, ix.
20. Huard and Grmek (1966), 26–30.
21. Hall (1957).
22. Teodorico, *Cyrurgia,* ed. Campbell and Colton, 1:149; Siraisi (1990), 170–171.
23. In *Ars chirurgica,* 1546, f. 303.
24. Ibid., f. 331r–v.
25. Ibid., f. 336v.
26. Nicaise (1893), 2–4.
27. Ibid., 206–208.
28. See Siraisi (1990), 169–170.
29. Nicaise (1890), 215–216.
30. Ibid., 167–173.
31. Siraisi (1990), 170–173.
32. Jones (1984), 99–102.
33. *Ars chirurgica,* 1546.
34. Jones (1984), 110–113.
35. Beck (1974).

36. Huard and Grmek (1966); Keil (1983–84).

11. The Regimens of Health

1. Littré, 6:466–662.
2. See Smith (1980).
3. Jaeger (1923).
4. Plutarch, *Opera moralia* (Paris, 1985), 2:93–135.
5. Kühn, 6:1–452; ed. K. Koch (Leipzig and Berlin, 1923).
6. Thorndike (1946).
7. Concerning the presence in the work of Galen of the six so-called nonnatural things, see García Ballester (1990), who provides all preceding bibliography.
8. Opsomer and Halleux (1985).
9. See Wickersheimer (1966); also Beccaria (1956). The two catalogs provide numerous examples.
10. [Canon of medicine], I, 3, 1 (ed. Venice, 1527, 43 and 43v).
11. Concerning the history of the text and its transmission, see Manzalaqui (1970–71); Ryan and Schmitt (1982).
12. Wickersheimer (1950).
13. Published during the Renaissance as the *Tacuinum sanitatis*, Strasbourg, 1531.
14. See the facsimile reproduction *Codex Vindobonensis series nova 644 der Osterreichischen Nationalbibliothek*, 2 vols. (Graz, 1967); also Opsomer (1991).
15. I consulted two manuscripts of the fifteenth century: ms. Vienna 5501, fol. 24r–37v (dated from 1447), and ms. Paris, Bibl. Arsenal, 972, fol. 134r–162v.
16. *Tractatus Rabbi Moysi de regimine sanitatis ad Soldanum Regem*, Augsburg, 1518 (= *Regimen of Health for the Sultan*).
17. See Sudhoff (1914–1920).
18. This definition, used by P. Laín Entralgo in his analysis of anatomical texts, is applied to the order of the information contained in a text. See Laín Entralgo (1987), 21.
19. See Thorndike and Kibre (1963), cols. 246, 513, 524, 598, 780.
20. Published by Roy (1913), 1:153–158.
21. *Liber conservacionis sanitatis senis*, ms. Paris, Bibl. Nat., Lat. 11015, fol. 32–41.
22. *De conservanda sanitate*. For the manuscripts, see Thorndike and Kibre (1963), col. 1413.
23. *Le Régime du corps*.
24. A critical edition of his text is forthcoming in *Arnaldi de Villanova opera medica omnia* (Barcelona, 1975 and following years).
25. For a summary of the contents, from a different point of view, see Demaitre (1980), 59–69.

26. His work has been confused with that of Arnald of Villanova.

27. Ms. Munich 7744, fol. 27r–41r, and Vienna 3011, fol. 127r–147r.

28. Maynus de Mayneriis, *Regimen sanitatis;* idem, *Praxis medicinalis,* 14.

29. Maynus de Mayneriis, *Regimen sanitatis ad dominum Antonium de Flisco,* ms. Paris, Bibl. Arsenal, 873, fol. 7r.

30. Maynus de Mayneriis, *Regimen sanitatis ad dominum Antonium,* 102.

31. Arnald of Villanova, *Speculum medicinae,* in *Opera omnia* (Venice, 1505), 13.5v.

32. Barnaba da Reggio, *Regimen sanitatis ad dominum Antonium,* ms. Paris, Bibl. Nat., Nouvelles acquisitions latines 1430, fol. 1v.

33. Arnald of Villanova, *Speculum medicinae,* 13.5v.

34. There are exceptions of slight importance. For instance, in the *Regimen sanitatis* of the Four Masters of Montpellier, mention is made of the lunar cycles (esp. the full moon) among the factors that have a harmful effect on the air (see Sudhoff [1923], 185). Other astrological elements can be found in a regimen written in French, the *Régime ordonné pour le gouvernement de la santé du corps selon la disposition de chascun,* ms. Paris, Bibl. Nat., Lat. 11299, fol. 1–18, and ms. Paris, Bibl. Arsenal, 2894, fol. 1–143v.

35. Maynus de Mayneriis, *Regimen sanitatis ad dominum Antonium,* fol. 4r.

36. Barnaba da Reggio, *Regimen sanitatis ad dominum Antonium,* fol. 1vb.

37. *Tractatus Rabbi Moysi,* 1v.

38. Maynus de Mayneriis, *Regimen sanitatis ad dominum Antonium,* fol. 5r.

39. *Regimen compilatus ab Angelo de Aquila,* ms. Paris, Bibl. Nat., Lat. 4120, fol. 91r.

40. See Maynus de Mayneriis, *Regimen sanitatis ad dominum Antonium,* fol. 5r.

41. Gerardo de Solo, *Regimen per dietam,* ms. Vienna, 5486, fol. 34v.

42. Chunrardus Erstensis, *Regimen sanitatis,* ms. Vienna 3011, fol. 307r.

43. Peter of Spain (Petrus Hispanus), *De conservanda sanitate,* ms. Vienna, 3011, fol. 127v.

44. Maynus de Mayneriis, *Praxis medicinalis,* 2.27.41.

45. Bernard de Gordon, *Regimen sanitatis,* ms. Cues 308, chap. 7, fol. 52va.

46. [Canon] (Venice, 1527), I, 3, 2, 1, 170.

47. Bernard de Gordon, *Regimen sanitatis,* fol. 52vb.

48. *Pantegni,* in Constantine of Africa, *Opera* (Basel, 1563), 5.12.20v.

49. Maynus de Mayneriis, *Regimen sanitatis ad dominum Antonium,* fol. 10r–v.

50. Bernard de Gordon, *Regimen sanitatis,* fol. 3ra.

51. Ibid., fol. 53a.

52. Maynus de Mayneriis, *Regimen sanitatis ad dominum Antonium,* fol. 9v.

53. Ibid., fol. 52v.

54. *Regimen compilatus ab Angelo de Aquila,* fol. 97r.

55. Barnaba da Reggio, *Regimen sanitatis ad dominum Antonium,* fol. 2va.

56. Arnald of Villanova, *Regimen sanitatis ad regem Aragonum,* in *Opera omnia* (Venice, 1505), 2.82v.

57. Bernard de Gordon, *Regimen sanitatis,* fol. 53ra.

58. According to Bernard de Gordon (see *Regimen sanitatis,* fol. 53ra), this was a "strong" form of exercise that should be left to the young and the dissolute. For Arnald, this form of exercise was not in keeping with royal authority. See above, n. 56.

59. Bernard de Gordon, *Regimen sanitatis,* fol. 35ra.

60. Ibid., fol. 53ra.

61. Ibid.

62. Ibid.

63. Johannes de Toleto, *De conservanda sanitate,* ms. Paris, Bibl. Nat., Nouvelles acquisitions latines 543, fol. 63v.

64. See Avicenna, [Canon of medicine], I, 3, 2, 7, 176; Rhazes, *Regimen ad Almansorem* (Basel, 1544), 4.4.91; Averroës, *Colliget* (Venice, 1574), 6.6.137.

65. Johannes de Toleto, *De conservanda sanitate,* fol. 63v.

66. Maynus de Mayneriis, *Regimen sanitatis ad dominum Antonium,* fol. 12r.

67. Jacques Despars, *Expositio supra librum Canonis Avicenna* (Lyons, 1498), fol. 179r.

68. Schipperges (1985).

69. Published by Stouff (1970), 235.

70. The first books of prescriptions were drawn up in the fourteenth century. There are numerous remarkable examples of these books in Italy, France, and Catalonia. See Ketchman Weaton (1983).

71. Arnald of Villanova, *Speculum medicinae,* 78.26v.

72. Maynus de Mayneriis, *Regimen sanitatis ad dominum Antonium,* fol. 18r.

73. Avicenna, [Canon of medicine], I, 3, 2, 7, 175.

74. *Secretum secretorum cum glosis et notulis fratris Rogeri,* ed. R. Steele (Oxford, 1920), 2.4.68–69.

75. *Commentum supra regimen sanitatis Salernitanum, Praxis medicinalis,* 89.

76. Maynus de Mayneriis, *Regimen sanitatis ad dominum Antonium,* fol. 20v.

77. *Commentum super regimen,* 89.

78. See *Regimen sanitatis,* ms. Munich, 363, fol. 75r.

79. Ariès and Duby (1985).

80. Arnald of Villanova, *Regimen sanitatis ad regem Aragonum,* 4.82v.

81. *Regimen compilatus ab Angelo de Aquila,* fol. 97v.

82. Arnald of Villanova, *Speculum medicinae,* 83.

83. These effects are explained in the *Problemata* by pseudo-Aristotle, part. 27, 1–3 and 6–11, a text often used by the authors of the Middle Ages.

84. Bernard de Gordon, *Regimen sanitatis,* fol. 49vb.

85. Maynus de Mayneriis, *Regimen sanitatis ad dominum Antonium,* 1.4.5.

86. Bernard de Gordon, *Regimen sanitatis,* fol. 50ra.

87. Maynus de Mayneriis, *Regimen sanitatis ad dominum Antonium,* 1.4.5.
88. Bernard de Gordon, *Regimen sanitatis,* fol. 6ovb.
89. Ibid.
90. *Regimen sanitatis,* 1.5; *Praxis medicinalis, 7.*
91. Ibid.
92. Ibid.
93. Ibid.
94. Ibid., fol. 61ra.

12. Diseases in Europe

1. We can only hypothesize that the "domestication" of fire by mankind, known in Europe as far back as 400,000 years ago, must have made it possible to ward off predators and, through the cooking of food, prevent a certain number of parasites.

2. Accidents represented 10 percent of the causes of death among the Eskimos of Greenland in the middle of the nineteenth century; 80 percent were hunting accidents.

3. See in particular Sigerist (1951); Brothwell and Sandison (1967); Steinbock (1976); Grmek (1983b); Capasso (1985); Ortner and Putschar (1985). The term "pathocenosis" was coined by Grmek in 1969 to designate the structured set of pathological states present within a certain population at a given point in time. In a stable ecological situation, the pathocenosis tends toward a state of equilibrium.

4. Note that smallpox and measles were not known to the physicians of ancient Greece.

5. Grmek (1983b), 42.

6. The summary presented here is largely borrowed from Grmek (1983b) and Corvisier (1985).

7. Concerning malaria in antiquity, see Grmek (1983b) and, especially, Jones (1909), Celli (1925), and Bruce-Chwatt and De Zulueta (1980).

8. *Aphorismi,* 6.46.

9. Corvisier (1985), 118–121.

10. Grmek (1983b), 248–249.

11. Ibid., 461–462.

12. The bibliography concerning the plague of Athens is quite rich; see especially Page (1953); MacArthur (1958); Scarborough (1970); Longrigg (1980); Holladay (1988).

13. Krause (1825); Haeser (1875). See Grmek (1983b).

14. For epidemics in Italy during ancient times, see also Corradi (1865) and Grimm (1965).

15. Schnurrer (1823); Haeser (1875).

16. Grmek (1991b).

17. See especially Schmitt (1936); Gilliam (1961); Litmann (1973).

18. See Sabbah (1982).

19. *De re rustica,* 1.12.2.

20. For the outbreak of leprosy in Europe, see Jeanselme (1931); Grmek (1983b); Manchester (1984).

21. Shrewsbury (1949).

22. Biraben (1975); Allen (1979); Bratton (1981).

23. Chaumartin (1946); Wickersheimer (1966).

24. Proust (1893).

25. Wickersheimer (1966).

26. The existence of crossover immunities between leprosy and tuberculosis gave rise to the hypothesis that leprosy would be eliminated by a sharp increase in tuberculosis. See Grmek (1969 and 1978), and (1983b), 298; Manchester (1984). For the history of leprosy, see also Brody (1974); Bériac (1988).

27. Biraben (1975–76) (with bibliography). Among the most recent publications, see McNeill (1976); Bulst (1979); Williman (1983); Gottfried (1983).

28. Grmek (1980).

Bibliography

Anthologies

Agrimi, J., and C. Crisciani, eds. (1980). *Malato, medico e medicina nel Medioevo* (anthology of essays). Turin.

Brock, A. J. (1929). *Greek Medicine; Being Extracts Illustrative of Medical Writers from Hippocrates to Galen.* London and Toronto.

Cohen, M. R., and I. E. Drabkin (1958). *A Source Book in Greek Science,* 2d ed. Cambridge, Mass.

Corner, G. W. (1927). *Anatomical Texts of the Earlier Middle Ages.* Washington.

Diels, H. (1879). *Doxographi Graeci.* Berlin.

Diels, H., and W. Kranz (1951). *Die Fragmente der Vorsokratiker,* 6th ed., 3 vols. Berlin.

Dumont, J.-P. (1988). *Les Présocratiques.* Paris.

Firpo, L. (1972). *Medicina medievale: Testi dell'Alto Medioevo.* Turin.

Freeman, K. (1946). *The Pre-Socratic Philosophers: A Companion to Diels.* Oxford.

Ideler, J.-L. (1841–1842). *Physici et medici Graeci minores,* 2 vols. Berlin. (Repr., Amsterdam, 1963.)

Kollesch, J., and D. Nickel (1979). *Die antike Heilkunst.* Leipzig.

Manuli, P. (1980). *Medicina e antropologia nella tradizione antica* (anthology of essays). Turin.

Müri, W. (1962). *Der Arzt im Altertum,* 3d ed. Munich.

Pasquinelli, A. (1958). *I presocratici: Frammenti e testimonianze.* Turin.

Pazzini, A., ed. (1958). *Corpus scriptorum medicorum infimae latinitatis et prioris medii aevi.* Rome.

———, ed. (1971). *Crestomazia della letteratura medica in volgare dei due primi secoli della lingua.*

Rose, V. (1870). *Anecdota Graeca et Graecolatina.* Berlin. (Repr., Amsterdam, 1963.)

Sachau, E. (1870). *Inedita Syriaca.* Vienna.

Theil, P. (1965). *L'Esprit éternel de la médecine: Anthologie des écrits médicaux anciens,* vol. 1, *L'Antiquité occidentale.* Paris.

Primary Sources

Abano, Pietro. See Peter of Abano

'Abd al-Latif al-Bagdadi (1162–1231)

The Eastern Key, ed. and trans. K. H. Zand, J. A. Videan, and I. E. Videan. London, 1965.
[Treatise on diabetes], ed. H. J. Thies. Bonn, 1971.

Abraham ibn Ezra (ca. 1090–1167)

Book of Medical Experiments, ed. and trans. J. O. Leibowitz and S. Marcus. Jerusalem, 1984.

Abu'l-Qasim az-Zahrawi (ca. 936–ca. 1013)

The Compilation (of Medical Knowledge) for Those Who Cannot Themselves Practice Medicine, book 30, *Surgical Operations and Instruments*, ed. and trans. M. S. Spink and G. L. Lewis. Berkeley and Los Angeles, 1973.

Abu Sa'id ibn Bahtisu' (d. 1058)

[Concerning the treatment of diseases of the body and the soul], ed. F. Klein-Franke. Beirut, 1977.

Aetius of Amida (6th c.)

Libri medicinales, ed. A. Olivieri. Vols. 1–4, Leipzig and Berlin, 1935. Vols. 5–8, Berlin, 1950.

Agnellus of Ravenna (6th or 7th c.)

Commentaria in librum de sectis Galeni, ed. and trans. L. G. Westerink. Buffalo, 1981.

Albertus Magnus (1193–1280)

Opera omnia, ed. A. Borgnet. Paris, 1890–1899.

Albucasis (ca. 936–ca. 1013)

On Surgery and Instruments, ed. M. S. Spink and G. L. Lewis. Berkeley and Los Angeles, 1973.

Alderotti, Taddeo. See Taddeo Alderotti

Aldobrandino of Siena (d. 1287)

Le Régime du corps, ed. L. Landouzy and R. Pepin. Paris, 1911.

Alexander of Thralles (525–ca. 605)

Libri duodecim de re medica (Therapeutica), ed. T. Puschmann. Vienna, 1878–1879. (Repr., Amsterdam, 1963.)

ʿAli ibn al-ʿAbbas al-Magusi (late 10th c.)

[Complete exposition of the medical art, or, Royal book]. Bulaq, 1877. Anatomical portion, ed. P. De Koning, in *Three Arabic Treatises of Anatomy,* Leiden, 1896. Lat. trans., Constantine of Africa, *Pantegni,* Lyons, 1515, and Basel, 1536; Stephen of Pisa (known as Stephen of Antioch), *Regalis dispositio,* Venice, 1492.

Alphanus of Salerno (11th c.)

De quattuor humoribus, ed. P. Capparoni. Rome, 1928.
See also Nemesius of Emesa; Salerno (school of)

Anonymus Londinensis

Anonymi Londinensis ex Aristotelis iatricis Menoniis et aliis medicis eclogae, ed. and trans. W. H. S. Jones. London, 1947.

Anonymus Parisinus

De morbis acutis et chronicis, ed. and trans. I. Garofalo and B. Fuchs. Leiden, 1997.

Anthimus (6th century)

De observatione ciborum ad Theodoricum regem Francorum epistula, ed. and trans. H. S. Weber, Leiden, 1924.

Antoine Ricart (d. 1422)

De quantitatibus et proportionibus humorum, ed. J.-M. Dureau-Lapeyssonie. Paris, 1966.

Antonio Guaineri (d. ca. 1445)

Opera omnia. Venice, 1508.
De peste, in Agrimi and Crisciani (1980).
De pleuresi. Lyons, 1525.

Antonius Musa (1st c. B.C.)

De herba vettonica, ed. E. Howald and H. E. Sigerist. Leipzig and Berlin 1927.

Apollonios of Kition (1st c. B.C.)

Commentarius in Hippocratem de articulis, ed. H. Schöne. Leipzig, 1896.

Pseudo-Apuleius (4th c.)

Codex Casinensis 97. Repr. F. W. Hunger, Leiden, 1935.
Herbarius, ed. E. Howald and H. E. Sigerist. Leipzig and Berlin, 1927.

Archigenes (2d c.)

Fragmenta medica, ed. C. Brescia. Naples, 1955.

Arderne, John. See John Arderne

Aretaeus the Cappadocian (1st c.)

*De causis et signis acutorum et diuturnorum morborum: De curatione acutorum et diutur-
norum morborum,* trans. F. Adams. London, 1856.

Aristotle (384–322 B.C.)

De generatione animalium, ed. and trans. A. L. Peck. London and Cambridge, Mass.,
   1953, 2d ed.
Historia animalium, ed. and trans. A. L. Peck. London and Cambridge, Mass., 1965–
   1970. Trans.: D. W. Thompson. Oxford, 1910.
De motu animalium, ed. and trans. M. Nussbaum. Princeton, 1978.
De partibus animalium, ed. and trans. A. L. Peck. London and Cambridge, Mass.,
   1968, 4th ed. Trans. D. M. Balme. Oxford, 1972.
Parva naturalia, ed. D. Ross. Oxford, 1955.
Problemata, ed. and trans. W. H. S. Hett. London, 1957–1961.

Arnald of Villanova (ca. 1240–1311)

Opera medica omnia, ed. M. R. McVaugh, L. Demaitre, P. Gil Sotres, J. A. Paniagua, García Ballester, E. Sanchez Salor, R. J. Durling, and others. Barcelona, 1975–1990.
Opera omnia. Venice, 1505; Basel, 1585.

"Articella"

Latin collection of medical treatises, used as a textbook. The first editions contain: *Liber Johannitii qui dicitur Ysagoge; De pulsibus Philareti; De urinis Theophili; Aphorismi Hippocratis in ordine collecti; Aphorismi eiusdem cum commento Galeni; Liber pronosticorum Hippocratis; Liber regiminis acutorum Hippocratis; Liber epidemiarum Hippocratis; Liber Hippocratis qui intitulatur de natura fetus; Liber Galeni qui dicitur Tegni sive Ars parva; Gentilis de Fulgineo de divisione librorum Galeni; Libellus de lege Hippocratis et libellus qui dicitur iusiurandum.* Venice, 1483; Lyons, 1525.

Asclepiades of Bithynia (late 2d c. B.C.)

Fragmenta, trans. R. M. Green. New Haven, 1955.

Avenzoar. See Ibn Zuhr

Averroës (Ibn Rushd, 1126–1198)

Colliget seu de medicina libri septem [The generalities of medicine], ed. J. M. Forneas Besteiro and C. Alvarez de Morales. Madrid, 1987.
[Commentary on the Cantica of Avicenna]. Venice, 1484.

Avicenna (Ibn Sina, 980–1037)

Book of the Cures (of the Soul), book 6, *Of the Soul,* trans. E. A. Van Dyck. Verona, 1906.
[Canon of medicine], ed. A. H. Hakeem. New Delhi, 1982. Eng. trans. of the first book, O. C. Gruber, London, 1930, and M. H. Shah, Karachi, 1966.
Poem on Medicine, trans. H. C. Krueger. Springfield, 1963.

Bacon, Roger (1214–1294)

Opera hactenus inedita, ed. R. Steele, 16 fascicles. Oxford, 1905–1940 (see in particular fasc. 9, *De retardatione accidentium senectutis cum aliis opusculis de rebus medicinalibus,* ed. A. G. Little and E. Withington, 1928).
Opus majus, trans. R. B. Burke. Philadelphia, 1928.

Bartholomaeus of Salerno (12th c.)

Practica, ed. S. De Renzi, in *Collectio Salernitana*, vol. 4. Naples, 1856.
See also Salerno (school of)

Benzi, Ugo. See Ugo Benzi

Bernard de Gordon (d. ca. 1320)

De conservatione vitae humanae (added to *Lilium medicinae*). Lyons, 1574.
Practica dicta Lilium medicinae. Naples, 1480, and Venice, 1496.

al-Biruni (973–1048)

Book of Medicinal Drugs, ed. and trans. H. M. Said, *Al-Biruni's Book on Pharmacy and Materia Medica*. Karachi, 1973.
[Book of stones], ed. F. Krenkow. Hyderabad, 1936–37.
Chronology of Ancient Peoples, trans. E. Sachau. London, 1879.
[Letter containing a catalog of the works of Rhazes], ed. P. Kraus. Paris, 1936.
[Selected works], ed. G. Strohmaier. Leipzig, 1991.
[al-Biruni and Ibn Sina,] [Questions and answers], ed. S. H. Nasr and M. Mohaghegh. Teheran, 1972.

Bonvesin de la Riva (13th c.)

De magnalibus Mediolani: Le meraviglie di Milano. Milan, 1974.

Bruno de Longoburgo (13th c.)

Cyrurgia magna, ed. S. P. Hall. Oxford, 1957.

Caelius Aurelianus (5th c.)

Capsula eburnea.
Gynaecia (Lat. text), ed. M. F. Drabkin and I. E. Drabkin. Baltimore, 1951.
De morbis acutis [= *Celeres passiones*]: *De morbis diuturnis* [= *Tardae passiones*], ed. and trans. I. E. Drabkin. Chicago, 1950.
Prognostica Ypocratis, ed. K. Sudhoff, in *Archiv für Geschichte der Medizin*, 1916, and H. E. Sigerist, in *Archiv für Geschichte der Medizin*, 1921.

Cassiodorus (ca. 480–ca. 575)

De institutione divinarum litterarum. In J. P. Migne, ed., *Patrologia Latina*, vol. 70.

Cassius Felix (5th c.)

De medicina, ed. V. Rose. Leipzig, 1879.

Celsus (Aulus Cornelius Celsus, 1st c. A.D.)

De medicina, ed. and trans. W. G. Spencer. London and Cambridge, Mass., 1935–1938.

Constantine of Africa (ca. 1015–1087)

De anatomia, ed. V. Angrisani. Rome, 1968.

Breviarium dictum viaticum (trans. of the treatise by Ibn al-Gazzar). Lyons, 1511 and 1515 (in Rhazis, *Opera parva*).

Liber de chirurgia, ed. M. T. Malato and L. Loria. Rome, 1960.

Liber de coitu, ed. E. Montero-Cartelle. Santiago de Compostela, 1983.

De melancholia (trans. of the treatise by Ishaq ibn 'Imran), ed. K. Garbers. Hamburg, 1977. Ed. M. T. Malato and U. De Martini. Rome, 1959.

Opera conquisita undique magni studio. Basel, 1536 and 1539.

Pantegni (trans. of the treatise by 'Ali ibn al-'Abbas al-Magusi). Lyons, 1515, and Basel, 1536.

De urinis (trans. of the treatise by Ishaq al-Isra'ili), ed. E. Fontana. Pisa, 1966.

Ysagoge Johannitii ad Tegni Galeni (trans. of the treatise by Hunayn ibn Ishaq). Leipzig, 1497 (see Articella); modern ed., G. Maurach, in *Sudhoffs Archiv für Geschichte der Medizin*, 1978.

Copho (11th c.)

Anatomia porci, trans. T. N. Haviland. In *Wiener tierärztliche Wochenschrift*, 1960.

Ars medendi. Hagenau, 1532.

Despars, Jacques. See Jacques Despars

Diocles of Carystos (4th c. B.C.)

Ad Antigonum regem epistula de tuenda valetudine, ed. W. Jaeger. Berlin, 1938. (Repr., 1963.)

Fragmenta, ed. M. Wellmann. Berlin, 1901.

Dioscorides (1st c.)

Codex Neapolitanus. Photographic reproduction by C. Bertelli, S. Lilla, and G. Orofino. Rome and Graz, 1992.

Codex Vindobonensis med. gr. 1. Photographic reproduction by H. Gerstinger. Graz, 1970.
De materia medica, trans. R. T. Gunther. London, 1959.

Dominicus Gundisalvi (12th c.)

De divisione philosophiae, ed. L. Baur. In *Beiträge zur Geschichte der Philosophie des Mittelalters.* Münster, 1903.

Erasistratus (ca. 330–ca. 250 B.C.)

Fragmenta, ed. and comm. I. Garofalo. Pisa, 1988.

Erotian (1st c.)

Vocum hippocraticarum collectio, ed. E. Nachmanson. Göteborg and Uppsala, 1918.

al-Farabi (ca. 870–950)

[Philosophical works], ed. F. Dieterici. Leiden, 1890–1892. 2d ed., ed. A. Badawi, Benghazi, 1980.

Galen (129–ca. 210) [including the pseudo-Galenic works]

Opera omnia, ed. C. G. Kühn, 20 vols. Leipzig, 1821–1833. (Repr., Hildesheim, 1964–65).
Administrationes anatomicae. Vols. 1–9, Kühn, 2:215–731; trans. C. Singer, London, 1956. Vols. 9–15, ed. and trans. W. L. H. Duckworth, M. C. Lyons, and B. Towers, Cambridge, 1962.
An in arteriis natura sanguis contineatur. Kühn, 4:703–736. Ed. and trans. D. J. Furley and J. S. Wilkie. Princeton, 1984.
De animi cuiuslibet peccatorum dignotione et curatione, trans. P. W. Harkins. Columbus, 1963.
De bono habitu. Kühn, 4:750–756. Trans. R. J. Penella. Rheinisch Museum Philologie, 1977.
De captionibus penes dictione [= De sophismatis]. Kühn, 14:582–598. Ed. and trans. R. B. Edlow. Leiden, 1977.
De causis respirationis. Kühn, 4:465–469. Trans. D. J. Furley and J. S. Wilkie. Princeton, 1984.
De cognoscendis curandisque animi morbis, trans. P. W. Harkins. Columbus, 1963.
De cuiuslibet animi peccatorum dignotione et medela. Kühn, 5:58–103. Trans. P. W. Harkins. Columbus, 1963.

De curandi ratione per venae sectionem. Kühn, 11:250–316. Trans. P. Brain. Cambridge, Mass., 1986.

De diaeta in morbis acutis secundum Hippocratem. Kühn, 19:182–221. Trans. (of the Arabic text) M. C. Lyons. Berlin, 1969.

De dignotione ex insomniis. Kühn, 6:832–835. Trans. S. M. Oberhelman. In *Journal of the History of Medicine,* 1983.

De elementis ex Hippocratis sententia, ed. and trans. P. De Lacy. Berlin, 1996.

De examinando medico, ed. (of the Arabic text) and trans. A. Z. Iskandar. Berlin, 1988.

De experientia medica, ed. (of the Arabic text) and trans. R. Walzer. Oxford, 1944. Also trans. R. Walzer and M. Frede. Indianapolis, 1984.

De facultatibus naturalibus. Kühn, 2:1–214. Ed. and trans. A. J. Brock. Cambridge, Mass., 1979, 6th ed.

De locis affectis. Kühn, 8:1–452. Trans. R. E. Siegel. Basel and New York, 1976.

De marcore [= *De marasmo*]. Kühn, 7:666–704. Trans. C. Theoharides. In *Journal of the History of Medicine,* 1971.

De motu musculorum. Kühn, 4:367–464. Trans. C. M. Goss. In *American Journal of Anatomy,* 1968.

De musculorum dissectione. Kühn, 18(B):926–1026. Trans. C. M. Goss. In *Anatomical Records,* 1963.

De nervorum dissectione. Kühn, 2:831–856. Trans. C. M. Goss. In *American Journal of Anatomy,* 1966. Ed. (of the Arabic text) and trans. E. S. Smith. Ann Arbor, 1978.

De optima corporis nostri constitutione. Kühn, 4:737–749. Trans. R. J. Penella. In *Bulletin of the History of Medicine,* 1973.

De ossibus ad tirones. Kühn, 2:732–778. Ed. and trans. M. G. Moore. Ann Arbor, 1969. Trans. C. M. Goss and E. G. Chodkowski. In *American Journal of Anatomy,* 1984.

De partibus artis medicativae, ed. (of the Arabic text) and trans. M. C. Lyons (based on the Latin text, ed. H. Schöne). Berlin, 1969.

De placitis Hippocratis et Platonis. Kühn, 5:181–805. Ed. and trans. P. De Lacy. Berlin, 1978–1984.

De praenotione ad Epigenem. Kühn, 14:599–673. Ed. and trans. V. Nutton. Berlin, 1979.

De propriorum animi cuiuslibet affectuum dignotione et curatione. Kühn, 5:1–57. Trans. P. W. Harkins. Columbus, 1963.

De sanitate tuenda. Kühn, 6:1–452. Trans. R. M. Green. Springfield, 1951.

De secretis mulierum: De secretis virorum, trans. (of the Arabic text) M. Levey. In *Janus,* 1968.

De sectis ad eos qui introducuntur. Kühn, 1:64–105. Trans. R. Walzer and M. Frede. Indianapolis, 1984.

De semine. Kühn, 4:512–651. Ed. and trans. P. De Lacy. Berlin, 1992.

De tremore, palpitatione, convulsione et rigore. Kühn, 7:584–642. Trans. D. Sider and

M. McVaugh. In *Transactions and Studies of the College of Physicians of Philadelphia*, 1979.

De tumoribus praeter naturam. Kühn, 7:705–732. Ed. and trans. J. Reedy. Michigan, 1968.

De usu partium corporis humani. Kühn, 3:1–939. Trans. M. T. May. Ithaca, 1968.

De usu pulsuum. Kühn, 5:149–180. Trans. D. J. Furley and J. S. Wilkie. Princeton, 1984.

De usu respirationis. Kühn, 4:470–511. Ed. and trans. D. J. Furley and J. S. Wilkie. Princeton, 1984.

De venae sectione adversus Erasistrateos Romae degentes. Kühn, 11:187–249. Trans. P. Brain. Cambridge, Mass., 1986.

De venae sectione adversus Erasistratum. Kühn, 11:147–186. Trans. P. Brain. Cambridge, Mass., 1986.

De venarum arteriarumque dissectione. Kühn, 2:779–830. Trans. C. M. Goss. In *Anatomical Records*, 1961. Ed. (of the Arabic text) and trans. E. S. Smith. Ann Arbor, 1978.

In Hippocratis de aere, aquis et locis. Unpublished Arabic text, ms. Cairo, Tal ʿat Tibb 550. Ed. (of the Hebrew text) and trans. A. Wasserstein. Jerusalem, 1982.

In Hippocratis de officina medici commentarii III. Kühn, 18(B):629–925. Ed. (of the Arabic text) and trans. M. C. Lyons. Berlin, 1963.

In Platonis Timaeum commentarius, ed. (of the Arabic text) and trans. P. Kraus and R. Walzer. London, 1951.

Institutio logica, trans. J. S. Kiefer. Baltimore, 1964.

Methodus medendi. Kühn, 10:1–1021. Trans. R. J. Hankinson. Oxford, 1991.

Subfiguratio empirica, ed. J. Atzpodien. Husum, 1986.

Gariopontus (11th c.)

Passionarius. Lyons, 1526.

Gentile da Foligno (d. 1348)

Consilia. Pavia, 1488, and Venice, 1502.

Expositiones . . . cum textu Avicennae. Venice, 1492.

Expositio et quaestiones subtilissimae super primo libro Microtechni Galeni. Venice, 1576.

Tractatus de pestilentia et causis eius et remediis, ed. K. Sudhoff. In *Archiv für Geschichte der Medizin*, 1911.

Gerson, Jean. See Jean Gerson

Gilbertus Anglicus (Gilbert of Aquila, 13th c.)

Compendium medicinae, tam morborum universalium quam particularium. Lyons, 1510.

Experimenta, ed. P. Pansier. In *Janus*, 1903.

Gilles de Corbeil (ca. 1140–1224)

Carmina medica, ed. L. Choulant. Leipzig, 1826.

Guaineri, Antonio. See Antonio Guaineri

Guglielmo de Saliceto (ca. 1210–ca. 1280)

Cirurgia. Piacenza, 1476, and Venice, 1490.
Summa conservationis et curationis corporis. Piacenza, 1475, and Venice, 1489.

Guido da Vigevano (14th c.)

Anatomia, ed. E. Wickersheimer. Paris, 1926.
Liber conservacionis sanitatis senis (Ms. Parisinus lat. 1015).

Guillaume de Saint-Thierry (12th c.)

De natura corporis et animae, ed. G. Rialdi. Pisa, 1967. Also ed. M. Lemoine. Paris, 1988.

Gundisalvi, Dominicus. See Dominicus Gundisalvi

Guy de Chauliac (d. 1368)

Inventarium sive collectorium in parte chirurgicali medicinae [= *Chirurgia magna*, or, *Ars chirurgica Guidonis Cauliaci*]. Venice, 1498 and 1546 (both also include treatises on surgery by Bruno, Teodorico, Rolando, Ruggiero, Lanfranchi, and Leonardo Bertapaglia). Ed. E. Nicaise, Paris, 1890.

Heinrich von Pfalzpeint (or Pfolspeundt, 15th c.)

[Book of surgery], ed. H. Haeser and A. Middeldorpf. Berlin, 1868.

Henri de Mondeville (ca. 1270–ca. 1330)

Cyrurgia, ed. J. L. Pagel. Berlin, 1892.

Herophilus (ca. 330–ca. 260 B.C.)

Fragmenta, ed., trans., and comm. H. von Staden. Cambridge and New York, 1989.

Hildegard von Bingen (1098–1179)

Liber compositae medicinae [= *Causae et curae*], ed. P. Kaiser. Leipzig, 1903.
Liber simplicis medicinae [= *Physica*], ed. C. Daremberg and F. A. Reuss. In J. P. Migne, ed., *Patrologia Latina*, vol. 197.

Hippocrates (460–377 B.C.)

Opera omnia, ed. É. Littré, 10 vols. Paris, 1839–1861. (Repr., Amsterdam, 1973–1978.)
Opera selecta. Ed. and trans. W. H. S. Jones, Cambridge, Mass., and London, 1923–1931 (Loeb, 1, 2, and 4); W. H. S. Jones and E. T. Withington, Cambridge, Mass., and London, 1928 (Loeb, 3); P. Potter, Cambridge, Mass., and London, 1988 (Loeb, 5 and 6).
De aere, aquis, lucis, ed. H. Diller. Berlin, 1970.
De arte, ed. J. Jouanna. Paris, 1988.
De diaeta [*Regimen*], ed. R. Joly with S. Byl. Berlin, 1984.
De morbis II, ed. J. Jouanna. Paris, 1983.
De natura hominis, ed. J. Jouanna. Berlin, 1975.
De prisca medicina, ed. J. Jouanna. Paris, 1990.

Hugh of Saint-Victor (ca. 1096–1141)

Didascalicon, ed. C. H. Buttimer. Washington, 1939. Trans. J. Taylor. New York, 1961.

Humbert de Romans (13th c.)

De eruditione praedicatorum, book 2, *De modo prompte cudendi sermones circa omne hominum genus.* In *Bibliotheca Maxima Patrum,* 25, Rome, 1739.

Hunayn ibn Ishaq (Johannitius, 809–877)

Questions about Medicine, trans. P. Ghalioungui. Cairo, 1980.
Extracts of the work cited above, known primarily in the Latin version by Constantine of Africa: *Ysagoge Johannitii ad Tegni Galeni.* Leipzig, 1497 (see Articella). Modern ed., G. Maurach, in *Sudhoffs Archiv für Geschichte der Medizin,* 1978, 148–174.
[On the Syriac and Arabic translations of Galen], ed. G. Bergsträsser. Leipzig, 1925.

Ibn Abi Usaybi'a (1203–1270)

[Sources of information concerning the categories of physicians], ed. A. Müller. Cairo, 1882.

Ibn Butlan (d. ca. 1063)

[Banquet of physicians], ed. F. Klein-Franke. Wiesbaden, 1985.
Codex Vindobonensis series nova 644 (Tacuinum sanitatis). Reproduction, Graz, 1967.
Tacuinum sanitatis, ed. H. Elkhadem. Louvain, 1990.

Ibn Gulgul (10th c.)

[Categories of physicians and scholars], ed. F. Sayyid. Cairo, 1955.

Ibn Gumay' (d. 1198)

Treatise to Salah ad-Din on the Revival of the Art of Medicine, ed. and trans. H. Fähndrich. Wiesbaden, 1983.

Ibn Hindu (11th c.)

[Key of medicine], ed. M. Mohaghegh and M. T. Daneshpajuh. Teheran, 1989.

Ibn Ridwan (d. 1068)

On the Prevention of Bodily Ills in Egypt, ed. and trans. A. S. Gamal and W. S. Dols. Berkeley, 1984.
[Useful book on the methods of teaching medicine], ed. J. Grand'Henry. Louvain-la-Neuve, 1984.
[The way to happiness through the medical art], ed. A. Dietrich. Göttingen, 1982.

Ibn Rushd. See Averroës

Ibn Sina. See Avicenna

Ibn Zuhr (Avenzoar, ca. 1092–ca. 1162)

[Preparation of life by therapy and regimen], Lat. trans. Al-Teisir. Venice, 1490.

Ishaq ibn 'Imran (10th c.)

Maqala fi l-malihuliya [= *Constantini Africani libri duo de melancholia*], ed. K. Garbers. Hamburg, 1977.

Isidore of Seville (ca. 570–636)

Etymologiarum sive Originum libri XX, ed. W. M. Lindsay. Oxford, 1911.
Liber IV: De medicina, trans. W. D. Sharpe. Philadelphia, 1964.

Jacopo da Forli (d. 1413)

In Hippocratis aphorismos et Galeni super eisdem commentarios expositio. Venice, 1547.

Jacques Despars (15th c.)

Expositio supra librum Canonis Avicenne. Lyons, 1498.

Jan Yperman (d. 1330)

De cyrurgie (in Flemish), ed. C. Broeckx. Antwerp, 1866. Ed. E. C. Van Lersum. Leiden, 1912.

Jean de Bourgogne (d. 1372)

De epidemia, ed. G. Guttmann. Berlin, 1903. Ed. K. Sudhoff. In *Archiv für Geschichte der Medizin,* 1912.

Jean Gerson (1362–1428)

Decene quaestiones de medicorum statu, ed. R. Peitz. Pattensen, 1978.
De erroribus circa artem magicam: Harangua pro licentiandis in medicina. In *Opera omnia,* 1:210–219. Antwerp, 1706.
Oratio pro licentiandis in medicina. In *Opera omnia,* 4:712–717. Antwerp, 1706.

Johannes Mesue. See Yuhanna ibn Masawayh

Johannitius. See Hunayn ibn Ishaq

Johann von Ketham (15th c.)

Fasciculus medicine, ed. C. Singer. Florence, 1925.

John Arderne (b. 1307)

De arte phisicali et de cirurgia, trans. D'Arcy Power. London, 1922.
De fistula in ano. Medieval Eng. trans., ed. D'Arcy Power. London, 1910.

John of Alexandria (7th c.)

Commentaria in librum de sectis Galeni, ed. C. D. Pritchet. Leiden, 1982.

al-Kindi (9th c.)

Medical Formulary, ed. and trans. M. Levey. Madison and London, 1966.

Lanfranchi (13th c.)

Chirurgia magna, trans. R. von Fleischhacker. London, 1894.

Maimonides (Rabbi Mose ben Maimon, 1135–1204)

[Aphorisms], ed. (in part) P. Kahle. Leipzig and Berlin, 1934. Hebrew text *(Pirke Moshe bi-refu'ah)* ed. S. Muntner. Jerusalem, 1959.
Regimen of Health for the Sultan, trans. A. Bar-Sela, H. Hoff, and E. Faris. Philadelphia, 1964.

Marcellus de Bordeaux (5th c.)

De medicamentis, ed. E. Liechtenhan, J. Kollesch, and D. Nickel, 2 vols. Berlin, 1968.

Matthaeus Platearius (d. 1161)

Circa instans [= *Liber de simplici medicina*]. Venice, 1497.
See also Salerno (school of)

Maynus de Mayneriis (d. ca. 1364)

Praxis medicinalis. Lyons, 1586 (erroneously attributed to Arnald of Villanova).
De preservatione ab epydimia, ed. R. Simonini. Modena, 1923.
Regimen sanitatis. Louvain, 1482, and Lyons, 1586.

Michele Savonarola (ca. 1384–ca. 1467)

De cura languoris animi ex morbo venientis, ed. C. Menini. Ferrara, 1956.

Ad mulieres Ferrarienses de regimine pregnantium, ed. L. Belloni. Milan, 1952.
Practica maior. Venice, 1547 and 1559.
De preservatione a peste et eius cura, ad civitatem Ferrarie, ed. K. Sudhoff. In *Archiv für Geschichte der Medizin,* 1925.

Mondino de' Liuzzi (ca. 1275–1326)

Anathomia, trans. C. Singer. Florence, 1924.

Mustio (6th c.)

Gynaecia, ed. V. Rose. Leipzig, 1882.

Nemesius of Emesa (4th c.)

De natura hominis, ed. W. Telfer. London, 1955. Ed. M. Morani. Leipzig, 1987.

Nicander of Colophon (2d c. B.C.)

Theriaka and *Alexipharmaka,* ed. and trans. A. S. F. Gow and A. F. Scholfield. Cambridge, 1953. Corr. P. Knoefel. Lewiston, 1991.

Nicholas of Damascus (64 B.C.–A.D. 14)

De plantis, ed. (in five languages) H. J. Drossaart Lulofs and E. L. J. Poortman. Amsterdam, 1989.

Nicholas of Salerno (12th c.)

Antidotarium. Venice, 1471. Repr. and comm. D. Goltz. In *Mittelalterliche Pharmazie und Medizin.* Stuttgart, 1976.

Opicino de' Canistris (13th c.)

De laudibus civitatis Ticinensis: Il libro delle lodi della città di Pavia. Pavia, 1984.

Oribasius (4th c.)

Collectiones medicae, ed. J. Raeder, 4 vols. Leipzig and Berlin, 1928–1933. (Repr., Amsterdam, 1964.) Trans. of book 47 *(De laqueis),* C. L. Day. Lawrence, Kans., 1967.
Oribasius latinus, ed. H. Morland. Oslo, 1940.

Synopsis ad Eustathium: Libri ad Eunapium, ed. J. Raeder. Leipzig and Berlin, 1926. (Repr., Amsterdam, 1964.)

Paul of Aegina (Paulus Aegineta, 7th c.)

Epitomae medicae, trans. and comm. F. Adams *(The Seven Books of Paulus Aegineta),* 3 vols. London, 1844–1847.

Petrarca, Francesco (Petrarch, 1304–1374)

Invectiva contra medicum, ed. P. G. Ricci and B. Martinelli. Rome, 1987.

Pfalzpeint, Heinrich von. See Heinrich von Pfalzpeint

Philaretes (7th c.)

De pulsibus, ed. and comm. J. A. Pithis. Husum, 1983.

Philomenos (2d c.)

De venenatis animalibus eorumque remediis, ed. M. Wellmann. Leipzig and Berlin, 1908.

Peter Comestor (d. 1198)

Sermo XLII Synodicus. In J. P. Migne, ed., *Patrologia Latina,* vol. 198.

Peter of Abano (ca. 1250–1316)

Conciliator differentiarum philosophorum et praecipue medicorum. Venice, 1476 and 1565. (Repr., Padua, 1985.)
De venenis. Mantua, 1473, and Padua, 1473. Ed. and comm. A. Benedicenti. Florence, 1949.

Peter of Spain (Petrus Hispanus, ca. 1220–1277)

Summule logicales, ed. I. M. Bochenski. Turin, 1947. Ed. L. M. De Rijk. Assen, 1972.
Thesaurus pauperum, ed. M. H. da Rocha Pereira. In *Obras Médicas de Pedro Hispano.* Coimbra, 1973.

Pietro da Tossignano (14th c.)

Consilium pro peste evitanda, ed. C. Singer. Florence, 1925.

Pietro Torrigiano (b. ca. 1275)

Plusquam commentum in Microtegni Galeni. Bologna, 1489, and Venice, 1557.

Platearius, Matthaeus. See Matthaeus Platearius

Plato (ca. 428–347 B.C.)

Timaeus, trans. F. M. Cornford. London, 1937. Trans. D. Lee. London, 1977.

Pliny the Elder (A.D. 23–79)

Historia naturalis, ed. and trans. H. Rackham, W. H. S. Jones, and D. E. Eichholz,
    10 vols. Cambridge, Mass., and London, 1938–1963.

Plutarch (ca. A.D. 48–ca. 125)

De tuenda sanitate praecepta, ed. J. Defradas and R. Klaer. Paris, 1985.

Praxagoras (4th c.)

Fragmenta, ed. and trans. F. Steckerl. Leiden, 1958.

Priscianus, Theodorus. See Theodorus Priscianus

Qusta ibn Luqa (10th c.)

[Book on infection], ed. H. Fähndrich. Stuttgart, 1987.

ar-Razi, Muhammad ibn Zakariya' (Rhazes, 865–925)

Anatomy, ed. P. De Koning. In *Three Arabic Treatises of Anatomy.* Leiden, 1896.
Book for the Salih al-Mansur. Numerous editions of the Lat. trans. *(Regimen ad Alman-*
    sorem), esp. book 9 [Special pathology a capite ad calcem]. First ed., Nonus
    Almansoris, Venice, 1483.
Book of Guidance, trans. A. J. Arberry. London, 1950.
Book of Smallpox and Measles, trans. W. A. Greenhill. London, 1848.
Book That Contains All. Hyderabad, 1955 and foll. years.

[Introduction to the medical art], ed. M. C. Vazquez de Benito. Salamanca, 1979.
Thirty-Three Clinical Observations, ed. and trans. E. Meyerhof. In *Isis*, 1935.

Rhazes. See ar-Razi

Ricart, Antoine. See Antoine Ricart

Rolando di Parma (13th c.)

Codex Casanatensis Lat. 1382. Photographic reproduction by G. Carbonelli. Rome, 1928.
Libellus de cyrurgia. Venice, 1498 and 1546.

Rufus of Ephesus (1st c.)

Opera, ed. C. Daremberg and E. Ruelle. Paris, 1879. (Repr., Amsterdam, 1963.)
De corporis humani appellationibus, ed. G. Kowalski. Göttingen, 1960.
De ictero (Lat. and Arabic texts), ed. M. Ullmann. Wiesbaden, 1983.
De melancholia, It. trans. A. Sacino. Rome, 1969.
Observationes medicae (Arabic text), ed. M. Ullmann, *Rufus von Ephesos Krankenjour-nale*. Wiesbaden, 1978.
De podagra (Lat. text), ed. H. Morland. Oslo, 1933.
Quaestiones medicinales, trans. A. Brock. In *Greek Medicine*. London and Toronto, 1929.

Ruggero di Parma (Rogerius Frugardi, 12th c.)

Cyrurgia, ed. K. Sudhoff. In *Beiträge zur Geschichte der Chirurgie im Mittelalter*, vol. 2. Leipzig, 1918.

Salerno (school of)

Regimen sanitatis Salernitanum. Pisa, 1484.
De Renzi, S., ed. *Collectio Salernitana: Ossia documenti inediti e trattati di medicina appartenenti alla Scuola Salernitana*, 5 vols. Naples, 1852–1859.
Giacosa, P. *Magistri Salernitani nondum editi*. Turin, 1901.
Lawn, B. *I Quesiti Salernitani*. Salerno, 1969.
———. *The Prose Salernitan Questions*. London, 1979.

Savonarola, Michele. See Michele Savonarola

Scribonius Largus (1st c.)

Compositiones, ed. S. Sconocchia. Leipzig, 1983.

Secreta secretorum (Pseudo-Aristotle)

Sirr al-asrar, ed. and trans. R. Steele. Oxford, 1920.

Serenus, Quintus (ca. 3d c.)

Liber medicinalis, ed. F. Vollmer. Leipzig and Berlin, 1916.

Sergius of Reshayna (6th c.)

[Two medical treatises], ed. E. Sachau, Inedita Syriaca. Vienna, 1870.

Soranos of Ephesus (1st c.)

Gynaecia, trans. O. Temkin. Baltimore, 1956. (Repr., Baltimore, 1992.)

Stephen of Alexandria (Stephen of Athens, 7th c.)

Commentaria in Galeni librum therapeuticum ad Glauconem, ed. F. R. Dietz. Königsberg, 1834.
Commentaria in Hippocratis aphorismos, ed. and trans. L. G. Westerink. Berlin, 1985–1996.
Commentaria in Hippocratis prognosticon, ed. and trans. J. M. Duffy. Berlin, 1983.

"Suda"

Suidae Lexicon, ed. A. Adler, 5 vols. Leipzig, 1928–1938. (Repr., Stuttgart, 1971–1977.)

Taddeo Alderotti (1223–ca. 1295)

De conservatione sanitatis. Bologna, 1477.
Consilia, ed. G. M. Nardi. Turin, 1937.
Expositiones in arduum aphorismorum Ippocratis volumen. Venice, 1527.
In Micratechnem Galeni commentaria. Naples, 1522.

Teodorico Borgognoni (d. 1298)

Cyrurgia, trans. E. Campbell and J. Colton, 2 vols. New York, 1955–1960.

Theodorus Priscianus (5th c.)

Euporiston, ed. V. Rose. Leipzig, 1894.

Theophanes Chrysobalantes (Theophanes Nonnos, 10th c.)

Epitome de curatione morborum Graece ac Latine, ed. I. S. Bernard. Gotha and Amsterdam, 1794–1795.

Theophilos Protospatharios (7th c.)

De corporis humani fabrica, ed. W. A. Greenhill. Oxford, 1842.
De urinis, ed. F. Morel. Paris, 1608. Ed. U. Bussemeker. In *Revue de philologie,* 1845. See Articella.

Theophrastus (372–287 B.C.)

Opera quae supersunt omnia, ed. F. Wimmer. Paris, 1866. (Repr., Frankfurt, 1964.)
Fragmenta et testimonia, ed. W. W. Fortenbaugh. Leiden, 1992.
Historia plantarum, ed. and trans. A. Hort. London and Cambridge, Mass., 1916.
Metaphysica, ed. and trans. M. Van Raalte. Leiden, 1993.
De sensibus, ed. and trans. G. M. Stratton. New York, 1964.

Ugo Benzi (1376–1439)

Consilia medica. Bologna, 1482.
Expositio super Aphorismos Hippocratis. Venice, 1517.

Ugolino da Montecatini (15th c.)

De balneis, ed. G. M. Nardi. Florence, 1950.

Ursus of Salerno (12th c.)

Aphorismi cum commentariis, ed. R. Creutz. In *Quellen und Studien für Geschichte der Naturwissenschaften und Medizin,* 1936.
De commixtionibus elementorum libellus, ed. W. Stürner. Stuttgart, 1976.
Compendium de urinis, ed. P. Giacosa. Turin, 1901.
See also Salerno (school of)

Vindicianus (4th c.)

Epistula ad Pentadium, ed. R. Peiper. In *Philologus,* 1874. Ed. V. Rose. In *Theodori Prisciani Euporiston.* Leipzig, 1894.
Gynaecia, ed. K. Sudhoff. In *Archiv für Geschichte der Medizin,* 1915. Ed. J. Schipper. Leipzig, 1921.

Walafrid Strabo (d. 849)

Hortulus, trans. R. Payne and W. Bunt. Pittsburgh, 1968.

William of Conches (b. 1080)

Philosophia mundi. Basel, 1531. In the form of a dialogue, *Dragmaticon philosophine,* Strasbourg, 1567 (repr., Frankfurt, 1967, and New York, 1968).

Yperman, Jan. See Jan Yperman

Yuhanna ibn Masawayh (Johannes Mesue, ca. 777–857)

Le Livre des axiomes médicaux [*Medical aphorisms*], ed. (of the Arabic text), medieval Lat. trans., and Fr. trans. D. Jacquart and G. Troupeau. Geneva, 1980.

Secondary Sources

Ackerknecht, E. H. (1955). *A Short History of Medicine.* New York. (Rev. ed., Baltimore, 1982.)
——— (1963). *Geschichte und Geographie der wichtigsten Krankheiten.* Stuttgart.
Adam, P. (1982). *Charité et assistance en Alsace au Moyen Age.* Strasbourg.
Affleck, G. (1947). *The History of Physical Education.* Philadelphia.
Agrimi, J., and C. Crisciani (1978a). "Malattia, malato, medico nell'ideologia medievale," in *Storia della sanità in Italia: Metodo e indicazioni di ricerca* (Rome), pp. 163–185.
——— (1978b). *Medicina del corpo e medicina dell'anima: Note sul sapere del medico fino all'inizio del secolo XIII.* Milan.
——— (1988). *Edocere medicos: Medicina scolastica nei secoli XIII–XV.* Milan and Naples.
——— (1990). "Per una ricerca su Experimentum-Experimenta: Riflessione epistemologica e tradizione medica," in Janni and Mazzini (1990).
——— (1992). "Immagini e ruoli della 'vetula' fra sapere medico e antropologia religiosa (sec. XIII–XV)," in *I poteri carismatici e informali* (Palermo), pp. 224–261.

———— (1994). *Les Consilia médicaux*. Turnhout. (*Typologie des sources du Moyen Age occidental*, fasc. 69.)

Albert, M. (1894). *Les Médecins grecs à Rome*. Paris.

Alberzoni, M. P., and O. Grassi, eds. (1989). *La carità a Milano nei secoli XII–XV.* Milan.

Albini, G. (1982). *Guerra, fame, peste: Crisi di mortalità e sistema sanitario nella Lombardia tardomedievale*. Bologna.

Allbutt, T. C. (1921). *Greek Medicine in Rome*. London. (Repr., New York, 1970.)

Allen, P. (1979). "The Justinianic Plague," *Byzantion* 49: 5–20.

Alston, M. N. (1944). "The Attitude of the Church towards Dissection before 1500," *Bulletin of the History of Medicine* 16: 221–238.

Alverny, M. T. d' (1982). "Translations and Translators," in R. L. Benson and G. Constable, eds., *Renaissance and Renewal in the Twelfth Century* (Oxford), pp. 421–462.

———— (1985). "Pietro d'Abano traducteur de Galien," *Medioevo* 11: 19–64.

Amacher, M. P. (1964). "Galen's Experiment on the Arterial Pulse and the Experiment Repeated," *Sudhoffs Archiv für Geschichte der Medizin* 48: 177–180.

Amundsen, D. W. (1978). "Medieval Canon Law on Medical and Surgical Practice by the Clergy," *Bulletin of the History of Medicine* 46: 22–44.

———— (1979). "Medicine and Surgery as Art or Craft: The Role of Schematic Literature in the Separation of Medicine and Surgery in the Late Middle Ages," *Transactions and Studies of the College of Physicians of Philadelphia*, 5th ser., 43–57.

———— (1982). "Medicine and Faith in Early Christianity," *Bulletin of the History of Medicine* 61: 326–350.

———— (1986). "The Medieval Catholic Tradition," in Numbers and Amundsen (1986), 65–107.

Amundsen, D. W., and G. B. Ferngren (1982). "Philanthropy in Medicine: Some Historical Perspectives," in Shelp (1982), 1–31.

———— (1986). "The Early Christian Tradition," in Numbers and Amundsen (1986), 40–64.

Anderson, M. E. (1953). *The Human Body in the Philosophy of St. Thomas Aquinas*. Washington.

André, J. (1981). *L'Alimentation et la cuisine à Rome*. Paris.

———— (1985). *Les Noms de plantes dans la Rome antique*. Paris.

———— (1991). *Le Vocabulaire latin de l'anatomie*. Paris.

Angel, J. L. (1972). "Ecology and Population in the Eastern Mediterranean," *World Archaeology* 4: 88–105.

Annawati, G. C. (1950). *Essai de bibliographie avicennienne*. Cairo.

Arbesmann, R. (1954). "The Concept of 'Christus medicus' in St. Augustine," *Traditio* 10: 1–28.

Ariès, P. (1975). *Essais sur l'histoire de la mort en Occident: Du Moyen Age à nos jours.* Paris.

——— (1977). *L'Homme devant la mort.* Paris.

Artelt, W. (1937). *Studien zur Geschichte der Begriffe "Heilmittel" und "Gift": Urzeit, Homer, Corpus hippocraticum.* Leipzig. (Repr., Darmstadt, 1968.)

——— (1940). *Die ältesten Nachrichten über die Sektion menschlicher Leichen im mittelalterlichen Abendland.* Berlin.

——— (1949). *Einführung in die Medizinhistorik.* Stuttgart.

——— (1953–1966). *Index zur Geschichte der Medizin, Naturwissenschaft und Technik,* 2 vols. Munich.

Ascheri, M. (1982). *I "consilia" dei giuristi medievali: Per un repertorio incipitario computerizzato.* Siena.

Assereto, G. (1983). "Pauperismo ed assistenza: Messa a punto di studi recenti," *Archivo storico italiano* 141: 253–271.

Avril, J. (1982). "La Pastorale des malades et des mourants aux XIIe et XIIIe siècles," in Braert and Verbeke (1982), 88–106.

Ayache, L. (1992). *Hippocrate.* Paris.

Baader, G. (1978). "Die Schule von Salerno," *Medizinhistorisches Journal* 3: 124–145.

——— (1981). "Galen im mittelalterlichen Abendland," in Nutton (1981). 213–228.

——— (1984). "Early Medieval Latin Adaptations of Byzantine Medicine in Western Europe," *Dumbarton Oaks Papers* 38: 251–259.

Baader, G., and G. Keil (1978). "Mittelalterliche Diagnostik," in Habricht, Marguth, and Wolf (1978), 121–144.

———, ed. (1982). *Medizin im mittelalterlichen Abendland.* Darmstadt.

Baader, G., and R. Winau, eds. (1989). *Die hippokratischen Epidemien: Theorie, Praxis, Tradition* (Verhandlungen des Ve Colloque hippocratique, Berlin, 1984). Stuttgart.

Baas, J. H. (1876). *Grundriss der Geschichte der Medizin und des heilenden Standes.* Stuttgart. (Eng. trans., New York, 1889.)

Balducelli, R. (1951). *Il concetto teologico di carità attraverso le maggiori interpretazioni patristiche e medievali di "I ad Cor. XIII."* Rome and New York.

Baldwin, J. W. (1970). *Masters, Princes, and Merchants: The Social Views of Peter the Chanter and His Circle,* 2 vols. Princeton.

Bariéty, M., and C. Coury (1963). *Histoire de la médecine.* Paris.

Barnes, J., J. Brunschwig, and M. Scholfield, eds. (1982). *Science and Speculation: Studies in Hellenistic Theory and Practice.* Cambridge and Paris.

Baroncelli, F., and G. Assereto (1980). "Pauperismo e religione nell'Italia moderna," *Società e storia* 7: 169–201.

Barry, J., and C. Jones, eds. (1991). *Medicine and Charity before the Welfare State.* London and New York.

Baumstark, A. (1922). *Geschichte der syrischen Literatur.* Bonn.

Bazàn, B. C., J. W. Wippel, G. Fransen, and D. Jacquart (1985). *Les Questions disputées et les questions quodlibétiques dans les facultés de théologie, de droit et de médecine.* Turnhout. (Typologie des sources du Moyen Age occidental, fasc. 44–45.)

Bean, W. B. (1981). "Changing Patterns of Ideas about Disease," in Rothschild (1981), 25–51.

Beaujouan, G. (1972). "Manuscrits médicaux du Moyen Age conservés en Espagne," *Mélanges de la Casa de Vélazquez* 8: 161–221.

——— (1975). "Réflexions sur les rapports entre théorie et pratique au Moyen Age," in J. E. Murdoch and E. Sylla, eds., *The Cultural Context of Medieval Learning* (Boston and Dordrecht), pp. 440–443.

———, ed. (1966). *Médecine humaine et vétérinaire à la fin du Moyen Age.* Geneva and Paris.

Beccaria, A. (1956). *I codici di medicina del periodo presalernitano (secolo IX, X et XI).* Rome.

——— (1959, 1961, 1971). "Sulle tracce di un antico canone latino di Ippocrate e di Galeno," *Italia medioevale e umanistica* 2 (1959): 1–56; 4 (1961): 1–75; 14 (1971): 1–23.

Beck, R. T. (1974). *The Cutting Edge: Early History of the Surgeons of London.* London.

Becker, M. B. (1974). "Aspects of Lay Piety in Early Renaissance Florence," in C. Trinkhaus and H. A. Oberman, eds., *The Pursuit of Holiness in Late Medieval and Renaissance Religion* (Leiden), pp. 177–199.

Benedetti, A. (1969). *Traumatologia al tempo di Ippocrate.* Rome.

Benedum, J. (1977). "Griechische Arztinschriften aus Kos," *Zeitschrift für Papyrologie und Epigraphie* 25: 272–274.

——— (1978). "Der Badearzt Asklepiades und seine bithynische Heimat," *Gesnerus* 35: 20–43.

Benton, J. F. (1982). "New Light on the 'Patria' of Arnald of Villanova," *Viator* 13: 245–257.

Benveniste, É. (1945). "La Doctrine médicale des Indo-Européens," *Revue de l'histoire des religions* 130: 5–12.

Berghoff, E. (1947). *Entwicklungsgeschichte des Krankheitsbegriffes.* Vienna.

Bergsträsser, G. (1913). *Hunain ibn Ishaq und seine Schule.* Leiden.

Bériac, F. (1988). *Histoire des lépreux au Moyen Age: Une société d'exclus.* Paris.

Bernabeo, R. (1987). "Le scuole della farmacologia romana," in Zanca (1987), 63–100.

Bertier, J. (1972). *Mnésithée et Dieuchès.* Leiden.

Biraben, J.-N. (1975–1976). *Les Hommes et la peste dans les pays européens et méditerranéens,* 2 vols. Paris and The Hague.

Birkenmajer, A. (1970). "Le Rôle joué par les médecins et les naturalistes dans la réception d'Aristote aux XIIe et XIIIe siècles" (1930), in *Études d'histoire des sciences et de la philosophie du Moyen Age* (Wrocław), pp. 73–87.

Bliquez, L. J., and A. Kazhdan (1984). "Four Testimonia to Human Dissection in Byzantine Times," *Bulletin of the History of Medicine* 58: 554–561.

Bloch, H. (1986). *Monte Cassino in the Middle Ages*. Rome.

Boncompagni, R. (1972). "Concezione della malattia e senso dell'individualità nei testi cnidi del 'Corpus hippocraticum,'" *Parole del passato* 27: 209–238.

Bonenfant, P. (1965). *Hôpitaux et bienfaisance publique dans les anciens Pays-Bas des origines à la fin du XVIIIe siècle*. Brussels.

Bono, J. J. (1984). "Medical Spirits and the Medieval Language of Life," *Traditio* 40: 91–130.

Bonser, W. (1963). *The Medical Background of Anglo-Saxon England*. London.

Bonuzzi, L. (1987). "Gli dei greci e i mali degli uomini," in Zanca (1987), 37–61.

Boulle, L., M. D. Grmek, et al. (1982). *Laennec: Catalogue des manuscrits scientifiques*. Paris.

Bourgeois, A. (1972). *Lépreux et maladreries du Pas-de-Calais*. Arras.

Bourgey, L. (1953). *Observation et expérience chez les médecins de la Collection hippocratique*. Paris.

Bourgey, L., and J. Jouanna, eds. (1975). *La Collection hippocratique et son rôle dans l'histoire de la médecine* (proceedings of the first Hippocratic Colloquium, Strasbourg, 1972). Leiden.

Bousquet, J. (1956). "Inscriptions de Delphes (7: Delphes et les Asclépiades)," *Bulletin de correspondance hellénique* 80: 579–591.

Braert, H., and W. Verbeke, eds. (1982). *Death in the Middle Ages*. Louvain.

Brain, P. (1982). "The Hippocratic Physician and His Drugs: A Reinterpretation of 'Aporieisthai' and 'Diamartanein' in Chapter 2 of Peri Aeron, Hydaton, Topon," *Classical Philology* 77: 48–51.

——— (1986). *Galen on Bloodletting*. Cambridge, Mass.

Brandenburg, D. (1973). *Medizinisches in Tausendundeiner Nacht*. Stuttgart.

——— (1976). *Medizinisches bei Herodot*. Berlin.

Bratton, T. L. (1981). "The Identity of the Plague of Justinian," *Transactions and Studies of the College of Physicians of Philadelphia* 3: 113–124, 174–180.

Brecher, K., E. Lieber, and A. E. Lieber (1978). "A Near-Eastern Sighting of the Supernova Explosion of 1054," *Nature* 273 (5665): 728–730.

Bressan, E. (1981). *"L'hospitale" e i poveri: La storiografia sull'assistenza, L'Italia e il caso "lombardo."* Milan.

Bretzl, H. (1903). *Botanische Forschungen des Alexanderzuges*. Leipzig.

Briau, R. (1855). *La Chirurgie de Paul d'Égine*. Paris.

Brodman, E. (1954). *The Development of Medical Bibliography*. Baltimore.

Brody, S. N. (1974). *The Disease of the Soul: Leprosy in Medieval Literature*. Ithaca and London.

Brothwell, D., and A. T. Sandison (1967). *Diseases in Antiquity*. Springfield.

Brown, E. A. R. (1981). "Death and the Human Body in the Later Middle Ages: The Legislation of Boniface VIII on the Division of the Corpse," *Viator* 12: 21–270.

———— (1990). "Authority, the Family, and the Dead in Late Medieval France," *French Historical Studies* 16: 803–832.

Browne, E. G. (1921). *Arabian Medicine.* Cambridge.

Browning, R. (1985). "A Further Testimony to Human Dissection in the Byzantine World," *Bulletin of the History of Medicine* 59: 518–521.

Bruce-Chwatt, L. J., and J. De Zulueta (1980). *The Rise and Fall of Malaria in Europe.* Oxford.

Brunet, P., and A. Mieli (1935). *Histoire des sciences: Antiquité.* Paris.

Brunn, L. von (1946–47). "Hippokrates und die meteorologische Medizin," *Gesnerus* 3: 151–173, and 4: 1–18, 65–85.

Brusatin, M. (1981). *Il muro della peste: Spazio della pietà e governo del lazzaretto.* Venice.

Büchi, J. (1982). *Die Entwicklung der Rezept-und Arzneibuchliteratur,* vol. 1, *Altertum und Mittelalter.* Zurich.

Buck, C. D. (1949). *A Dictionary of Related Indo-European Synonyms.* Chicago.

Bulgakov, P. G. (1972). *Zhizn' i trudy Beruni.* Tashkent.

Bullough, V. L. (1966). *The Development of Medicine as a Profession: The Contribution of the Medieval University to Modern Medicine.* Basel and New York.

Bulst, N. (1979). "Der schwarze Tod: Demographische, wirtschafts-und kultur-geschichtliche Aspekte der Pestkatastrophe von 1347–1352—Bilanz neueren Forschung," *Saeculum* 30: 45–67.

Bürgel, J. C. (1968). "Averroes 'Contra Galenum,'" *Nachrichten der Akademie der Wissenschaften in Göttingen, I: Philosophisch-Historische Klasse* 9 (1967): 263–340.

———— (1973). "Psychosomatic Methods of Cures in the Islamic Middle Ages," *Humaniora Islamica* 1: 157–172.

Burnett, C., and D. Jacquart, eds. (1994). *Constantine the African and 'Ali ibn al-'Abbas al-Magusi, The Pantegni, and Related Texts.* Leiden, New York, and Cologne.

Busacchi, V., and R. Bernabeo (1978). *Storia della medicina.* Bologna.

Bussy, J. (1990). *L'Occidente cristiano, 1400–1700.* Turin.

Byl, S. (1980). *Recherches sur les grands traités biologiques d'Aristote: Sources écrites et préjugés.* Brussels.

———— (1988). "Rheumatism and Gout in the Corpus Hippocraticum," *Antiquité classique* 57: 89–102.

———— (1990). "Étiologie divine dans l'Antiquité classique," in *Actes du XXXIIe Congrès de la Société Internationale d'histoire de la médecine* (Antwerp), pp. 51–62.

———— (1992). "Néologismes et premières attestations de noms de maladies, symptômes et syndromes dans le Corpus hippocraticum," in Gourevitch, ed. (1992), 77–94.

Bylebyl, J. J. (1990). "The Medical Meaning of 'Physica,'" in McVaugh and Siraisi (1990), 16–41.

Bynum, W. F., and V. Nutton, eds. (1981). *Theories of Fever from Antiquity to the Enlightenment.* London.

Caille, J. (1978). *Hôpitaux et charité publique à Narbonne au Moyen Age.* Toulouse.

Cambiano, G. (1982). "Patologia e metafora politica: Alcmeone, Platone e Corpus hippocraticum," *Elenchos* 3: 219–236.

Campbell, A. M. (1931). *The Black Death and Men of Learning.* New York.

Campese, S., P. Manuli, and G. Sissa (1983). *Madre materia.* Turin.

Canguilhem, G. (1972). *Le Normal et le Pathologique,* 4th ed. Paris.

Capasso, L. (1985). *L'origine delle malattie.* Chieti.

Capitani, U. (1991). "I Sesti e la medicina," in Mudry and Pigeaud (1991), 95–123.

Caplan, A., H. T. Engelhardt, and J. J. McCartney, eds. (1981). *Concepts of Health and Disease: Interdisciplinary Perspectives.* Reading, Mass.

Capriglione, J. C. (1985). *Prassagora di Cos.* Naples.

Caroti, S. (1976). "Nicole Oresme, Quaestio contra divinatores horoscopios," *Archives d'histoire doctrinale et littéraire du Moyen Age* 43: 201–310.

Carpentier, E. (1962). *Une ville devant la peste: Orvieto et la Peste Noire de 1348.* Paris.

Castelli, G. (1938). *Gli antichi ospedali e l'unificazione ospedaliera milanese del XV secolo.* Milan.

Castiglioni, A. (1927). *Storia della medicina.* Milan. (3d rev. ed., 2 vols., Milan and Verona, 1948; Eng. trans., New York, 1941, rev. ed., 1947.)

Catahier, P. (1989). *Histoire de la découverte de la petite circulation sanguine.* Paris.

Cattaneo, E. (1984). "Il vescovo 'promotor charitatis' nella città medievale," *Ravennatensia* 10: 13–29.

Caturegli, G. (1966). *La farmacologia celsiana.* Pisa.

Celli, A. (1925). *Malaria e colonizzazione nell'Agro Romano dai più antichi tempi ai nostri giorni.* Florence (Eng. trans., *History of Malaria in the Roman Campagna from Ancient Times,* London, 1933.)

Champier, S. (1506). *De medicinae claris scriptoribus.* Lyons.

Chantraine, P. (1968). *Dictionnaire étymologique de la langue grecque: Histoire des mots.* Paris.

Chaumartin, H. (1946). *Le Mal des ardents et le Feu de Saint-Antoine.* Vienna.

Chiellini Nari, M. (1991). "Le opere di misericordia per immagini," in *La conversione alla povertà,* pp. 415–445.

Choulant, J. L. (1828). *Handbuch der Bücherkunde für die ältere Medizin.* Leipzig. (Rev. ed., Leipzig, 1841; repr., Graz, 1956.)

Cipolla, C. M. (1976). *Public Health and the Medical Profession in the Renaissance.* Cambridge.

——— (1981). *Fighting the Plague in Seventeenth-Century Italy.* Madison, Wisc.

——— (1986). *Contro un nemico invisibile: Epidemie e strutture sanitarie nell'Italia del Rinascimento.* Bologna.

Clarke, E. (1963). "Apoplexy in the Hippocratic Writings," *Bulletin of the History of Medicine* 37: 301–314.

———, ed. (1971). *Modern Methods in the History of Medicine.* London.

Clay, R. M. (1909). *The Medieval Hospitals of England.* London.

Clements, F. E. (1932). "Primitive Concepts of Disease," *Publications of the American Association of Archaeology and Ethnology* 32: 185–252.

Cohn-Haft, L. (1956). *The Public Physicians of Ancient Greece.* Northampton, Mass.

Collectif (1978). *Assistance et charité* (Cahiers de Fanjeaux 13). Toulouse.

——— (1987). *Santé, médecine et assistance au Moyen Age* (proceedings of the 110th National Congress of Learned Societies). Paris.

——— (1990). *Città e servizi sociali nell'Italia dei secoli XII–XV* (proceedings of the twelfth scholarly conference, Centro di studi di storia e d'arte). Pistoia.

——— (1991). *La conversione alla povertà nell'Italia dei secoli XII–XIV* (proceedings of the twenty-seventh International History Conference, Todi, 1990). Spoleto.

Colnat, A. (1937). *Les Épidémies et l'histoire.* Paris.

Coopland, G. W. (1952). *Nicole Oresme and the Astrologers.* Liverpool.

Corner, G. W. (1937a). "On Early Salernitan Surgery and Especially the 'Bamberg Surgery,'" *Bulletin of the History of Medicine.* 5: 1–32.

——— (1937b). "Salernitan Surgery in the Twelfth Century," *British Journal of Surgery* 25: 84–99.

Corradi, A. (1865–1894). *Annali delle epidemie occorse in Italia dalle prime memorie fino al 1850,* 8 vols. Bologna. (Repr., 5 vols., Bologna, 1972–1973.)

Corsi, P., and P. Weindling, eds. (1983). *Information Sources in the History of Science and Medicine.* London.

Corvisier, J.-N. (1985). *Santé et société en grèce ancienne.* Paris.

——— (1991). *Aux origines du miracle grec.* Paris.

Cosmacini, G. (1988). *Storia della medicina e della sanità in Italia.* Rome and Bari.

Coury, C. (1967). "The Basic Principles of Medicine in the Primitive Mind," *Medical History* 5: 111–127.

——— (1968). "Le Signe du doigt hippocratique," *Pagine di storia della medicina* 12: 3–12.

Cranz, F. E., and P. O. Kristeller, eds. (1980). *Catalogus Translationum et Commentariorum: Medieval and Renaissance Latin Translations and Commentaries, Annotated Lists and Guides.* Washington.

Creutz, R. (1936). "Die medizinisch-naturphilosophischen Aphorismen und Kommentare des Magister Urso Salernitanus," *Quellen und Studien zur Geschichte der Naturwissenschaften und Medizin* 5 (fasc. 1): 1–192.

Crisciani, C. (1978). "Exemplum Christi e sapere: Sull'epistemologia di Arnaldo da Villanova," *Archives internationales d'histoire des sciences* 28: 245–315.

——— (1983a). "Doctus et expertus: La formazione del medico tra Due e Trecento," *Per una storia del costume educativo (Età classica e Medioevo): Quaderni della Fondazione Giangiacomo Feltrinelli,* 23.

——— (1983b). "Valeurs éthiques et savoir médical entre le XIIe et le XIVe siècle: Problèmes et thèmes d'une recherche," *History and Philosophy of the Life Sciences* 5: 33–52.

—— (1990a). "History, Novelty, and Progress in Scholastic Medicine," *Osiris,* 2d ser., 6: 118–139.

—— (1990b). "Il medico cristiano nel Medioevo," *Kos,* new ser., 57.

Crombie, A. C. (1962). *Robert Grosseteste and the Origins of Experimental Science, 1100–1700.* Oxford.

——, ed. (1963). *Scientific Change: Symposium on the History of Science* (Oxford, 1961). London.

Crombie, A. C., and J. O. North (1970). "Roger Bacon," in Gillispie (1970–1980), 1: 377–385.

Crombie, A. C., and N. Siraisi, eds. (1987). *The Rational Arts of Living.* Northampton, Mass.

Crotti Pasi, R. (1992). "Il sistema caritativo-assistenziale: Strutture e forme di intervento," in *Storia di Pavia,* vol. 3, book 1. Milan.

Cunningham, A. (1982). "Two Legacies of the Late Alexandrian School," *Nihon Schigaku Zassi* 28: 400–424.

Currer, C., and M. Stacey, eds. (1986). *Concepts of Health, Illness and Disease: A Comparative Perspective.* Leamington Spa.

Da Costa Roque, M. (1979). *As pestes medievais europeias e o "Regimento proueytoso contra ha pestenença," Lisboa, Valentim Fernandes (1495–1496).* Paris.

Daremberg, C. (1853). *Notices et extraits des manuscrits médicaux grecs, latins et français, des principales bibliothèques de l'Europe,* vol. 1, *Manuscrits grecs d'Angleterre.* Paris.

—— (1862). *La Médecine: Histoire et doctrines.* Paris. (Repr., New York, 1976.)

—— (1870). *Histoire des sciences médicales, comprenant l'anatomie, la physiologie, la médecine, la chirurgie et les doctrines de pathologie générale,* 2 vols. Paris.

Dechambre, A. (1864–1884). *Dictionnaire encyclopédique des sciences médicales,* 100 vols. Paris.

Degen, R. (1986). "An Unknown Manuscript of the Book of Epidemics of Hippocrates," *Zeitschrift für Geschichte der arabisch-islamischen Wissenschaften* 3: 269–279.

—— (1989). "Zur arabischen Überlieferung von Galens Erklärung des Buches 'Über die Diät der akuten Krankheiten,'" *Zeitschrift für Geschichte der arabisch-islamischen Wissenschaften* 5: 184–195.

Deichgräber, K. (1930). *Die griechische Empirikerschule: Sammlung der Fragmente und Darstellung der Lehre.* Berlin. (Repr., Berlin, 1965.)

—— (1933). *Die Epidemien und das Corpus Hippocraticum.* Berlin. (2d ed., Berlin, 1971, with concluding note and supplement.)

De Koning, P. (1896). *Trois traités d'anatomie arabes par Muhammad Zakariya al-Razi, Ali ibn al-Abbas and Ali ibn Sina.* Leiden.

Delaunay, P. (1948). *La Médecine et l'eglise.* Paris.

Delaveau, P. (1982). *Histoire et renouveau des plantes médicinales.* Paris.

Dell'Anna, G. (1990). *Nicolaus de Paganica, "Compendium medicinalis astrologiae."* Galatina.

Della Peruta, F., ed. (1984). *Malattia e medicina* (= *Annali della Storia d'Italia*, vol. 3). Turin.

Delmas, B. (1966). "Le Chancelier Jacques Angeli et la médecine à Montpellier au milieu du XVe siècle," in *École nationale des chartes: Positions des thèses* (Paris), pp. 23–28.

Demaitre, L. E. (1975). "Theory and Practice in Medical Education at the University of Montpellier in the Thirteenth and Fourteenth Centuries," *Journal of the History of Medicine* 30: 102–123.

—— (1976). "Scholasticism in Compendia of Practical Medicine, 1250–1450," *Manuscripta* 20: 81–95.

—— (1980). *Doctor Bernard de Gordon, Professor and Practitioner.* Toronto.

Demaitre, L. E., and A. A. Travill (1980). "Human Embryology and Development in the Works of Albertus Magnus," in Weisheipl (1980), pp. 405–440.

Denifle, H., and Chatelain, A. (1891). Chartularium Universitatis Parisiensis, 2 vol., Paris.

De Renzi, S. (1852–1859). *Collectio Salernitana,* 5 vols. Naples.

—— (1857). *Storia documentata della Scuola medica di Salerno.* Naples.

Derrida, J. (1968). "La Pharmacie de Platon," *Tel Quel,* nos. 32–33.

De Spiegeler, P. (1987). *Les Hôpitaux et l'assistance à liège: Aspects institutionnels et sociaux.* Paris.

Dezeimeris, E. (1824). "Des principes du méthodisme, considérés comme source de la doctrine physiologique," *Journal complémentaire du dictionnaire des sciences médicales,* 3–17 and 80–88.

De Zulueta, J. (1973). "Malaria and Mediterranean History," *Parassitologia* 15: 1–15.

Di Benedetto, V. (1980). "Cos e Cnido," in Grmek, ed. (1980), 97–112.

—— (1986). *Il medico e la malattia: La scienza di Ippocrate.* Turin.

Diels, H. (1893). "Über das physikalische System des Straton," *Sitzungsberichte der Kgl. Preussischen Akadaemie der Wissenschaften,* 101–127. (New ed. in H. Diels, *Kleine Schriften zur Geschichte der antiken Philosophie,* Hildesheim, 1969.)

—— (1905–1906). *Die Handschriften der antiken Ärzte,* parts 1 and 2 *(Abhandlungen der Königlich-Preussischen Akademie der Wissenschaften, Philosophisch-historische Klasse).* Berlin.

—— (1907). *Bericht über den Stand des interakademischen Corpus medicorum antiquorum und Erster Nachtrag zu den in den Abhandlungen 1905 und 1906 veröffentlichten Katalogen: Die Handschriften der antiken Ärzte,* parts 1 and 2. Berlin.

Diepgen, P. (1937). *Die Frauenheilkunde der alten Welt.* Munich.

—— (1940). "Das Krankheitsgift in der Geschichte der Medizin," *Deutsche Medizinische Wochenschrift,* 1374–1378.

—— (1949–1955). *Geschichte der Medizin: Die historische Entwicklung der Heilkunde und des ärztlichen Lebens,* 3 vols. Berlin.

—— (1958). *Über den Einfluss der autoritativen Theologie auf die Medizin des Mittelalters.* Mainz and Wiesbaden.

Diepgen, P., G. P. Gruber, and H. Schadewaldt (1969). "Der Krankheitsbegriff, seine Geschichte und Problematik," in *Handbuch der allgemeinen Pathologie*, vol. 1. (Berlin), pp. 1–50.

Dierbach, J. H. (1824). *Die Arzneimittel des Hippokrates oder Versuch einer systematischen Aufzählung der in allen hippokratischen Schriften vorkommenden Medikamente.* Leipzig. (Repr., Hildesheim, 1969.)

Dietrich, A. (1966). *Medicinalia Arabica: Studien über arabische medizinische Handschriften in türkischen und syrischen Bibliotheken.* Göttingen.

——— (1988). *Dioscurides triumphans.* Göttingen. (Abhandlungen der Akademie der Wissenschaften in Göttingen, Philosophisch-Historische Klasse, 3d ser., n. 173.)

Diller, H. (1932). "Opsis adèlon ta fainomena," *Hermes* 67: 14–42.

——— (1934). *Wanderarzt und Aetiologe: Studien zur hippokratischen Schrift Peri aeron, hydaton, topon.* Leipzig.

——— (1973). *Kleine Schriften zur antiken Medizin.* Berlin and New York.

Dodds, E. R. (1959). *The Greeks and the Irrational.* Berkeley.

Dols, M. W. (1987). "The Origins of the Islamic Hospital: Myth and Reality," *Bulletin of the History of Medicine* 61: 367–390.

——— (1988). "Galen and Islamic Psychiatry," in Manuli and Vegetti (1988), 243–280.

Dols, M. W., and A. S. Gamal (1984). *Medieval Islamic Medicine: Ibn Ridwan's Treatise "On the Prevention of Bodily Ills in Egypt."* Berkeley.

Donini, P. (1984). "Problemi del pensiero scientifico a Roma: Il primo e il secondo secolo d.C.," in Giannantoni and Vegetti (1984), 353–374.

Dorvault, M. (1867). *L'Officine ou répertoire général de pharmacie pratique.* Paris.

Dousset, J. C. (1985). *Histoire des médicaments des origines à nos jours.* Paris.

Drachmann, A. G. (1948). *Ktesibios, Philon, and Hero: A Study in Ancient Pneumatics.* Copenhagen.

Ducatillon, J. (1977). *Polémiques dans la Collection hippocratique.* Lille and Paris.

Duffy, J. (1985). "Byzantine Medicine in the Sixth and Seventh Centuries: Aspects of Teaching and Practice," in Scarborough (1985). 21–27.

Duminil, M.-P. (1983). *Le Sang, les vaisseaux, le coeur dans la Collection hippocratique: Anatomie et physiologie.* Paris.

Dureau-Lapeyssonie, J. M. (1966). "L'oeuvre d'Antoine Ricart, médecin catalan du XVe siècle," in Beaujouan (1966), 171–368.

Durling, R. J. (1961). "A Chronological Census of Renaissance Editions and Translations of Galen," *Journal of the Warburg and Courtauld Institutes* 24: 230–305.

——— (1967–1981). "Corrigenda and Addenda to Diels' Galenica," *Traditio* 23: 461–476; 37: 373–381.

Eamon, W., and G. Keil (1987). "'Plebs amat empirica': Nicholas of Poland and His Critique of the Medieval Medical Establishment," *Sudhoffs Archiv für Geschichte der Medizin* 71: 180–196.

Eastwood, B. S. (1982). "The Place of Medicine in a Hierarchy of Knowledge," *Sudhoffs Archiv für Geschichte der Medizin* 66: 20–37.

Edelstein, L. (1933). "Empirie und Skepsis in der Lehre der griechischen Empiriker-schule," *Quellen und Studien zur Geschichte der Naturwissenschaften und Medizin* 3: 45–53. (Repr. in Flashar [1971], 296–307.)

——— (1952). "The Relation of Ancient Philosophy to Medicine," *Bulletin of the History of Medicine* 26: 299–316.

——— (1967). *Ancient Medicine*. Baltimore.

Elford, D. (1988). "William of Conches," in P. Dronke, ed., *A History of Twelfth-Century Western Philosophy* (Cambridge), pp. 308–327.

Elgood, C. (1966). *Safavid Surgery*. London.

——— (1969). *Safavid Medical Practice*. Hertford.

Elliott, J. S. (1914). *Outlines of Greek and Roman Medicine*. London.

Engelhardt, H. T. (1975). "The Concept of Health and Disease," in Engelhardt and Spicker (1975), 125–141.

Engelhardt, H. T., and S. F. Spicker, eds. (1975). *Evaluation and Explanation in Biomedical Sciences*. Dordrecht.

Englert, L. (1929). "Untersuchungen zu Galens Schrift Thrasybulos," in K. Sudhoff and H. E. Sigerist, eds., *Studien zur Geschichte der Medizin*, vol. 18. Leipzig.

Ey, H. (1981). *Naissance de la médecine*. Paris.

Fabricius, C. (1972). *Galens Exzerpte aus älteren Pharmakologen*. Berlin and New York.

Federici-Vescovini, G. (1983). "L'astrologia tra magia, religione e scienza," in G. Federici-Vescovini, ed., *"Arti" e filosofia nel secolo XIV* (Florence), pp. 171–193.

——— (1987). "Peter of Abano and Astrology," in *Astrology, Science, and Society* (Woodbridge), pp. 19–39.

Ferngren, G. B. (1982). "A Roman Declamation on Vivisection," *Transactions and Studies of the College of Physicians in Philadelphia*, 5th ser. 4 (4): 272–290.

——— (1992). "Early Christianity as a Religion of Healing," *Bulletin of the History of Medicine* 66: 1–15.

Ferrari, G. A. (1984). "Meccanica 'allargata,'" in Giannantoni and Vegetti (1984), 225–286.

——— (1985). "Macchina e artificio," in Vegetti (1985), 163–179.

Feugère, M., E. Künzl, and U. Weisser (1985). "Les aiguilles à cataracte de Mont-bellet (Saône-et-Loire)," *Jahrbuch des Römish-Germanischen Zentralmuseums Mainz* 32: 436–508.

Flashar, H. (1966). *Melancholie und Melancholiker in den medizinischen Theorien der Antike*. Berlin.

———, ed. (1971). *Antike Medizin*. Darmstadt.

Fleck, L. (1935). *Entstehung und Entwicklung einer wissenschaftlichen Tatsache*. Basel. (New ed., Frankfurt, 1980.)

Flint, V. J. (1989). "The Early Medieval 'Medicus,' the Saint and the Enchanter," *Social History of Medicine* 2: 127–145.

Fortenbaugh, W. W. (1992). *Theophrastus of Eresus: Sources for His Life, Writings, Thought, and Influence,* 2 vols. Leiden.

Foucault, M. (1961). *Histoire de la folie à l'âge classique: Folie et déraison.* Paris.

—————— (1969). *L'Archéologie du savoir.* Paris.

—————— (1972). *The Birth of Clinics.* New York. (Originally *Naissance de la clinique: Une archéologie du regard médical,* Paris.)

Fraser, P. M. (1969). "The Career of Erasistratus of Ceos," *Rendiconti dell'Istituto lombardo, Classe lettere* 103: 518–537.

—————— (1972). *Ptolemaic Alexandria,* 3 vols. Oxford.

Frede, M. (1982). "The Method of the So-Called Methodical School of Medicine," in Barnes, Brunschwig, and Scholfield (1982), 1–23.

—————— (1987). *Essays in Ancient Philosophy.* Minneapolis.

Freind, J. (1725–1726). *The History of Physick, from the Time of Galen to the Beginning of the Sixteenth Century,* 2 vols. London. (4th ed., London, 1750.)

French, R. (1979). "A Note on the Anatomical Accessus of the Middle Ages," *Medical History* 23: 461–468.

French, R., and F. Greenaway (1986). *Science in the Early Roman Empire: Pliny the Elder, His Sources and Influence.* London and Sydney.

Fruton, J. S. (1992). *A Skeptical Biochemist.* Cambridge, Mass.

Furley, D. J., and J. S. Wilkie (1984). *Galen on Respiration and the Arteries.* Princeton.

Gai, L. (1977). *Interventi rinascimentali nello spedale del Ceppo, Contributi per la storia dello spedale del Ceppo di Pistoia.* Pistoia.

García Ballester, L. (1972). *Galeno en la sociedad y en la ciencia de su tiempo.* Madrid.

—————— (1982). "Arnau de Vilanova (c. 1240–1311) y la reforma de los estudios médicos en Montpellier (1309): El Hipócrates latín y la introducción del nuevo Galeno," *Dynamis* 2: 97–158.

—————— (1988). *La medicina a la València medieval: Medicina y societat en un país medieval mediterrani.* Valencia.

—————— (1990). "On the Origin of the 'Six Non-Natural Things' in Galen," in Harig and Kollesch (1990).

García Ballester, L., and P. Gil-Sotres (1986). *Teorías sobre la fiebre y averroismo medico en Montpellier: Bernardo de Gordon y Arnau de Vilanova.* Santander and Pamplona.

García Ballester, L., et al. (1994). *Practical Medicine from Salerno to Black Death.* Cambridge.

Garin, E. (1979). "Problemi di religione e filosofia nella cultura fiorentina del Quattrocento," in *La cultura filosofica del Rinascimento italiano* (Florence), pp. 127–142.

Garofalo, I. (1988). *Erasistrati fragmenta.* Pisa.

—————— (1992). "Prolegomena all'edizione dell'Anonymus Parisinus Darembergi sive Fuchsii," in Garzya (1992), 91–106.

Garrison, F. H. (1913). *An Introduction to the History of Medicine.* Philadelphia. (4th rev. ed., Philadelphia and London, 1929.)

Garrison, F. H., and L. T. Morton (1983). *A Medical Bibliography.* London.

Garzya, A., ed. (1989). *Contributi alla cultura greca nell'Italia meridionale,* vol. 1 (*Hellenica et Byzantina Neapolitana,* 13). Naples.

——— (1992). *Tradizione e ecdotica dei testi medici tardoantichi e bizantini* (proceedings of the International Convention, Anacapri, 1990). Naples.

Gazza, V. (1955–56). "Prescrizioni mediche nei papiri dell'Egitto greco-romano," *Aegyptus* 35: 86–110; 36: 73–114.

Geremek, B. (1980). "Povertà," in *Enciclopedia Einaudi,* vol. 10. Turin.

——— (1987). *La Potence ou la pitié.* Paris.

Geymonat, L., ed. (1970–1976). *Storia del pensiero filosofico e scientifico,* 7 books in 8 vols., Milan.

Giannantoni, G., and M. Vegetti, eds. (1984). *La scienza ellenistica* (proceedings of the three days of study held at Pavia, 1982). Naples.

Gil, J. S. (1990). "The Translators of the Period of D. Raymundo: Their Personalities and Translations (1125–1187)," in Hamesse and Fattori (1990), 109–119.

——— (1990). "Los evacuantes particulares: Ventosas, escarificaciones, sanguijuelas y cauterios en la terapéutica de la Baja Edad Media," *Medicina y Historia* 34: 1–16.

Gilliam, J. F. (1961). "The Plague under Marcus Aurelius," *American Journal of Philology* 82: 225–251.

Gillispie, C. C., ed. (1970–1980). *Dictionary of Scientific Biography,* 16 vols. New York.

Gillmeister, H. (1988). "Medieval Sport: Modern Methods of Research—Recent Results and Perspectives," *International Journal of Sports History* 5: 53–68.

Gil Sotres, P. (1986). *Scripta minora de flebotomia en la tradición del siglo XIII.* Santander and Pamplona.

Ginouvès, R., A.-M. Guimier-Sorbets, J. Jouanna, and L. Villard, eds. (1994). *L'Eau, la santé et la maladie dans le monde grec.* Paris.

Girard, M. C. (1988). *Connaissance et méconnaissance de l'hellébore dans l'antiquité.* Quebec.

——— (1990). *"L'Hellébore: Panacée ou placebo,"* in Potter, Maloney, and Desautels (1990), 393–405.

Gohlmann, W. E. (1974). *The Life of Ibn Sina.* Albany, N.Y.

Gonthier, N. (1978). *Lyons et ses pauvres au Moyen Age (1350–1500).* Lyons.

Goodman, L. E. (1992). *Avicenna.* London.

Gottfried, R. S. (1983). *The Black Death, Natural and Human Disaster in Medieval Europe.* New York and London.

Gourevitch, D. (1984). *Le Triangle hippocratique dans le monde gréco-romain: Le Malade, sa maladie et son médecin.* Rome.

——— (1987a). "Asclépiade de Bithynie dans Pline: Problèmes de chronologie," in Pigeaud and Orose (1987), 67–81.

——— (1987b). "L'Esthétique médicale de Galien," *Les Études classiques* 55: 267–290.

——— (1988a). "Galien, médecin décideur," *Prospective et santé: La Clinique demain* 46: 81–88.

——— (1988b). "Introduction," in Soranos d'Éphèse, *Maladies des femmes*, vol. 1, book 1, ed. P. Bourguière, D. Gourevitch, and Y. Malinas (Paris), pp. i–xlvi.

——— (1991). "La Pratique méthodique: Définition de la maladie, indication et traitement," in Mudry and Pigeaud (1991), 51–81.

——— (1992). "Comment parlent d'elles-mêmes les sectes médicales à Rome? Comment en parle-t-on?" *Revue de philologie* 66: 29–35.

———, ed. (1992). *Maladie et maladies: Histoire et conceptualisation (Mélanges en l'honneur de M. Grmek).* Geneva.

Gourevitch, M. (1964). "Esquisse d'une mythologie de la santé et de la maladie," *Encéphale* 2: 437–477.

Grabmann, M. (1909–1911). *Die Geschichte der scholastischen Methode.* Freiburg.

Granshaw, L., and R. Porter, eds. (1989). *The Hospital in History.* London and New York.

Gregory, T. (1975). "La Nouvelle Idée de la nature et du savoir scientifique au XIIe siècle," in J. E. Murdoch and E. D. Sylla, eds., *The Cultural Context of Medieval Learning* (Dordrecht and Boston), pp. 193–218.

Grensemann, H. (1975). *Knidische Medizin*, part 1, *Die Testimonien zur ältesten knidischen Lehre und Analysen knidischer Schriften im Corpus hippocraticum.* Berlin.

——— (1987). *Knidische Medizin*, part 2, *Versuch einer weiteren Analyse der Schicht A in den pseudohippokratischen Schriften "De Mulieribus I und II."* Stuttgart.

Grimm, J. (1965). *Die literarische Darstellung der Pest in der Antike und in der Romania.* Munich.

Grisnaschi, M. (1976). "L'Origine et les métamorphoses du Sirr al-asrar," *Archives d'histoire doctrinale et littéraire du Moyen Age* 43: 7–112.

——— (1980). "La Diffusion du 'Secretum secretorum' (Sirr al-asrar) dans l'Europe occidentale," *Archives d'histoire doctrinale et littéraire du Moyen Age* 47: 1–70.

Grmek, M. D. (1965). "Prolégomènes à une histoire générale des sciences," *Annales: Economies, sociétés, civilisations* 20: 138–146.

——— (1967). "Bolest [disease]," in *Medicinska Enciklopedija*, vol. 1 (Zagreb), pp. 490–529.

——— (1969). "Préliminaires d'une étude historique des maladies," *Annales: Economies, sociétés, civilisations* 24: 1437–1483.

——— (1979). "Définition du domaine propre de l'histoire des sciences et considérations sur ses rapports avec la philosophie des sciences," *History and Philosophy of the Life Sciences* 1: 3–12.

——— (1980). "Le Concept d'infection dans l'Antiquité et au Moyen Age: Les Anciennes mesures sociales contre les maladies contagieuses et la fondation de la première quarantaine à Dubrovnik (1377)," *Rad Jugoslavenske Akademije* 384: 9–55.

——— (1982). "Le Médecin au service de l'hôpital médiéval en Europe occidentale," *History and Philosophy of the Life Sciences* 4: 25–64.

——— (1983a). "Ancienneté de la chirurgie hippocratique," in Lasserre and Mudry (1983), 285–295.

——— (1983b). *Les Maladies à l'aube de la civilisation occidentale.* Paris.

——— (1984a). "Les Vicissitudes des notions d'infection, de contagion et de germe dans la médecine antique," *Mémoires du Centre Jean-Palerne* 5: 53–70.

——— (1984b). "Vestigia della chirurgia greca: Il codice di Niceta e suoi discendenti," *Kos* 1: 52–60.

——— (1989). *Diseases of the Ancient World*, trans. Mireille Muellner and Leonard Muellner. Baltimore and London.

——— (1990a). "L'Expérimentation biologique quantitative dans l'Antiquité," in *La Première Révolution biologique* (Paris), pp. 17–43.

——— (1990b). *La Première Révolution biologique: Réflexions sur la physiologie et la médecine du XVIIe siècle.* Paris.

——— (1990c). "La Vie mouvementée de Jacques de Plaisance, médecin du roi, lecteur universitaire et évêque de Zagreb," *Croatica Christiana* 27: 31–50.

——— (1991a). "Ideas on Heredity in Greek and Roman Antiquity," *Physis* 28: 11–34.

——— (1991b). "The Four Humours," *Encyclopaedia Moderna* 12: 14–17.

———, ed. (1980). *Hippocratica* (proceedings of the third Hippocratic Colloquium, Paris, 1978). Paris.

Grmek, M. D., and D. Gourevitch (1985). "Les Expériences pharmacologiques dans l'Antiquité," *Archives internationales d'histoire des sciences* 35: 3–27.

——— (1986). "Medice, cura te ipsum: Les maladies de Galien," in *Études de lettres* (Lausanne), pp. 45–64.

——— (1988). "L'École médicale de Quintus et de Numisianus," *Mémoires du Centre Jean-Palerne* 8: 43–60.

——— (1994). "Aux sources de la doctrine médicale de Galien: L'Enseignement de Marinus Quintus et Numisianus," in *Aufstieg und Niedergang der römischen Welt*, 37, 2 (Berlin), pp. 1491–1528.

Grmek, M. D., and R. Wittern (1977). "Die Nierenkrankheit des attischen Strategen Nikias und die Nierenleiden im 'Corpus hippocraticum,'" *Archives internationales d'histoire des sciences* 26: 3–22.

Grmek, M. D., R. S. Cohen, and G. Cimino, eds. (1981). *On Scientific Discovery: The Erice Lectures 1977.* Dordrecht and Boston.

Guglielmi, N. (1971). "Modos de marginalidad en la edad media: Extranjería, pobreza, enfermedad," *Anales de historia Antigua y Medieval* 16: 7–94.

Gundert, B. (1992). "Parts and Their Roles in Hippocratic Medicine," *Isis* 83: 453–465.

Gurdjian, E. S. (1973). *Head Injury from Antiquity to the Present.* Springfield.

Gurlt, E. J. (1898). *Geschichte der Chirurgie und ihrer Ausübung.* Berlin.

Haase, W., ed. (1993–94). *Aufstieg und Niedergang der römischen Welt,* 37, 2 (Berlin).

Habricht, C., F. Marguth, and J. H. Wolf, eds. (1978). *Medizinische Diagnostik in Geschichte und Gegenwart (Festschrift Goerke).* Munich.

Haeser, H. (1845). *Lehrbuch der Geschichte der Medizin und der Volkskrankheiten.* Jena. (3d rev. ed., 3 vols., Jena, 1875–1882.)

Hahm, D. E. (1977). *The Origins of Stoic Cosmology.* Columbus.

Hall, A. R. (1983). "On Whiggism," *History of Science* 21: 45–59.

Hall, S. P. (1957). "The *Cyrurgia magna* of Brunus Longoburgensis: A Critical Edition" (D. Phil. thesis). St. Hilda's College, Oxford.

Hamesse, J., and M. Fattori, eds. (1990). *Rencontres de cultures dans la philosophie médiévale: Traductions et traducteurs de l'Antiquité tardive au XIVe siècle* (proceedings of the International Colloquium of Cassino, 1989). Louvain.

Hankinson, R. J. (1987). "Causes and Empiricism: A Problem in the Interpretation of Later Greek Medical Method," *Phronesis* 32: 329–348.

Harig, G. (1974). *Bestimmung der Intensität im medizinischen System Galens: Ein Beitrag zur theoretischen Pharmakologie, Nosologie und Therapie in der galenischen Medizin.* Berlin.

——— (1980). "Anfänge der theoretischen Pharmakologie im Corpus hippocraticum," in Grmek, ed. (1980), 223–245.

Harig, G., and J. Kollesch, eds. (1990). *Galen und das hellenische Erbe.* Berlin.

Harris, C. R. S. (1973). *The Heart and the Vascular System in Ancient Greek Medicine (from Alcmaeon to Galen).* Oxford.

Hau, F. R. (1975). "Razis Gutachten über Rosenschnupfen," *Medizinhistorisches Journal* 10: 94–102.

——— (1983). "Die Medizinische Geschichtsschreibung im islamischen Mittelalter," *Clio Medica* 18: 69–80.

Hecker, J. F. K. (1822–1829). *Geschichte der Heilkunde nach den Quellen bearbeitet,* 2 vols. Berlin.

Heger, H. (1967). *Die Melancholie bei den französischen Lyrikern des Spätmittelalters.* Bonn.

Heinimann, F. (1961). "Eine vorplatonische Theorie der 'techne,'" *Museum Helveticum* 18: 105–130.

Henschen, F. (1962). *The History and Geography of Diseases.* New York.

Herberger, M. (1981). *Dogmatik: Zur Geschichte von Begriff und Methode in Medizin und Jurisprudenz.* Frankfurt.

Herrlinger, R. (1967). *Geschichte der medizinischen Abbildung,* vol. 1, *Von der Antike bis um 1600.* Munich.

Herter, H. (1963a). "Die kulturhistorische Theorie der hippokratischen Schrift 'Von der alten Medizin,'" *Maia* 15: 464–483.

——— (1963b). "Die Treffkunst des Arztes in hippokratischer und platonischer Sicht," *Sudhoffs Archiv für Geschichte der Medizin* 47: 247–290.

—————— (1976). "The Problematic Mention of Hippocrates in Plato's 'Phaedrus,'" *Illinois Classical Studies* 1: 22–42.

Herzlich, C. (1969). *Santé et maladie: Analyse d'une représentation sociale.* Paris.

Herzog, R. (1931). *Die Wunderheilungen von Epidauros.* Leipzig.

Hewson, M. A. (1975). *Giles of Rome and the Medieval Theory of Conception.* London.

Hoeppli, R. (1959). *Parasites and Parasitic Infections in Early Medicine and Science.* Singapore.

Hohlweg, A. (1988). "Medizinischer 'Enzyklopädismus' und das 'ponema iatrikon' des Michael Psellos," *Byzantinische Zeitschrift* 81: 39–49.

Holladay, A. J. (1988). "New Developments in the Problem of the Athenian Plague," *Classical Quarterly,* new ser., 38: 247–250.

Horden, P. (1988). "A Discipline of Relevance: The Historiography of the Later Medieval Hospital," *Social History of Medicine* 1: 359–374.

Horstmanshoff, H. F. J. (1989). *Di pijlen van de pest: Pestilenties in de griekse wereld (800–400 v.C.).* Amsterdam.

Huard, P., and M. D. Grmek (1960). *Le Premier Manuscrit chirurgical turc, rédigé par Charaf éd-Din (1465).* Paris.

—————— (1966). *Mille ans de chirurgie en Occident: Ve–XVe siècle.* Paris.

Hugonnard-Roche, H. (1984). "La Classification des sciences de Gundissalinus et l'influence d'Avicenne," in Jolivet and Rashed (1984), 41–75.

Hunger, H. (1978). *Die hochsprachliche profane Literatur der Byzantiner,* 2 vols. Munich.

Hunt, R. W. (1950). "Stephen of Antioch," *Medieval and Renaissance Studies* 2: 172–173.

Ieraci Bio, A. M. (1989). "La Trasmissione della letteratura medica greca nell'Italia meridionale fra X e XV secolo," in *Garzya* (1989), 133–257.

Ilberg, J. (1905). "Aus Galen's Praxis," *Neue Jahrbücher für das klassische Altertum* 15: 276–312. (Repr. in Flashar [1971], 59–75.)

—————— (1925). *Die Ärzteschule von Knidos.* Leipzig.

Imbert, J. (1947). *Les Hôpitaux en droit canonique.* Paris.

——————, ed. (1982). *Histoire des hôpitaux en France.* Toulouse.

Imhof, A. E. (1983). *Der Mensch und sein Körper von der Antike bis heute.* Munich.

Ioannidi, H. (1983). "Les Notions de partie du corps et d'organe," in Lasserre and Mudry (1983), 327–339.

Iskandar, A. Z. (1974). "Ibn al-Nafis," in Gillispie (1970–1980), 9: 602–606.

—————— (1976). "An Attempted Reconstruction of the Late Alexandrian Curriculum," *Medical History* 20: 235–258.

—————— (1978). "Hunayn ibn Ishaq," in Gillispie (1970–1980), 15: 241–243.

—————— (1984). *A Descriptive List of Arabic Manuscripts on Medicine and Science at the University of California, Los Angeles.* Leiden.

Isnardi Parente, M. (1989). *Stoici antichi,* 2 vols. Turin.

Jackson, R. (1988). *Doctors and Diseases in the Roman Empire.* London.

———— (1990). "Roman Doctors and Their Instruments: Recent Research into Ancient Practice," *Journal of Roman Archaeology* 3: 5–27.

Jacob, F. (1970). *La Logique du vivant: Une histoire de l'hérédité.* Paris.

Jacquart, D. (1981). *Le Milieu médical en France du XIIe au XVe siècle.* Geneva.

———— (1983). "La Réflexion médicale médiévale et l'apport arabe," in Postel and Quétel (1983), 43–53.

———— (1985). "Le Crâne et ses déformations dans les écrits médicaux du Moyen Age," *Histoire et archéologie: Les Dossiers* 97: 48–52.

———— (1986). "A l'aube de la renaissance médicale des XIe–XIIe siècles: 'L'Isagoge Iohannitii' et son traducteur," *Bibliothèque de l'École des chartes* 144: 209–240.

———— (1988). "Aristotelian Thought in Salerno," in P. Dronke, ed., *A History of Twelfth-Century Western Philosophy* (Cambridge), pp. 407–428.

———— (1990a). "Principales étapes dans la transmission des textes de médecine (XIe and XIVe siècles)," in Hamesse and Fattori (1990), 251–271.

———— (1990b). "Theory, Everyday Practice, and Three Fifteenth-Century Physicians," *Osiris*, 2d ser., 6: 140–160.

———— (1990c). "L'Enseignement de la médecine: Quelques termes fondamentaux," in Weijers (1990), 104–120.

———— (1992). "'Theorica' et 'Practica' dans l'enseignement de la médecine à Salerne au XIIe siècle," in Weijers, ed., *Vocabulaire des écoles et des méthodes d'enseignement au Moyen Age* (Turnhout), pp. 102–110.

———— (1994). "Medical Practice in Paris in the First Half of the Fourteenth Century," in García Ballester et al. (1994), 186–210.

Jacquart, D., and F. Micheau (1990). *La Médecine arabe et l'Occident médiéval.* Paris.

Jacquart, D., and C. Thomasset (1981). "Albert le Grand et les problèmes de la sexualité," *History and Philosophy of the Life Sciences* 3: 73–93.

———— (1985). *Sexualité et savoir médical au Moyen Age.* Paris. (Eng. trans., Oxford and Princeton, 1988.)

Jaeger, W. (1913). "Das Pneuma im Lykeion," *Hermes* 48: 29–74. (Repr. in Jaeger, *Scripta minora,* vol. 1, Rome, 1960.)

———— (1923). *Aristoteles: Grundlegung einer Geschichte seiner Entwicklung.* Berlin.

———— (1938). *Diokles von Karystos.* Berlin. (New ed., Berlin, 1963.)

Jagailloux, S. (1986). *La Médicalisation de l'Égypte au XIXe siècle (1798–1918).* Paris.

Janni, P., and I. Mazzini, eds. (1990). *Presenza del lessico greco e latino nelle lingue contemporanee.* Macerata.

Jeanselme, E. (1931). "Comment l'Europe au Moyen Age se protégea contre la lèpre," *Bulletin de la Société française d'histoire de la médecine* 25: 1–155.

Jetter, D. (1966–1987). *Geschichte des Hospitals:* vol. 1, *Westdeutschland von den Anfängen bis 1850;* vol. 2, *Zur typologie des Irrenhauses in Frankreich und Deutschland, 1780–1840;* vol. 3, *Nordamerika (Kolonialzeit);* vol. 4, *Spanien von den Anfängen bis um 1500;* vol. 5, *Wien von den Anfängen bis um 1500;* vol. 6, *Santiago, Toledo, Granada.* Wiesbaden.

———— (1973). *Grundzüge der Hospitalgeschichte.* Darmstadt.

———— (1978). "Klosterhospitäler: St. Gallen, Cluny, Escorial," *Sudhoffs Archiv für Geschichte der Medizin* 62: 313–337.

———— (1986). *Das europäische Hospital von der Spätantike bis 1800.* Cologne.

Johnstone, P. (1981). "Galen in Arabic: The Transformation of Galenic Pharmacology," in Nutton (1981), 197–212.

Jolivet, J., and R. Rashed, eds. (1984). *Études sur Avicenne.* Paris.

Joly, H. (1974). *Le Renversement platonicien: Logos, Epistèmè, Polis.* Paris.

Joly, R. (1960). *Recherches sur le traité pseudo-hippocratique "Du régime."* Paris.

———— (1961a). "La Question hippocratique et le témoignage du Phèdre," *Revue des études grecques* 74: 69–92.

———— (1961b). "Platon et la médecine," *Bulletin de l'Association Guillaume Budé,* 435–451.

———— (1966). *Le Niveau de la science hippocratique.* Paris.

———— (1983). "Hippocrates and the School of Cos. between Myth and Skepticism," in M. Ruse, ed., *Nature Animated II* (Dordrecht), pp. 29–47.

————, ed. (1977). *Corpus hippocraticum* (proceedings of the second Hippocratic Colloquium, Mons, 1975). Mons.

Jones, P. M. (1984). *Medieval Medical Miniatures.* Austin.

Jones, W. H. S. (1909). *Malaria and Greek History.* Manchester.

———— (1946). *Philosophy and Medicine in Ancient Greece.* Baltimore.

Joos, P. (1957). "Zufall, Kunst und Natur bei den Hippokratikern," *Janus* 46: 238–252.

Jordan, M. D. (1987). "Medicine as Science in the Early Commentaries on 'Johannitius,'" *Traditio* 43: 121–145.

———— (1990). "The Construction of a Philosophical Medicine: Exegesis and Argument in Salernitan Teaching on the Soul," in McVaugh and Siraisi (1990), 42–61.

Jouanna, J. (1966). "La Théorie de l'intelligence et de l'âme dans le traité hippocratique du Régime: Ses rapports avec Empédocle et le 'Timée' de Platon," *Revue des études grecques* 79: xv–xviii.

———— (1974). *Hippocrate: Pour une archéologie de l'école de Cnide.* Paris.

———— (1977). "La Collection hippocratique et Platon (Phèdre 269c–272a)," *Revue des études grecques* 90: 15–28.

———— (1978). "Le Médecin modèle du législateur dans les Lois," *Ktema* 3: 77–91.

———— (1980). "La Problématique du changement dans le Régime des maladies aiguës et chez Thucydide (livre VI)," in Grmek, ed. (1980), 299–319.

———— (1987). "Médecine hippocratique et tragédie grecque," *Anthropologie et Théâtre antique: Cahiers du Gita* 3: 109–131.

———— (1988a). "Ippocrate e il sacro," *Koinonia* 12: 91–113.

———— (1988b). "La Maladie sauvage dans la Collection hippocratique et la tragédie grecque," *Métis* 3: 343–360.

———— (1989). "Hippocrate de Cos et le sacré," *Journal des savants,* 3–22.

———— (1992). *Hippocrate.* Paris.

Joubaud, C. (1991). *Le Corps humain dans la philosophie platonicienne: Étude à partir du Timée.* Paris.

Judson, H. F. (1979). *The Eighth Day of Creation: Makers of the Revolution in Biology.* London.

Karimov, U. I. (1980). "O medicinskom nasledii Ibn Siny," in B. A. Baratov, ed., *Abu Ali Ibn Sina: K 1000-letiju so dnja rozdenija.* Tashkent.

Keenan, M. E. (1936). "Augustine and the Medical Profession," *Transactions and Proceedings of the American Philological Association,* 67.

Keil, G. (1983–84). "Mittelalterliche Chirurgie," *Acta Medicae Historiae Patavina* 30: 45–64.

Keil, G., and W. Loechel (1975). "Gestaltwandel und Zersetzung: Roger-Urtext und Roger-Glosse vom 12. bis ins 16. Jahrhundert," in A. Buck, ed., *Der Kommentar in der Renaissance* (Wiesbaden), pp. 209–224.

Ketchman Weaton, B. (1983). *Savoring the Past.* Philadelphia.

Kibre, P. (1978). "Arts and Medicine in the Universities of the Later Middle Ages," in J. Paques and J. Ijsewjn, eds., *The Universities in the Late Middle Ages* (Louvain), pp. 213–227. (Repr. in P. Kibre, *Studies in Medieval Science,* London, 1984.)

———— (1985). *Hippocrates Latinus: A Repertorium of Hippocratic Writings in the Latin Middle Ages.* New York.

Kibre, P., and I. A. Kelter (1987). "Galen's Methodus medendi in the Middle Ages," *History and Philosophy of the Life Sciences* 9: 17–36.

Kibre, P., and N. G. Siraisi (1975). "Matheolus of Perugia's Commentary on the Preface to the Aphorisms of Hippocrates," *Bulletin of the History of Medicine* 49: 405–428.

King, L. (1954). "What Is Disease?" *Philosophy of Science* 21: 193–203.

Klein-Franke, F. (1982). "Vorlesungen über die Medizin im Islam," *Sudhoffs Archiv für Geschichte der Medizin,* vol. 23.

———— (1984). *Iatromathematics in Islam: A Study on Yuhanna Ibn as Salt's Book on Astrological Medicine.* Hildesheim, Zurich, and New York.

Klibansky, R., E. Panofsky, and F. Saxl (1964). *Saturn and Melancholy.* London.

Knoefel, P. (1991). *Nicander Restored.* Lewiston.

Knowles, D., and N. Hadcok (1971). *Medieval Religious Houses: England and Wales.* London.

Kölbing, H. M. (1985). *Die ärztliche Therapie.* Darmstadt.

Kollesch, J. (1973). *Untersuchungen zu den pseudogalenischen Definitiones medicae.* Berlin.

———— (1977). "Die Stellung der knidischen Heilkunde in der Wissenschaftlichen Medizin der Griechen," in Joly (1977), 106–122.

———— (1987). "Galens Auseinandersetzung mit der Aristotelischen Samenlehre," in Wiesner (1987), 2: 17–26.

———— (1989). "Knidos als Zentrum der frühen wissenschaftlichen Medizin im antiken Griechenland," *Gesnerus* 46: 11–28.

Kollesch, J., and D. Nickel, eds. (1993). *Galen und das hellenistische Erbe.* Stuttgart.

Kornexl, E. (1970). *Begriff und Einschätzung der Gesundheit des Körpers in der griechischen Literatur von ihren Anfängen bis zum Hellenismus.* Innsbruck and Munich.

Koyré, A. (1966). *Études d'histoire de la pensée scientifique.* Paris.

Kräupl Taylor, F. (1979). *The Concept of Illness, Disease, and Morbus.* Cambridge, London, and New York.

Krause, C. F. T. (1825). *Ueber das Alter der Menschenpocken und anderer exanthematischer Krankheiten.* Hannover.

Kristeller, P. O. (1978). "Philosophy and Medicine in Medieval and Renaissance Italy," in Spicker (1978).

———— (1986). *Studi sulla Scuola medica salernitana.* Naples.

Kritikos, P. G., and S. N. Papadaki (1969). "Contribution à l'histoire de la pharmacie chez les Byzantins," in *Die Vorträge der Hauptversammlung der Internationalen Gesellschaft für Geschichte der Pharmazie in Athen 1967* (Stuttgart), pp. 13–78.

Kudlien, F. (1962). "Poseidonios und die Ärzteschule der Pneumatiker," *Hermes* 90: 419–429.

———— (1963). "Probleme um Diokles von Karystos," *Sudhoffs Archiv für Geschichte der Medizin* 47: 456–464. (Repr. in Flashar [1971], 192–201.)

———— (1964a). "Herophilos und der Beginn der medizinischen Skepsis," *Gesnerus* 21: 1–13. (Repr. in Flashar [1971], 280–295.)

———— (1964b). *Untersuchungen zu Aretaios von Kappadokien.* Mainz and Wiesbaden.

———— (1967). *Der Beginn des medizinischen Denkens bei den Griechen.* Zurich and Stuttgart.

———— (1968a). "Anatomie," in Pauly-Wissowa, *Real. Enzyklopädie,* suppl. 11 (Stuttgart), cols. 78–94.

———— (1968b). "Pneumatische Ärzte," in Pauly-Wissowa, *Real. Enzyklopädie,* suppl. 11 (Stuttgart), cols. 1097–1108.

———— (1968c). "Early Greek Primitive Medicine," *Clio Medica* 3: 305–336.

———— (1969). "Antike Anatomie und menschlicher Leichnam," *Hermes* 97: 78–94.

———— (1971a). "Probleme um Diokles von Karystos," in Flashar (1971).

———— (1971b). "Herophilos und des Beginn der medizinischen Skepsis," in Flashar (1971).

———— (1973). "The Old Greek Concept of 'Relative' Health," *Journal of the History of the Behavioral Sciences* 9: 53–59.

———— (1976). "Medicine as a 'Liberal Art' and the Question of the Physician's Income," *Journal of the History of Medicine* 31: 448–459.

———— (1977a). "Das Göttliche und die Natur im hippokratischen Prognostikon," *Hermes* 105: 268–274.

———— (1977b). "Bemerkungen zu W. D. Smith's These über die knidische Ärzteschule," in Joly (1977), 95–103.

———— (1979). *Der griechische Arzt im Zeitalter des Hellenismus: Seine Stellung in Staat und Gesellschaft.* Mainz and Wiesbaden.

Kudlien, F., and R. J. Durling, eds. (1991). *Galen's Method of Healing.* Leiden.

Kühn, H. J. (1956). *System- und Methodenprobleme im Corpus hippocraticum.* Wiesbaden.

Kuhn, T. (1962). *The Structure of Scientific Revolutions.* Chicago.

Kuhne, R. (1989). "El Kitab al-dury, prototipo árabe de la Capsula eburnea y representante más genuino de la tradición de los Secreta Hippocratis," *Al-Qantara* 10: 3–20, 291–327.

Künzl, E. (1983). *Medizinische Instrumente aus Sepulkralfunden der römischen Kaiserzeit.* Cologne.

Kuttner, S. (1952). "Pabst Honorius III und das Studium des Zivilrechts," in *Festschrift für Martin Wolf,* Tübingen.

Laignel-Lavastine, M., and B. Guégan, eds. (1936–1949). *Histoire générale de la médecine, de la pharmacie, de l'art dentaire et de l'art vétérinaire,* 3 vols. Paris.

Laín Entralgo, P. (1961). *Enfermedad y pecado.* Barcelona.

———— (1961). *La historia clínica: Historia y teoria del relato patográfico.* Barcelona.

———— (1987). *El cuerpo humano: Oriente y Grecia Antigua.* Madrid.

————, ed. (1972–1975). *Historia universal de la medicina,* 7 vols. Barcelona.

Lallemand, L. (1906). *Histoire générale de la charité,* vol. 3, *Le Moyen Age.* Paris.

Lanata, G. (1967). *Medicina magica e religione popolare in Grecia fino all'età di Ippocrate.* Rome.

Langholf, V. (1986). "Kallimachos, Komödie und hippokratische Frage," *Medizinhistorisches Journal* 21: 3–30.

———— (1990). *Medical Theories in Hippokrates: Early Texts and the "Epidemics."* Berlin.

Lanza, D., and M. Vegetti (1971). *Opere biologiche di Aristotele.* Turin.

Laplantine, F. (1986). *Anthropologie de la maladie.* Paris.

Lasserre, F., and P. Mudry, eds. (1983). *Formes de pensée dans la Collection hippocratique* (proceedings of the fourth Hippocratic Colloquium, Lausanne, 1981). Geneva.

Latronico, N. (1956). *La medicina degli antichi.* Milan.

Laurie, H. C. R. (1991). *The Making of Romance: Three Studies.* Geneva.

Le Clerc, D. (1696). *Histoire de la médecine, où l'on voit l'origine et le progrès de cet art.* Geneva. (Rev. ed., Amsterdam, 1702.)

Leclerc, L. (1876). *Histoire de la médecine arabe.* Paris.

Le Goff, J., and J.-C. Sournia, eds. (1985). *Les Maladies ont une histoire.* Paris.

Le Grand, L. (1901). *Statuts d'hôtels-Dieu et de léproseries.* Paris.

Leitner, H. (1973). *Bibliography to the Ancient Medical Authors.* Berne.

Lemay, R. (1962). *Abu Ma'shar and Latin Aristotelianism in the Twelfth Century.* Beirut.

Lemerle, P. (1971). *Le Premier Humanisme byzantin: Notes et remarques sur enseignement et culture à Byzance des origines au Xe siècle.* Paris.

Léonard, J. (1981). *La Médecine entre les pouvoirs et les savoirs: Histoire intellectuelle et politique de la médecine française au XIXe siècle.* Paris.

Lesky, E. (1950). *Die Zeugungs- und Vererbungslehre der Antike und ihr Nachwirken.* Mainz and Wiesbaden.

LeVay, D. (1990). *The History of Orthopaedics.* Carnforth.

Leven, K.-H. (1987). "Die 'Justinianische Pest,'" *Jahrbuch des Instituts für Geschichte der Medizin der Robert Bosch Stiftung* 6: 137–161.

——— (1990). "Das Bild der byzantinischen Medizin in der Satire 'Timarion,'" *Gesnerus* 47: 247–262.

Levey, M. (1973). *Early Arabic Pharmacology: An Introduction Based on Ancient and Medieval Sources.* Leiden.

Libera, A. de (1989). *La Philosophie médiévale.* Paris.

——— (1991). *Penser au Moyen Age.* Paris.

Lichtenthaeler, C. (1948–1963). *La Médecine hippocratique,* 9 vols. Lausanne, Neuchâtel, and Geneva.

——— (1975). *Geschichte der Medizin,* 2 vols. Cologne and Lövenich.

——— (1984). *Der Eid des Hippokrates: Ursprung und Bedeutung.* Cologne.

Lieber, E. (1981). "Galen in Hebrew: The Transmission of Galen's Works in the Medieval Islamic World," in Nutton (1981), 171–180.

Lindberg, D. C. (1983). *Roger Bacon's Philosophy of Nature.* Oxford.

Litmann, R. J., and M. L. Litman (1973). "Galen and the Antonine Plague," *American Journal of Philology* 94: 243–255.

Littré, É., ed. (1839–1861). *Oeuvres complètes d'Hippocrate (Opera Omnia Hippocratis),* 10 vols. Paris.

——— (1872). *Médecine et médecins.* Paris.

Lloyd, G. E. R. (1964a). "Experiment in Early Greek Philosophy and Medicine," *Proceedings of the Cambridge Philological Society,* new ser., 10: 50–72. (Repr. in Lloyd [1991], 70–99.)

——— (1964b). "The Hot and the Cold, the Dry and the Wet in the Greek Philosophy," *Journal of Hellenic Studies* 84: 92–106.

——— (1975a). "A Note on Erasistratus of Ceos," *Journal of Hellenic Studies* 95: 172–175.

——— (1975b). "The Hippocratic Question," *Classical Quarterly,* new ser., 25: 171–192.

——— (1979). *Magic, Reason, and Experience.* Cambridge.

——— (1987). *The Revolutions of Wisdom.* Berkeley.

——— (1991). *Methods and Problems in Greek Science: Selected Papers.* Cambridge.

——— (1992). "The Transformations of Ancient Medicine," *Bulletin of the History of Medicine* 66: 114–132.

Lockwood, D. P. (1951). *Ugo Benzi, Medieval Philosopher and Physician, 1376–1439.* Chicago.

Long, A., and D. Sedley (1989). *The Hellenistic Philosophers,* 2 vols. Cambridge.

Longere, J. (1975). *Oeuvres oratoires de maîtres parisiens au XIIe siècle,* vol. 2. Paris.

Longrigg, J. (1963). "Philosophy and Medicine," *Harvard Studies in Classical Philology* 67: 147–175.

——— (1980). "The Great Plague of Athens," *History of Science* 18: 209–225.

——— (1983). "Hippocrates, Ancient Medicine, and Its Intellectual Context," in Lasserre and Mudry (1983), 249–256.

——— (1993). *Greek Rational Medicine: Philosophy and Medicine from Alcmaeon to Alexandrians.* London and New York.

Lonie, I. M. (1964). "Erasistratus, the Erasistrateans, and Aristotle," *Bulletin of the History of Medicine* 38: 426–443.

——— (1965). "The Cnidian Treatises of the Corpus Hippocraticum," *Classical Quarterly* 15: 1–30.

——— (1973). "The Paradoxical Text 'On the Hearth,'" *Medical History* 17: 1–15, 136–153.

——— (1978). "Cos versus Cnidus and the Historians," *History of Science* 16: 42–75, 77–92.

——— (1981a). *The Hippocratic Treatises "On Generation," "On the Nature of the Child," "Diseases IV."* Berlin.

——— (1981b). "Fever Pathology in the Sixteenth Century: Tradition and Innovation," in Bynum and Nutton (1981), 19–44.

López Férez, J. A., ed. (1992). *Tratados hipocráticos* (proceedings of the seventh Hippocratic Colloquium, Madrid, 1990). Madrid.

Lorenz, G. (1990). *Antike Krankenbehandlung in historisch-vergleichender Sicht: Studien zum konkret-anschaulichen Denken.* Heidelberg.

Louis, P. (1990). *Vie d'Aristote.* Paris.

Löwy, I. (1990). *The Polish School of Philosophy of Medicine.* Dordrecht.

Lush, B., et al. (1961). *Concepts of Medicine.* Oxford.

MacArthur, M. D. (1958). "The Plague of Athens," *Bulletin of the History of Medicine* 32: 242–246.

MacBrooks, E. C., and P. Cranefield, eds. (1959). *Historical Development of Physiological Thought.* New York.

MacKinney, L. C. (1934). "Tenth-Century Medicine as Seen in the 'Historia' of Richer of Rheims," *Bulletin of the Institute of the History of Medicine* 2: 347–375.

——— (1952). "Medical Ethics and Etiquette in the Early Middle Ages: The Persistence of Hippocratic Ideals," *Bulletin of the History of Medicine* 20: 1–31.

——— (1962). "The Beginnings of Western Scientific Anatomy: New Evidence and a Revision in Interpretation of Mondeville's Role," *Medical History* 6: 233–239.

——— (1965). *Medical Illustrations in Medieval Manuscripts.* London.

Majno, G. (1975). *The Healing Hand: Man and Wound in the Ancient World.* Cambridge, Mass.

Major, R. H. (1954). *A History of Medicine*, 2 vols. Springfield.

Malagola, C. (1888). *Statuti delle Università et dei Collegi dello Studio bolognese*. Bologna.

Mâle, E. (1922). *L'Art religieux de la fin du Moyen Age en France*. Paris.

Maloney, G., and R. Savoie (1982). *Cinq cents ans de bibliographie hippocratique (1472–1982)*. Quebec.

Manchester, K. (1984). "Tuberculosis and Leprosy in Antiquity: An Interpretation," *Medical History* 28: 162–173.

Manetti, D. (1986). "Note di lettura nell'Anonimo Londinense," *Zeitschrift für Papyrologie und Epigraphik* 63: 57–74.

Mani, N. (1991). "Die wissenschaftlichen Grundlagen der Chirurgie bei Galen," in Kudlien and Durling (1991), 26–49.

Mansfeld, J. (1971). *The Pseudo-Hippocratic Tract Peri hebdomadon cg. 1–11 and Greek Philosophy*. Assen.

——— (1980). "Plato and the Method of Hippocrates," *Greek, Roman and Byzantine Studies* 21: 341–362.

Mantegazza, M. (1989). "Per una nuova lettura della farmacologia antica a partire dall'opera di Dioscoride," in *Le piante medicinali e il loro impiego in farmacia nel corso dei secoli: Atti del Congresso Internazionale di Storia della farmacia* (Piacenza), pp. 29–35.

Manuli, P. (1980). *Medicina e antropologia nella tradizione antica*. Turin.

——— (1985). "Medico e malattia," in Vegetti (1985), 229–245.

Manuli, P., and M. Vegetti (1977). *Cuore, sangue e cervello: Biologia e antropologia nel pensiero antico*. Milan.

———, ed. (1988). *Le opere psicologiche di Galeno*. Naples.

Manzalaqui, M. (1970–71). "The Pseudo-Aristotelian Kitab Sirr al-Asrar," *Oriens* 23–24: 147–257.

Marcel, R. (1951). "Saint Socrate, patron de l'Humanisme," *Revue internationale de philosophie* 5: 135–143.

Marin, D. (1974). "Charitas," *Annali della Facoltà di Lettere e Filosofia dell'Università di Bari* 12: 159–234.

Marsden, E. W. (1968). *Greek and Roman Artillery: Historical Development*. Oxford.

Maurach, G. (1978). "Johannicius Isagoge ad Techne Galieni," *Sudhoffs Archiv für Geschichte der Medizin* 62: 148–174.

May, E. (1957). *La Médecine, son passé, son présent, son avenir*. Paris.

Mayr, E. (1982). *The Growth of Biological Thought: Diversity, Evolution, and Inheritance*. Cambridge, Mass.

Maziar Zafari, A., Nezami Aruzi, and Tschehar Maqaleh (1990). *Psychosomatische Aspekte in der mittelalterlichen Medizin Persiens*. Cologne.

Mazzi, M. S. (1978). *Salute e società nel Medioevo*. Florence.

Mazzini, I., and F. Fusco, eds. (1985). *I testi di medicina latini antichi: Problemi filologici e storici*. Rome.

Mazzini, I., and N. Palmieri (1991). "L'École médicale de Ravenne," in Mudry and Pigeaud (1991), 285–310.

McEvoy, J. (1982). *The Philosophy of Robert Grosseteste.* Oxford.

McNeill, W. H. (1976). *Plagues and Peoples.* Garden City, N.Y.

McVaugh, M. R. (1970). "Arnald of Villanova," in Gillispie (1970–1980), 1: 289–291.

―――― (1971). "The 'Experimenta' of Arnald of Villanova," *Journal of Medieval and Renaissance Studies* 1: 107–118.

―――― (1974). "The 'Humidum Radicale' in Thirteenth-Century Medicine," *Traditio* 30: 259–283.

―――― (1987). "The Two Faces of a Medical Career: Jordanus de Turre of Montpellier," in J. E. Murdoch and E. Grant, eds., *Mathematics and Its Applications to Science and Natural Philosophy in the Middle Ages* (Cambridge), pp. 301–324.

―――― (1990). "The Nature and Limits of Medical Certitude at Early Fourteenth-Century Montpellier," in McVaugh and Siraisi (1990), 62–84.

McVaugh, M. R., and N. G. Siraisi, eds. (1990). "Renaissance Medical Learning: Evolution of a Tradition," *Osiris,* 2d ser., 6.

Mehren, A. F. (1884). "Vues d'Avicenne sur l'astrologie et sur le rapport de la responsabilité humaine avec le destin," *Le Muséon* 3: 383–403.

Merlo, G. G., ed. (1988). *Esperienze religiose ed opere assistenziali nei secoli XI–XIII.* Turin.

Merton, R. K. (1973). *The Sociology of Science.* Chicago.

Mettler, C. C. (1947). *A History of Medicine.* Philadelphia.

Meunier, L. (1924). *Histoire de la médecine depuis ses origines jusqu'à nos jours.* Paris.

Meyerhof, M. (1929). "Autobiographische Bruckstücke aus arabischen Quellen," *Sudhoffs Archiv für Geschichte der Medizin* 22: 72–86.

―――― (1930). "Von Alexandrien nach Bagdad: Ein Beitrag zur Geschichte des philosophischen und medizinischen Unterrichts bei den Arabern," *Sitzungsberichte der Preussischen Akademie der Wissenschaften: Philosophisch-Historische Klasse,* 389–426.

―――― (1935a). "Ibn al-Nafîs (XIIIth Century) and His Theory of the Lesser Circulation," *Isis* 23: 100–120.

―――― (1935b). "Thirty-Three Clinical Observations by Rhazes (circa 900 A.D.)," *Isis* 23: 321–356.

―――― (1942). "Die literarischen Grundlagen der arabischen Heilmittellehre," *Ciba Zeitschrift* 85: 2961–2996.

―――― (1944). "La Surveillance des professions médicales et paramédicales chez les Arabes," *Bulletin de l'Institut d'Égypte* 26: 119–134. (Eng. trans. in P. Johnstone, ed., *Studies in Medieval Arabic Medicine,* London, 1984.)

Meyerhof, M., and J. Schacht (1968). *The Theologus Autodidactus of Ibn al-Nafîs.* Oxford.

Meyer-Steineg, T. (1913). *Ein Tag im Leben des Galen.* Jena.

Michalla, J. (1989). *Ägypten: Gesundheitsdienst seit dem Feldzug Napoleons.* Cologne.

Michaud-Quantin, P. (1966). "Les Petites Encyclopédies du XIIIe siècle," *Cahiers d'histoire mondiale* 9: 584–588.

Michler, M. (1968a). "Medical Ethics in Hippocratic Bone Surgery," *Bulletin of the History of Medicine* 42: 297–311.

———— (1968b). *Die Hellenistische Chirurgie,* part 1, *Die Alexandrinischen Chirurgen.* Wiesbaden.

———— (1969). *Das Spezialisierungsproblem und die antike Chirurgie.* Berne, Stuttgart, and Vienna.

Migliorini, P. (1991). "Elementi metodici in Teodoro Prisciano," in Mudry and Pigeaud (1991), 231–240.

Miller, H. W. (1962). "Aetiology of Disease in Plato's 'Timaeus,'" *Transactions and Proceedings of the American Philological Association* 93: 175–187.

Miller, J. I. (1969). *The Spice Trade of the Roman Empire.* Oxford.

Miller, T. S. (1978). "The Knights of Saint John and the Hospitals of the Latin West," *Speculum* 53: 709–733.

———— (1985). *The Birth of the Hospital in the Byzantine Empire.* Baltimore and London.

Milne, J. S. (1907). *Surgical Instruments in Greek and Roman Times.* London. (Repr., New York, 1970.)

Moisan, M. (1990a). *Lexique du vocabulaire botanique d'Hippocrate* (with the collaboration of G. Maloney and D. Grenier). Quebec.

———— (1990b). "Les Plantes narcotiques dans le 'Corpus hippocratique,'" in Potter, Maloney, and Desautels (1990), 381–391.

Mollat, M. (1978). *Les Pauvres au Moyen Age.* Paris.

———— (1982). "Complexité et ambiguïté des institutions hospitalières: Les Statuts d'hôpitaux (les modèles, leur diffusion et leur filiation)," in G. Politi, M. Rosa, and F. Della Peruta, eds., *Timore e carità: I poveri nell'Italia moderna* (Cremona), pp. 3–12.

Montalenti, G. (1962). "Storia della biologia e della medicina," in N. Abbagnano, ed., *Storia delle scienze,* vol. 3, book 1. Turin.

Montero-Cartelle, E. (1990). "Encuentro de culturas en Salerno: Constantino el Africano, traductor," in Hamesse and Fattori (1990), 65–88.

Moore, R. I. (1990). *The Formation of a Persecuting Society: Power and Deviance in Western Europe, 950–1250.* Cambridge, Mass.

Moraux, P. (1973–1984). *Der Aristotelismus bei den Griechen,* 2 vols. Berlin and New York.

———— (1985). *Galien de Pergame: Souvenirs d'un médecin.* Paris.

Morpurgo, P. (1990). *Filosofia della natura nella "Schola salernitana" del secolo XII.* Bologna.

Mudry, P. (1980). "Medicus amicus: Un trait romain dans la médecine antique," *Gesnerus* 37: 1–20.

———— (1982). *La Préface du "De Medicina" de Celse: Texte, traduction et commentaire.* Rome.

Mudry, P., and J. Pigeaud, eds. (1991). *Les Écoles médicales à Rome* (proceedings of the second International Colloquium on Ancient Latin Medical Texts, Lausanne, 1986). Geneva and Nantes.

Mueller, F. L. (1960). *Histoire de la psychologie de l'Antiquité à nos jours.* Paris.

Müller, I. von (1891). "Galen als Philologe," in *Verhandlungen der 41: Versammlung deutscher Philologen und Schulmänner.* Munich.

Mundy, J. H. (1966). "Charity and Social Work in Toulouse, 1100–1250," *Traditio* 13: 207–287.

Münster, L. (1955). "La medicina legale in Bologna dai suoi albori fino alla fine del secolo XIV," *Bollettino dell'Accademia Medica Pistoiese Filippo Pacini* 26: 257–271.

Murdoch, J. E. (1975). "From Social into Intellectual Factors: An Aspect of the Unitary Character of Late Medieval Learning," in J. E. Murdoch and E. D. Sylla, eds., *The Cultural Context of Medieval Learning* (Dordrecht and Boston), pp. 271–348.

Murdock, G. P. (1980). *Theories of Illness: A World Survey.* Pittsburgh.

Murray, A. (1974). "Religion among the Poor in Thirteenth-Century France: The Testimony of Humbert de Romans," *Traditio* 30: 285–324.

Musitelli, S. (1967). "Alle origini del 'Regimen Sanitatis,'" *Salerno* 1: 22–58.

Nardi, B. (1949). "L'Averroismo bolognese nel secolo XIII e Taddeo Alderotti," *Rivista di storia della filosofia* 4: 11–22.

Naso, I. (1982). *Medici e strutture sanitarie nella società tardo-medievale: Il Piemonte dei secoli XIV–XV.* Milan.

Nestle, W. (1940). *Vom Mythos zum Logos.* Stuttgart.

Neuburger, M. (1906–1911). *Geschichte der Medizin,* 2 vols. Stuttgart.

Newton, F. (1994). "Constantine the African and Monte Cassino: New Elements and the Text of the Isagoge," in Burnett and Jacquart (1994), pp. 16–47.

Nicaise, E. (1890). *La Grande Chirurgie de Guy de Chauliac, composée en l'an 1363.* Paris.

———— (1893). *Chirurgie de maître Henri de Mondeville, chirurgien de Philippe le Bel.* Paris.

Nickel, D. (1989). *Untersuchungen zur Embryologie Galens.* Berlin.

Nordenfelt, L., and B. I. B. Lindahl, eds. (1984). *Health, Disease, and Causal Explanation in Medicine.* Dordrecht.

Nordenskiöld, E. (1928). *The History of Biology.* New York.

Nörenberg, H.-W. (1968). *Das Göttliche und die Natur in der Schrift: "Über die heilige Krankheit."* Bonn.

Norman, J. M. (1991). *Garrison-Morton's Medical Bibliography.* Aldershot.

Nougaret, R. (1986). *Hôpitaux, Léproseries et Bodomies de Rodez, de la grande peste à l'hôpital général (vers 1340–1676).* Rodez.

Noye, I. (1977). "Maladie," in *Dictionnaire de spiritualité*, vol. 10, fasc. 44–45 (Paris), pp. 137–152.

Numbers, R. L., and D. W. Amundsen, eds. (1986). *Caring and Curing*. New York and London.

Nutton, V. (1973). "The Chronology of Galen's Earlier Career," *Classical Quarterly* 23: 158–171.

———— (1983). "The Seeds of Disease: An Explanation of Contagion and Infection from the Greeks to the Renaissance," *Medical History* 27: 1–34.

———— (1984). "Galen in the Eyes of His Contemporaries," *Bulletin of the History of Medicine* 58: 315–324.

———— (1985). "From Galen to Alexander: Aspects of Medicine and Medical Practice in Late Antiquity," in Scarborough (1985), 3–25.

————, ed. (1981). *Galen: Problems and Prospects* (collection of papers submitted at the 1979 Cambridge Conference on Galen). London.

O'Brien, D. (1981). *Pour interpréter Empédocle*. Paris.

Oesterle, H. J. (1980). "Vena basilica—Vena cephalica: Die Genese einer unverstandenen Terminologie," *Sudhoffs Archiv für Geschichte der Medizin* 64: 385–390.

Ogden, M. S. (1973). "The Galenic Works Cited by Guy de Chauliac's 'Chirurgia Magna,'" *Journal of the History of Medicine* 28: 24–33.

Oldoni, M. (1987). "La scuola medica di Salerno nella cultura europea fra XI e XIII secolo," *Quaderni medievali* 20: 74–94.

Olerud, A. (1951). *L'Idée de microcosmos et de macrocosmos dans le Timée de Platon*. Uppsala.

O'Neill, Y. V. (1970). "Another Look at the 'Anatomia porci,'" *Viator* 1: 115–124.

———— (1976). "Innocent III and the Evolution of Anatomy," *Medical History* 20: 415–431.

———— (1985). "Il corpo dello spirito: Medicina e cristianesimo," *Kos* 14: 18–32.

Opsomer, C. (1989). *Index de la pharmacopée du Ier au Xe siècle*, 2 vols. Hildesheim, Zurich, and New York.

———— (1991). *L'Art de vivre en santé: Images et recettes du Moyen Age*. "Le Tacuinum Sanitatis" (manuscript 1401) of the Bibliothèque de l'Université de Liège.

Opsomer, C., and R. Halleux (1985). "La Lettre d'Hippocrate à Antiochus et la lettre d'Hippocrate à Mécène," in Mazzini and Fusco (1985), 339–364.

Orofino, G. (1991). "Dioskurides war gegen Pflanzenbilder," *Die Waage* 4: 144–149.

———— (1992). "Il Dioscoride della Biblioteca Nazionale di Napoli: Le miniature," in *Dioscurides Neapolitanus: Biblioteca Nazionale di Napoli* (Rome and Graz), pp. 85–98.

Ortalli, E. (1965–1968). "La perizia medica a Bologna nei secoli XIII e XIV, Normativa e pratica di un Istituto giudiziario," *Atti e Memorie della Deputazione di Storia Patria per le Provincie di Romagna*, new ser., 17–19, 223–259.

Ortner, D. J., and W. G. J. Putschar (1985). *Identification of Pathological Conditions in Human Skeletal Remains*. Washington.

Ottosson, P. G. (1982). *Scholastic Medicine and Philosophy: A Study of Commentaries on Galen's "Tegni" (ca. 1300–1450).* Naples.

Page, D. L. (1953). "Thucydides' Description of the Great Plague of Athens," *Classical Quarterly* 47: 897–920.

Palmieri, N. (1981). "Un antico commento a Galeno," *Physis* 23: 197–296.

Paniagua, J. A. (1969). *El Maestro Arnau de Vilanova médico.* Valencia.

——— (1994). *Studia Arnaldiana.* Barcelona.

Paravicini-Bagliani, A. (1989). "L'Église médiévale et la renaissance de l'anatomie," *Revue médicale de la Suisse romande* 109: 987–991.

——— (1991). *Medicina e scienze della natura alla corte dei papi nel Duecento.* Spoleto.

Park, K. (1985). *Doctors and Medicine in Early Renaissance Florence.* Princeton.

Park, K., and J. Henderson (1991). "'The First Hospital among Christians': The Ospedale di Santa Maria Nuova in Early Sixteenth-Century Florence," *Medical History* 35: 164–188.

Pasca, M. (1987). *La Scuola medica salernitana: Storia, immagini, manoscritti dall'XI al XIII secolo.* Naples.

Paschetto, E. (1984). *Pietro d'Abano, medico e filosofo.* Florence.

Paterson, L. M. (1986). "Military Surgery: Knights, Sergeants, and Raimon of Avignon's Version of the 'Chirurgia' of Roger of Salerno (1180–1209)," in C. Harper-Bill and R. Harvey, eds., *The Ideals and Practice of Medieval Knighthood,* vol. 2 (Wolfeboro), pp. 117–146.

Patzelt, E. (1969). "Pauvreté et maladies," in *Povertà e ricchezza nella spiritualità dei secoli XI e XII* (Todi), pp. 165–187.

Pauly, A. (1874). *Bibliographie des sciences médicales.* Paris.

Pauly, A. F., and G. Wissowa (1893–1980). *Real-Enzyklopädie der klassischen Altertumswissenschaft.* Stuttgart. First ser., 1893 and following, 24 books in 49 vols.; second ser., 1903 and following, 10 books in 19 vols.; supplement, 15 vols.; index, 1 vol.

Pazzini, A. (1947). *Storia della medicina,* 2 vols. Milan. (Rev. ed., *Storia dell'arte sanitaria dalle origini ad oggi,* Turin, 1974.)

Pease, A. P. (1914). "Medical Allusions in the Works of St. Jerome," *Harvard Studies in Classical Philology* 25: 73–86.

Penella, R. J. (1990). *Greek Philosophers and Sophists in the Fourth Century A.D.: Studies in Eunapius of Sardis.* Leeds.

Penso, G. (1991). *La medicina medioevale.* Saronno.

Pentzopoulou-Valalas, T. (1990). "Experience and Causal Explanation in Medical Empiricism," in P. Nicolacopoulos, ed., *Greek Studies in the Philosophy and History of Science* (Dordrecht), pp. 91–107.

Pérez Tamayo, R. (1988). *El concepto de enfermedad,* 2 vols. Mexico.

Pesenti, T. (1982). "Generi e pubblico della letteratura medica padovana nel Tre e Quattrocento," in *Università e società nei secoli* (Pistoia), pp. 523–545.

——— (1984). *Professori e promotori di medicina nello Studio di Padova dal 1405 al 1509: Repertorio bio-bibliografico*. Padua.

——— (1989). "Arti e medicina: La formazione del curriculum medico," in L. Gargan and O. Limone, *Luoghi e metodi di insegnamento nell'Italia medioevale (secoli XII–XIV)* (study conference, Lecce-Otranto, 1986). Galatina.

Petrequin, J. E. (1877–78). *La Chirurgie d'Hippocrate*. Paris.

Pfaff, F. (1931). "Die nur arabische erhaltenen Teile der Epidemienkommentare des Galen und die Überlieferung des Corpus Hippocraticum," *Sitzungsberichte der Preussischen Akademie der Wissenschaften: Philosophisch-Historische Klasse*, 576–581.

Phillips, E. D. (1973). *Greek Medicine*. London.

Piazza, L. (1912). *Il De re medica di A.C. Celso nella medicina romana*. Catania.

Pigeaud, J. (1981). *La Maladie de l'âme: Étude sur la relation de l'âme et du corps dans la tradition médico-philosophique antique*. Paris.

——— (1982). "Les Mains des dieux: Quelques réflexions sur les problèmes du médicament dans l'Antiquité," *Littérature, médecine, société* 4: 53–73.

——— (1991). "Les Fondements du méthodisme," in Mudry and Pigeaud (1991), 7–50.

——— (1992). "La Médecine et ses origines," *Bulletin canadien d'histoire de la médecine* 9: 219–240.

Pigeaud, J., and J. Orose, eds. (1987). *Pline l'Ancien, témoin de son temps*. Salamanca and Nantes.

Pinault, J. R. (1992). *Hippocratic Lives and Legends*. Leiden.

Plamböck, G. (1964). *Dynamis im Corpus Hippocraticum*. Mainz and Wiesbaden.

Popper, K. R. (1959). *Logic of Scientific Discovery*. London.

Porter, R., and A. Wear (1987). *Problems and Methods in the History of Medicine*. London.

Postel, J., and C. Quétel, eds. (1983). *Nouvelle histoire de la psychiatrie*. Toulouse. (Rev. ed., Paris, 1993.)

Potter, P., G. Maloney, and J. Desautels, eds. (1990). *La Maladie et les maladies dans la Collection hippocratique* (proceedings of the sixth Hippocratic Colloquium, Quebec, 1987). Quebec.

Pouchelle, M. C. (1976). "La prise en charge de la mort," *Archives européennes de sociologie* 17: 249–278.

——— (1983). *Corps et Chirurgie à l'apogée du Moyen Age*. Paris.

Poulet, J., M. Martiny, and J. C. Sournia, eds. (1977–1980). *Histoire de la médecine, de la pharmacie, de l'art dentaire et de l'art vétérinaire*, 8 vols. Paris.

Pourriere, J. (1969). *Les Hôpitaux d'Aix-en-Provence au Moyen Age: XIIIe-XIVe-XVe siècles*. Aix-en-Provence.

Preiser, G. (1976). *Allgemeine Krankheitsbezeichnungen im Corpus Hippocraticum*. Berlin.

———— (1978). "Diagnosis und diagignoskein: Zum Krankenerkennen im Corpus Hippocraticum," in Habricht, Marguth, and Wolf (1978), 91–99.

Premuda, L. (1960). *Storia della medicina.* Padua.

Pressouyre, L. (1966). "Le Cosmos platonicien de la cathédrale d'Anagni," *Mélanges d'archéologie et d'histoire,* 78.

Preus, A. (1977). "Galen's Criticism of Aristotle's Conception Theory," *Journal of the History of Biology* 10: 65–85.

Proust, A. (1893). "Études d'hygiène: Épidémies anciennes et épidémies modernes," *Revue des deux mondes* 120: 641–680.

Puccinotti, F. (1850–1866). *Storia della medicina,* 3 vols. Livorno.

Puschmann, T., M. Neuburger, and J. Leopold, eds. (1901–1905). *Handbuch der Geschichte der Medizin,* 3 vols. Jena.

Quain, E. A. (1945). "The Medieval 'Accessus ad Auctores,'" *Traditio* 3: 215–265.

Rando, D. (1983). "'Laicus religiosus' tra strutture civili ed ecclesiastiche: L'ospedale di Ognissanti a Treviso," *Studi medievali* 24: 617–656.

Raschke, M. G. (1978). "New Studies in Roman Commerce with the East," in H. Temporini and W. Haase, eds., *Aufstieg und Niedergang der Römischen Welt,* 2d part, *Principat,* vol. 9, book 2, *Politische Geschichte,* 650–676, 904–1055.

Rather, L. J. (1959). "Towards a Philosophical Study of the Idea of Disease," in MacBrooks and Cranefield (1959), 351–373.

Rawson, E. (1982). "The Life and Death of Asclepiades of Bithynia," *Classical Quarterly,* new ser., 32: 358–370.

Rebouis, E. (1888). *Étude historique et critique sur la peste.* Paris.

Rechenauer, G. (1991). *Thukydides und die hippokratische Medizin: Naturwissenschaftliche Methodik als Modell für Geschichtsdeutung.* Hildesheim.

Redeker, F. (1917). *Die "Anatomia magistri Nicolai phisici" und ihr Verhältnis zur Anatomia Chophonis und Richardi.* Leipzig.

Reingold, N. (1981). "Science, Scientists, and Historians of Science," *History of Science* 19: 274–283.

Repici, L. (1988). *La natura e l'anima: Saggi su Stratone di Lampsaco.* Turin.

Reynolds, J. (1986). "The Elder Pliny and His Times," in French and Greenaway (1986), 1–10.

Reznek, L. (1987). *The Nature of Disease.* London and New York.

Richards, P. (1977). *The Medieval Leper and His Northern Heirs.* Cambridge and Totowa.

Riddle, J. M. (1974). "Theory and Practice in Medieval Medicine," *Viator* 5: 157–184.

———— (1980). "Dioscorides," in Cranz and Kristeller (1980), 4: 1–143.

———— (1985). *Dioscorides on Pharmacy and Medicine.* Austin.

Riese, W. (1953). *The Conception of Disease: Its History, Its Versions, and Its Nature.* New York.

Ritter, H., and M. Plessner (1962). *Das Ziel des Weisen von Pseudo-Magrīti.* London.

Robert, F. (1975). "La Prognose hippocratique dans les livres V et VII des Épidémies," in *Le Monde grec (Hommage à Claire Préaux)* (Brussels), pp. 257–270.

Romano, R. (1971). *Tra due crisi: l'Italia del Rinascimento.* Turin.

Romilly, J. de (1966). "Thucydide et l'idée de progrès," *Annali della Scuola normale superiore di Pisa (Lettere, storia e filosofia)* 35: 143–191.

——— (1976). "Alcibiade et le mélange entre jeunes et vieux: Politique et médecine," in *Mélanges Lesky, Wiener Studien*, new ser., 10 (89): 93–105.

——— (1990). *La Construction de la vérité chez Thucydide.* Paris.

Roselli, A. (1975). *La chirurgia ippocratica.* Florence.

Rosenberg, C. E. (1992). *Explaining Epidemics and Other Essays in the History of Medicine.* Cambridge.

Rosenthal, F. (1956). "An Ancient Commentary on the Hippocratic Oath," *Bulletin of the History of Medicine* 30: 52–87.

——— (1968). *A History of Muslim Historiography.* Leiden.

——— (1969). "The Defense of Medicine in the Medieval Muslim World," *Bulletin of the History of Medicine* 43: 524–540.

——— (1971). *The Herb Hashish versus Medieval Muslim Society.* Leiden.

Rossi, P., ed. (1988). *Storia della scienza moderna e contemporanea,* 3 books in 5 vols. Turin.

Rothschild, H., ed. (1981). *Biocultural Aspects of Disease.* New York.

Rothschuh, K. E. (1980). "Medicina historica: Zum Selbstverständnis der historischen Medizin," *Janus* 67: 7–19.

———, ed. (1975). *Was ist Krankheit? Erscheinung, Erklärung, Sinngebung.* Darmstadt.

Roussel, F. (1988). "Le Concept de mélancolie chez Aristote," *Revue d'histoire des sciences* 41: 229–330.

Roy, E. (1913). "Un régime de santé pour les petits enfants et l'hygiène de Gargantua," in *Mélanges Émile Picot,* vol. 1 (Paris), pp. 153–158.

Rubin, M. (1987). *Charity and Community in Medieval Cambridge.* Cambridge.

Ruska, J. (1922). "Al-Biruni als Quelle für das Leben und die Schriften al-Razi's," *Isis* 5: 26–50.

Russo, F. (1969). *Éléments de bibliographie de l'histoire des sciences et des techniques.* Paris.

Ryan, W. F., and C. B. Schmitt, eds. (1982). *Pseudo-Aristotle: The Secrets of Secrets— Sources and Influences.* London.

Sabbah, G. (1982). "La 'peste d'Amida' (Ammian Marcellin, 19, 4)," *Mémoires du Centre Jean-Palerne* 3: 131–157.

——— (1985). "Observations préliminaires à une nouvelle édition de Cassius Felix," in Mazzini and Fusco (1985), 279–312.

———, ed. (1991). *Le Latin médical: La Constitution d'un langage scientifique* (= *Mémoires du Centre Jean-Palerne* 10). Saint-Étienne.

Sabbah, G., K. Fischer, and P. Corsetti, eds. (1988). *Bibliographie des textes médicaux latins: Antiquité et haut Moyen Age.* Saint-Étienne.

Sadegh-Zadeh, K. (1977). "Krankheitsbegriffe und nosologische Systeme," *Metamedicine* 1: 4–41.

Sadek, M. H. (1983). *The Arabic Materia Medica of Dioscorides.* St. John Chrysostom.

Saffron, M. H. (1975). "Salernitan Anatomists," in Gillispie (1970–1980), 12: 80–83.

Saint-Denis, A. (1983). *L'Hôtel-Dieu de Laon, 1150–1300: Institution hospitalière et société aux XIIe et XIIIe siècles.* Nancy.

—— (1985). "Soins du corps et médecine contre la souffrance à l'hôtel-Dieu de Laon au XIIIe siècle," *Le Souci du corps* 8: 40–42.

Santi, F. (1987). "Il cadavere e Bonifacio VIII, tra Stefano Tempier e Avicenna: Intorno ad un saggio di Elizabeth Brown," *Studi Medievali,* 3d ser., 28: 861–878.

Sarton, G. (1918). "Le Nouvel Humanisme," *Scientia* 23: 161–175.

—— (1927–1948). *Introduction to the History of Science,* 3 books in 5 vols. Baltimore.

—— (1935). "The History of Science versus the History of Medicine," *Isis* 23: 313–320.

—— (1952–1959). *A History of Science,* 2 vols. Cambridge, Mass. (3d ed., Cambridge, 1960.)

—— (1954). *Galen of Pergamon.* Lawrence.

Saunier, A. (1986). "La Vie quotidienne dans les hôpitaux du Moyen Age," in Le Goff and Sournia (1985), 85–89.

Savage-Smith, E. (1987). "Drug Therapy of Eye Diseases in Seventeenth-Century Islamic Medicine: The Influence of the 'New Chemistry' of the Paracelsians," *Pharmacy in History* 29: 3–28.

Scarborough, J. (1969). *Roman Medicine.* London.

—— (1970). "Thucydides, Greek Medicine, and the Plague at Athens: A Summary of Possibilities," *Episteme* 4: 1–90.

—— (1975). "The Drug Lore of Asclepiades of Bithynia," *Pharmacy in History* 17: 43–57.

—— (1976). "Celsus on Human Vivisection at Ptolemaic Alexandria," *Clio Medica* 11: 25–38.

—— (1977–1979). "Nicander's Toxicology," *Pharmacy in History* 17: 3–23; 21: 3–34, 73–92.

—— (1978). "Theophrastus on Herbals and Herbal Remedies," *Journal of the History of Biology* 11: 353–385.

—— (1981). "The Galenic Question," *Sudhoffs Archiv für Geschichte der Medizin* 65: 1–31.

—— (1983). "Theoretical Assumptions in Hippocratic Pharmacology," in Lasserre and Mudry (1983), 307–325.

————— (1986). "Pharmacy in Pliny's 'Natural History,'" in French and Greenaway (1986), 59–85.

————— (1989). "Pharmaceutical Theory in Galen's Commentaries on the Hippocratic Epidemics: Some Observations on Roman Views of Greek Drug Lore," in Baader and Winau (1989), 270–282.

————— (1991). "The Pharmacy of Methodist Medicine: The Evidence of Soranus' Gynecology," in Mudry and Pigeaud (1991), 203–216.

—————, ed. (1985). Symposium on Byzantine Medicine (= Dumbarton Oaks Papers 38). Washington.

Scarborough, J., and V. Nutton (1982). "The 'Preface' of Dioscorides' 'Materia Medica': Introduction, Translation, and Commentary," Transactions and Studies of the College of Physicians of Philadelphia, 5th ser., 4: 187–227.

Schacht, J. (1936). "Über den Hellenismus in Baghdad und Cairo im 11. Jahrhundert," Zeitschrift der Deutschen Morgenländischen Gesellschaft 90: 536ff.

Schipperges, H. (1955). "Die frühen Uebersetzer der arabischen Medizin in chronologischer Sicht," Sudhoffs Archiv für Geschichte der Medizin 39: 53–93.

————— (1961). Ideologie und Historiographie des Arabismus. Wiesbaden. (Sudhoffs Archiv für Geschichte der Medizin 1.)

————— (1964a). Die Assimilation der arabischen Medizin durch das lateinische Mittelalter. Wiesbaden. (Sudhoffs Archiv für Geschichte der Medizin 3.)

————— (1964b). Die Benediktiner in der Medizin des frühen Mittelalters. Leipzig.

————— (1973). "Petrus Hispanus," in K. Fasmann, ed., Die Grossen der Weltgeschichte (Zurich), pp. 679–691.

————— (1976a). Arabische Medizin im lateinischen Mittelalter. Berlin.

————— (1976b). "Zur Bedeutung von 'physica' und zur Rolle des 'phisicus' in der abendländischen Wissenschaftsgeschichte," Sudhoffs Archiv für Geschichte der Medizin 60: 354–374.

————— (1982). "Zum topos von 'ratio et experimentum,'" in G. Keil, ed., Fachprosa-Studien: Beiträge zur mittelalterlichen Wissenschafts-und Geistesgeschichte (Berlin), pp. 25–36.

————— (1985). Der Garten der Gesundheit: Medizin im Mittelalter. Munich.

Schmitt, C. B. (1981). "Experience and Experiment: A Comparison of Zabarella's View with Galileo's in 'De motu,'" in C. B. Schmitt, Studies in Renaissance Philosophy and Science (London), pp. 80–138.

Schmitt, H. G. (1936). Die Pest des Galenos. Würzburg.

Schmitt, J. C. (1988). Religione, folklore e società nell'Occidente medievale. Bari.

Schnayder, J. (1973). "Der Begriff 'Dynamis' in den Werken des Theophrastos," Eos 61: 49–56.

Schnurrer, F. (1823). Die Krankheiten des Menschengeschlechts historisch und geographisch beobachtet. Tübingen.

Schöner, E. (1964). Das Viererschema in der antiken Humoralpathologie. Wiesbaden. (Sudhoffs Archiv für Geschichte der Medizin 4.)

Schuhl, P.-M. (1960). "Platon et la médecine," *Revue des études grecques* 83: 73–79.

Schürmann, A. (1991). *Griechische Mechanik und antike Wissenschaft*. Stuttgart.

Seidler, E. (1967). *Die Heilkunde des ausgehenden Mittelalters in Paris*. Wiesbaden. (*Sudhoffs Archiv für Geschichte der Medizin* 8.)

Semelaigne, A. (1869). *Études historiques sur l'aliénation mentale dans l'Antiquité*. Paris.

Semmler, J. (1986). "Die Sorge um den kranken Mitbruder im Benediktinerkloster des frühen und hohen Mittelalters," in Wunderli (1986), 45–59.

Sendrail, M., ed. (1980). *Histoire culturelle de la maladie*. Toulouse.

Senn, G. (1929). "Ueber Herkunft und Stil der Beschreibungen von Experimenten im Corpus Hippocraticum," *Sudhoffs Archiv für Geschichte der Medizin* 22: 217–289.

Sezgin, F. (1970). *Geschichte des arabischen Schrifttums*, vol. 3, *Medizin, Pharmazie, Zoologie, Tierheilkunde bis ca. 430 H*. Leiden.

———— (1971). *Geschichte des arabischen Schrifttums*, vol. 4, *Alchimie, Chemie, Botanik, Agrikultur bis ca. 430 H*. Leiden.

Shatzmiller, J. (1989). *Médecine et justice en Provence médiévale*. Aix-en-Provence.

Sheils, W. J., ed. (1982). *The Church and Healing*. Oxford.

Shelag, J. (1968). "Chronology of the Campaigns of Aelius Gallus and C. Petronius," *Journal of Roman Studies* 58: 71–84.

Shelp, E. E., ed. (1982). *Beneficence and Health Care*. Dordrecht.

———— (1985). *Virtue and Medicine: Explorations in the Character of Medicine*. Dordrecht.

Sherwin-White, S. M. (1978). *Ancient Cos*. Göttingen.

Shrewsbury, J. F. D. (1949). "The Yellow Plague," *Journal of the History of Medicine*, 5–47.

———— (1979). *A History of Bubonic Plague in the British Isles*. Cambridge.

Shryock, R. H. (1936). *The Development of Modern Medicine: An Interpretation of the Social and Scientific Factors Involved*. Philadelphia.

Siebenthal, W. von (1950). *Krankheit als Folge der Sünde*. Hannover.

Siegel, R. E. (1964). "Clinical Observation in Hippocrates: An Essay on the Evolution of the Diagnostic Art," *Journal of the Mt. Sinai Hospital* 31: 285–303.

———— (1968). *Galen's System of Physiology and Medicine*. Basel and New York.

Sigal, P. A. (1969). "Maladie, pèlerinage et guérison au XIIe siècle," *Annales: Economies, sociétés, civilisations* 24: 1522–1539.

Sigerist, H. E. (1931). *Einführung in die Medizin*. Leipzig.

———— (1935). "The History of Medicine and the History of Science," *Bulletin of the Institute of the History of Medicine*. 4: 1–3.

———— (1951–1961). *A History of Medicine*, 2 vols. New York.

———— (1958). "The Latin Medical Literature of the Early Middle Ages," *Journal of the History of Medicine* 13: 121–146.

———— (1960). *On the Sociology of Medicine*. New York.

Simon, B. (1978). *Mind and Madness in Ancient Greece*. Ithaca and London.

Singer, C., and E. A. Underwood (1962). *A Short History of Medicine.* Oxford.

Sinno, A. (1950). *Vicende della Scuola e dell'Almo Collegio Salernitano: Maestri finora ignorati.* Salerno.

Siraisi, N. G. (1980). "The Medical Learning of Albertus Magnus," in Weisheipl (1980), 379–404.

———— (1981). *Taddeo Alderotti and His Pupils: Two Generations of Italian Medical Learning.* Princeton.

———— (1987a). *Avicenna in Renaissance Italy: The Canon and Medical Teaching in Italian Universities after 1500.* Princeton.

———— (1987b). "Changing Concepts of the Organization of Medical Knowledge in the Italian Universities: Fourteenth to Sixteenth Centuries," in *La diffusione delle scienze islamiche nel Medio Evo europeo* (Accademia nazionale dei Lincei, international conference) (Rome), pp. 291–321.

———— (1990). *Medieval and Early Renaissance Medicine: An Introduction to Knowledge and Practice.* Chicago.

Skoda, F. (1988). *Médecine ancienne et Métaphore: Le Vocabulaire de l'anatomie et de la pathologie en grec ancien.* Paris.

Smith, W. D. (1965). "So-Called Possession in Pre-Christian Greece," *Transactions and Proceedings of the American Philological Association* 156: 403–426.

———— (1973). "Galen on Coans versus Cnidians," *Bulletin of the History of Medicine* 47: 569–578.

———— (1979). *The Hippocratic Tradition.* Ithaca and London.

———— (1980). "The Development of Classical Dietetic Theory," in Grmek, ed. (1980), 439–448.

———— (1982). "Erasistratus' Dietetic Medicine," *Bulletin of the History of Medicine* 56: 398–409.

———— (1989). "Notes on Ancient Medical Historiography," *Bulletin of the History of Medicine* 63: 73–109.

Solmsen, F. (1961). "Greek Philosophy and the Discovery of Nerves," *Museum Helveticum* 18: 150–197.

———— (1968). "The Vital Heat, the Inborn Pneuma, and the Aether," in *Kleine Schriften,* vol. 1. Hildesheim.

Sonderkamp, J. (1985). "Theophanes Nonnus: Medicine in the Circle of Constantine Porphyrogenitus," in Scarborough (1985), 29–41.

———— (1987). *Untersuchungen zur Überlieferung der Schriften des Theophanes Chrysobalantes (sog. Theophanes Nonnos).* Bonn.

Souques, A. (1936). *Étapes de la neurologie dans l'Antiquité grecque (d'Homère à Galien).* Paris.

Sournia, J.-C. (1991). *Histoire de la médecine et des médecins.* Paris.

———— (1992). *Histoire de la médecine.* Paris.

Southern, R. W. (1986). *Robert Grosseteste: The Growth of an English Mind in Medieval Europe.* Oxford.

Spicker, S. F., ed. (1978). *Organism, Medicine, and Metaphysics.* Dordrecht.

Spies, O., and H. Müller-Bütow (1971). *Anatomie und Chirurgie des Schädels, insbesondere der Hals-, Nasen- und Ohrenkrankheiten nach Ibn al-Quff*. Berlin.

Sprengel, K. (1792–1803). *Versuch einer pragmatischen Geschichte der Arzneykunde,* 5 vols. Halle. (Rev. ed., Halle, 1800–1803.)

Stannard, J. (1961). "Hippocratic Pharmacology," *Bulletin of the History of Medicine* 35: 497–518.

———— (1985). "Aspects of Byzantine Materia Medica," in Scarborough (1985), 205–211.

Starobinski, J. (1953). "Le Passé de la médecine," *Critique* 70: 256–270.

Steinbock, R. T. (1976). *Paleopathological Diagnosis and Interpretation: Bone Diseases in Ancient Human Populations*. Springfield.

Sticker, G. (1908–1910). *Abhandlungen aus der Seuchengeschichte und Seuchenlehre,* vols. 1 and 2. Giessen.

Stouff, L., ed. (1970). *Ravitaillement et alimentation en Provence aux XIVe et XVe siècles*. Paris.

Strohmaier, G. (1969). "Arabisch als Sprache der Wissenschaft in den frühen medizinischen Übersetzungen," *Mitteilungen des Instituts für Orientforschung* 15: 77–85.

———— (1974). "Hunayn ibn Ishaq et le serment hippocratique," *Arabica* 21: 321ff.

———— (1980). "Homer in Bagdad," *Byzantinoslavica* 41: 196–200.

———— (1987). "Von Alexandrien nach Bagdad—eine fiktive Schultradition," in Wiesner (1987), 2: 380–389.

———— (1989a). "Al-Mansûr und die frühe Rezeption der griechischen Alchemie: Ein Beitrag zur Rolle nichtliterarischer Kommunikation," *Zeitschrift für Geschichte der arabisch-islamischen Wissenschaften* 5: 169ff.

———— (1989b). "La Médecine grecque antique dans les traductions en langues orientales: Recherches et éditions de 1970 à aujourd'hui," *Centre Jean-Palerne, Université de Saint-Étienne: Lettre d'informations* 14: 12–32.

———— (1991). "La Tradition hippocratique en latin et en arabe," in Sabbah (1991), pp. 27–39.

Stückelberger, A. (1984). *Vestigia Democritea: Die Rezeption der Lehre von den Atomen in der antiken Naturwissenschaft und Medizin*. Basel.

Stürner, W. (1975). *Natur und Gesellschaft im Denken des Hoch- und Spätmittelalters*. Stuttgart.

Sudhoff, K. (1914–1918). *Beiträge zur Geschichte der Chirurgie im Mittelalter.* 2 vols. Leipzig.

———— (1914–1920). "Zum Regimen Sanitatis Salernitatum," *Archiv für Geschichte der Medizin* 7 (1914): 360–362; 8 (1915): 292–293; 9 (1916): 221–249; 10 (1917): 91–101; 12 (1920): 149–180.

———— (1916). "Die pseudohippokratische Krankheitsprognostik nach dem Auftreten von Hautausschlägen 'Secreta Hippocratis' oder 'Capsula eburnea' benannt," *Archiv für Geschichte der Medizin* 9: 79–116.

———— (1922). *Kurzes Handbuch der Geschichte der Medizin*. Berlin.

——— (1923). "Eine Diätregel für einen Bischoff aufgestellt von vier Professoren von Montpellier," *Archiv für Geschichte der Medizin* 14.

Susser, M. (1981). "Ethical Components of the Definition of Health," in Caplan, Engelhardt, and McCartney (1981), 93–105.

Tabanelli, M. (1956). *Chirurgia nell'antica Roma.* Turin.

——— (1958). *Lo strumento chirurgico e la sua storia.* Turin.

——— (1965). *La chirurgia italiana nell'alto medioevo,* 2 vols. Florence.

Talbot, C. H. (1967). *Medicine in Medieval England.* London.

Talbott, J. H. (1970). *A Bibliographical History of Medicine.* New York.

Taton, R., ed. (1957–1964). *Histoire générale des sciences,* 4 vols. Paris.

Temkin, O. (1928). "Die Krankheitsauffassung von Hippokrates und Sydenham in ihren Epidemien," *Sudhoffs Archiv für Geschichte der Medizin* 20: 327–352.

——— (1935a). "Celsus 'On Medicine' and the Ancient Medical Sects," *Bulletin of the Institute of the History of Medicine* 3: 249–264.

——— (1935b). "Studies on Late Alexandrian Medicine, I," *Bulletin of the Institute of the History of Medicine* 3: 405–430. (Repr. in O. Temkin, *The Double Face of Janus,* London and Baltimore, 1977, pp. 178–197.)

——— (1960). "The Byzantine Origin of the Names for the Basilic and Cephalic Veins," in *XVIIe Congrès international d'histoire de la médecine* (Athens and Kos), 1: 336–340.

——— (1961). "The Scientific Approach to Disease: Specific Entity and Individual Sickness," in Crombie (1963), 629–647. (Repr., in Caplan, Engelhardt, and McCartney [1981], 247–263.)

——— (1973). *Galenism: Rise and Decline of a Medical Philosophy.* Ithaca and London.

Temkin, O., and L. Temkin (1958). "Wunderlich versus Haeser: A Controversy over Medical History" *Bulletin of the History of Medicine* 32: 97–104.

Theodorides, J. (1986). *Histoire de la rage: Cave canem.* Paris.

Thivel, A. (1975). "Le 'Divin' dans la Collection hippocratique," in Bourgey and Jouanna (1975), 57–76.

——— (1981). *Cnide et Cos? Essai sur les doctrines médicales dans la Collection hippocratique.* Paris.

——— (1985). "Diagnostic et pronostic à l'époque d'Hippocrate et la nôtre," *Gesnerus* 42: 479–498.

Thomasset, C. (1982). *Une Vision du monde à la fin du XIIIe siècle: Commentaire du dialogue de Placides et Timéo.* Geneva.

Thorndike, L. (1923–1941). *A History of Magic and Experimental Science,* 8 vols. New York.

——— (1946). "Translation of Works of Galen from Greek by Niccolò da Reggio (circa 1308–1345)," *Byzantine Metabyzantina* 1: 213–235.

Thorndike, L., and P. Kibre. (1963). *A Catalogue of Incipits of Medieval Scientific Writings in Latin,* 2d ed. Cambridge, Mass.

Toledo-Pereyra, L. H. (1973). "Galen's Contribution to Surgery," *Journal of the History of Medicine* 28: 357–375.

Torfs, L. (1859). *Fastes des calamités publiques survenues dans les Pays-Bas*. Paris and Tournai.

Touwaide, A. (1984). "L'Authenticité et l'origine des deux traités de toxicologie attribués à Dioscoride, I: Historique de la question; II: Apport de l'histoire du texte grec," *Janus* 70: 1–53.

——— (1985). "Un recueil de pharmacologie du Xe siècle illustré au XIVe: Le Vaticanus gr. 284," *Scriptorium* 39: 13–56.

——— (1988). "Les Manuscrits grecs illustrés du traité de Dioscoride" in *Actes du XXXe Congrès international d'histoire de la médecine, Düsseldorf, 1986* (Düsseldorf), pp. 1148–1151.

——— (1990). "Le 'Traité de matière médicale' de Dioscoride: Pour une nouvelle lecture," *Bulletin du Cercle Benelux d'histoire de la pharmacie* 78: 32–39.

——— (1991a). "Les Poisons dans le monde antique et byzantin: Introduction à une analyse systémique," *Revue d'histoire de la pharmacie* 290: 265–281.

——— (1991b). "Nicandre, de la science à la poésie: Contribution à l'exégèse de la poésie médicale grecque," *Aevum* 65: 65–101.

——— (1992a). "Les Deux Traités de toxicologie attribués à Dioscoride," in Garzya (1992), 291–335.

——— (1992b). *Farmacopea araba medievale: Codice Ayasofia 3703*, 2 vols. Milan.

Trinkhaus, C. (1989). "Coluccio Salutati's Critique of Astrology in the Context of His Natural Philosophy," *Speculum* 64: 46–68.

Tuchman, B. W. (1978). *A Distant Mirror: The Calamitous 14th Century*. New York.

Ullmann, M. (1970). *Die Medizin im Islam*. Leiden and Cologne.

——— (1972). *Die Natur-und Geheimwissenschaften im Islam*. Leiden and Cologne.

——— (1977). "Die Tadkira des Ibn as-Suwaydi, eine wichtige Quelle zur Geschichte der griechisch-arabischen Medizin und Magie," *Der Islam* 54: 33–65.

——— (1978). *Islamic Medicine*. Edinburgh.

Ulman, J. (1965). *De la gymnastique aux sports modernes*. Paris.

Valensi, R. (1908). *Un Chirurgien arabe au Moyen Age: Albucasis*. Montpellier.

Vallance, J. T. (1990). *The Lost Theory of Asclepiades of Bithynia*. Oxford.

Van Brock, N. (1961). *Recherches sur le vocabulaire médical du grec ancien*. Paris.

Vauchez, A. (1978). "Assistance et charité en Occident (XIIIe–XVe siècles)," in V. Barbagli Bagnoli, ed., *Domanda e consumi, livelli e strutture, secc. XIII–XVIII* (Prato).

Vázquez Buján, M. E. (1991). "Isti methodici constabilitatem non habent: Remarques sur la persistance tardive du méthodisme," in Mudry and Pigeaud (1991), 241–254.

Vegetti, M. (1966–1969). "La medicina in Platone," *Rivista critica di storia della filosofia* 21 (1966): 3–39; 22 (1967): 251–270; 23 (1968): 251–267; 24 (1969): 3–22.

——— (1971). "I fondamenti teorici della biologia aristotelica nel 'De partibus animalium,'" in Lanza and Vegetti (1971), 489–554.

—— (1976). *Opere di Ippocrate*. Turin.

—— (1981). "Modelli di medicina in Galeno," in Nutton (1981).

—— (1983). *Tra Edipo et Euclide*. Milan.

—— (1986). *Il coltello e lo stilo*. Milan.

—— (1990). "I nervi dell'anima," *Biologica* 4: 11–28.

——, ed. (1985). *Il sapere degli antichi*. Turin.

Verbeke, G. (1945). *L'Évolution de la doctrine du pneuma*. Paris and Louvain.

Vereecke, L. (1990). "Medicina e morale in S. Antonino da Firenze (+ 1459)," in L. Vereecke, *Da Guglielmo d'Ockham a Sant'Alfonso de Liguori* (Milan), pp. 297–319.

Vernet, J. (1985). *Ce que la culture doit aux Arabes d'Espagne* (trans. from Spanish). Paris.

Viano, C. A. (1981). "Lo scetticismo antico e la medicina," in G. Giannantoni, ed., *Lo scetticismo antico*, vol. 2 (Naples), pp. 563–656.

—— (1984). "Perché non c'era sangue nelle arterie: La cecità epistemologica degli anatomisti antichi," in Giannantoni and Vegetti (1984), 297–352.

Villalba, J. de (1803). *Epidemiologia española, o historia cronológica de las pestes, contagios, epidemias y epizootias que han acaecido en España desde la venida de los cartaginesis hasto el año 1801*. Madrid.

Vintró, E. (1972). *Hipócrates y la nosología hippocrática*. Barcelona.

Vizgin, V. P. (1980). "Hippocratic Medicine as a Historical Source for Aristotle's Theory of the Dynameis," *Studies in the History of Medicine* 4: 1–12.

Voltaggio, F. (1992). *L'arte della guarigione nella cultura umana*. Turin.

Von Staden, H. (1975). "Experiment and Experience in Hellenistic Medicine," *Bulletin of the Institute of Classical Studies* 22: 178–199.

—— (1982). "Hairesis and Heresy: The Case of Haireseis Iatrikai," in B. F. Meyer and E. P. Sanders, ed., *Jewish and Christian Self-Definition*, vol. 3, *Self-Definition in the Graeco-Roman World* (London), pp. 76–100, 199–206.

—— (1988). "Cardiovascular Puzzles in Erasistratus and Herophilus," in *XXXI Congresso internazionale di storia della medicina* (Bologna).

—— (1989). *Herophilus: The Art of Medicine in Early Alexandria*. Cambridge and New York.

Vust-Mussard, M. (1970). "Remarques sur les livres I et III des Épidémies: Les Histoires de malades et le pronostic," *Études de lettres* 3: 65–76.

Wack, M. F. (1990). *Lovesickness in the Middle Ages: The "Viaticum" and Its Commentaries*. Philadelphia.

Watson, G. (1966). *Theriac and Mithridatium: A Study in Therapeutics*. London.

Weijers, O. (1987). *Terminologie des universités au Moyen Age*. Rome.

——, ed. (1990). *Méthodes et instruments du travail intellectuel au Moyen Age: Études sur le vocabulaire*. Turnhout.

Weisheipl, J. A. (1965). "Classification of the Sciences in Medieval Thought," *Medieval Studies* 27: 54–90.

——, ed. (1980). *Albertus Magnus and the Sciences*. Toronto.

Weisser, U. (1983). *Zeugung, Vererbung und pränatale Entwicklung in der Medizin des arabisch-islamischen Mittelalters.* Erlangen.

———— (1986). "Noch einmal zur Isagoge des Johannicius: Die Herkunft des lateinischen Lehrtextes," *Sudhoffs Archiv für Geschichte der Medizin* 70: 229–235.

———— (1991). "Zur Rezeption des 'Methodus medendi' im Continens des Rhazes," in Kudlien and Durling (1991), 141–145.

Wellmann, M. (1889). "Sextius Niger: Eine Quellenuntersuchung zu Dioscorides," *Hermes* 24: 530–569.

———— (1897). "Krateuas," *Abhandlungen der Königlichen Gesellschaft der Wissenschaften zu Göttingen, Philologisch-Historische Klasse*, new ser., 2 (1).

———— (1898). "Das älteste Kräuterbuch der Griechen," in *Festgabe für Franz Susemihl zur Geschichte griechischer Wissenschaft und Dichtung* (Leipzig), pp. 1–31.

———— (1901). *Fragmentsammlung der griechischen Aerzte*, vol. 1, *Die Fragmente der sikelischen Aerzte Akron, Philistion und des Diokles von Karystos.* Berlin.

———— (1905). "Empirische Schule," in Pauly and Wissowa (1893–1980). V, 2: 2516–2524.

———— (1914). *Die Schrift des Dioskurides: Ein Beitrag zur Geschichte der Medizin.* Berlin.

Wells, C. (1964). *Bones, Bodies, and Disease: Evidence of Disease and Abnormality in Early Man.* London.

West, S. (1973). "Cultural Interchange on a Water-Clock," *Classical Quarterly,* 61–64.

White, L. Jr. (1975). "Medical Astrologers and Late Medieval Technology," *Viator* 6: 295–308.

Wickersheimer, E. (1910). "Les Premières Dissections à la Faculté de médecine de Paris," *Bulletin de la Société de l'histoire de Paris et de l'Ile-de-France* 37: 159–169.

———— (1936). *Dictionnaire biographique des médecins en France au Moyen Age.* Geneva. (Repr., Geneva, 1979; D. Jacquart, supplement, Geneva, 1979.)

———— (1950). "Les Tacuini sanitatis et leur traduction allemande par Michel Herr," *Bibliothèque d'humanisme et Renaissance* 12: 85–97.

———— (1965). "Ignis sacer, ignis acer, ignis ager," *Actes du VIIIe Congrès international d'histoire des sciences, Florence,* 642–650.

———— (1966). *Les Manuscrits latins de médecine du Moyen Age dans les bibliothèques de France.* Paris.

Wiesner, J., ed. (1987). *Aristoteles, Werk und Wirkung: Paul Moraux gewidmet,* 2 vols. Berlin and New York.

Williman, D., ed. (1983). *The Black Death: The Impact of the Fourteenth-Century Plague.* Binghamton, N.Y.

Wilson, L. G. (1959). "Erasistratus, Galen, and the Pneuma," *Bulletin of the History of Medicine* 33: 293–314.

Wilson, N. G. (1980). "Medical History without Medicine," *Journal of the History of Medicine* 35: 5–7.

———— (1983a). *Scholars of Byzantium* London.

———— (1983b). "A Mysterious Byzantine Scriptorium: Ioannikios and His Colleagues," *Scrittura e Civiltà* 7: 161–176.

Wittern, R. (1978). "Zur Krankheitserkennung in der knidischen Schrift 'De internis affectionibus,'" in Habricht, Marguth, and Wolf (1978), 101–119.

Wöhrle, G. (1990). *Studien zur Theorie der antiken Gesundheitslehre.* Stuttgart.

Wolska-Conus, W. (1989). "Stéphanos d'Athènes et Stéphanos d'Alexandrie: Essai d'identification et de biographie," *Revue des études byzantines* 47: 5–89.

———— (1992). "Les Commentaires de Stéphanos d'Athènes au Prognostikon et aux Aphorismes d'Hippocrate: De Galien à la pratique scolaire d'Alexandrie," *Revue des études byzantines* 50: 5–86.

Wunderli, P., ed. (1986). *Der kranke Mensch in Mittelalter und Renaissance.* Düsseldorf.

Wunderlich, C. A. (1859). *Geschichte der Medizin.* Stuttgart.

Zanca, A., ed. (1987). *Il farmaco nei tempi dalle origini ai laboratori—Sui rimedi medicamenti e farmaci: Sulle teorie e pratiche della lotta degli uomini contro la malattie.* Parma.

Zarncke, F. (1879). "Der Priester Johannes," in *Abhandlungen der Philologisch-Historischen Klasse der königlich sächsischen Gesellschaft der Wissenschaften,* part 1, 8 (Leipzig).

Zimmermann, F. (1976). "Al-Farabi und die philosophische Kritik an Galen von Alexander zu Averroes," in A. Dietrich, ed., *Akten des VII: Kongresses für Arabistik und Islamwissenschaft* (Göttingen).

Zimmermann, G. (1973). *Ordensleben und Lebensstandard: Die "cura corporis" in den Ordensvorschriften des abendländischen Hochmittelalters.* Münster.

Contributors

Jole Agrimi
University of Pavia

Jean-Noël Biraben
Institut National d'Études Démographiques, Paris

Chiara Crisciani
University of Pavia

Bernardino Fantini
Institut Louis Jeantet d'Histoire de la Médecine, Geneva

Pedro Gil Sotres
University of Navarra, Pamplona

Danielle Gourevitch
École Pratique des Hautes Études, Paris

Mirko D. Grmek
École Pratique des Hautes Études, Paris

Danielle Jacquart
École Pratique des Hautes Études, Paris

Jacques Jouanna
University of Paris

Michael McVaugh
University of North Carolina, Chapel Hill

Gotthard Strohmaier
University of Berlin

Alain Touwaide
University of Barcelona

Mario Vegetti
University of Pavia

Index

469

Theory *(continued)*
  Herophilus of Chalcedon, 74, 89, 90; and iatrosophism, 143, 144; and Latin West, 201; and *Practica*, 232; and Rhazes, 157; and scholastic medicine, 214, 218, 219, 227, 229; and school of Salerno, 207. *See also* Practice; *specific schools*
Therapy: and Christian medicine, 181; and drugs, 259–272; and Erasistratus of Ceos, 74, 99–100; and Herophilus of Chalcedon, 89; and Hippocratic school, 36; and Homer, 323; and hospitals, 183, 191–192, 192; and Latin West, 201; and methodic medicine, 114–115; and plague, 195; and prehistory, 321; and scholastic medicine, 218; and school of Salerno, 207, 208; surgery as, 273–290. *See also* Practice
Thessalus of Thralles, 112
Thucydides, 38–39, 44, 67–68, 325
Timarion, 148
Tommaso del Garbo, 230
Translation, 162, 163, 198, 200, 202–205, 214–216, 236. *See also specific translators*
Trauma, 320, 347
Treatment. *See* Therapy
Trepanation, 321
Trivium, 212
Tuberculosis, 326–327, 350
Typhus, 325, 334

Ugo Benzi, 221–222
Ugo of Lucca, 281, 285
University medicine, 163, 210–223, 229, 300–302, 314. *See also* Scholastic medicine
University of Bologna, 210, 211, 212, 213, 216, 225, 231, 232–233

University of Montpellier, 210, 211, 212, 216, 217, 225
University of Padua, 233, 235
University of Paris, 210–211, 215–216, 220–221, 225, 230, 232
Urine, 131–132, 149, 208
Ursus of Salerno, 208–209; *De commixtionibus*, 208
Uterus, 57–58, 228. *See also* Gynecology

Vacuum, 95–96, 99
Vein: and Aristotle, 77; and Diocles of Carystos, 78; and Erasistratus of Ceos, 98–99; and Galen, 131, 216; and Herophilus of Chalcedon, 86, 87–88; and Hippocratic medicine, 57; and Praxagoras of Kos, 79. *See also* Artery; Vessel
Vessel, 57, 86. *See also* Artery; Vein
Vindicianus, 136
Vitamin, 328, 350
Vivisection, 86–87, 96, 108, 110. *See also* Dissection

Waste, 131–132, 151, 311–313. *See also* Evacuation
al-Watiq, 154
William of Conches: *Dragmaticon philosophiae*, 236; *Philosophia*, 236
Wunderlich, Carl August, 9

Xenodocheum, 184, 189

Yperman, Jan, 286
Yuhanna ibn Masawayh, 145, 149, 162, 165

Zeuxis, 91, 92, 109